Inherited Cardiac Diseases Predisposing to Sudden Death

Editors

RAFIK TADROS
JULIA CADRIN-TOURIGNY
JASON D. ROBERTS

CARDIAC ELECTROPHYSIOLOGY CLINICS

www.cardiacEP.theclinics.com

Consulting Editors
LUIGI DI BIASE
EMILY P. ZEITLER

September 2023 • Volume 15 • Number 3

ELSEVIER

1600 John F. Kennedy Boulevard • Suite 1800 • Philadelphia, Pennsylvania, 19103-2899

http://www.theclinics.com

CARDIAC ELECTROPHYSIOLOGY CLINICS Volume 15, Number 3
September 2023 ISSN 1877-9182, ISBN-13: 978-0-443-18334-8

Editor: Joanna Gascoine
Developmental Editor: Shivank Joshi

Cardiac Electrophysiology Clinics (ISSN 1877-9182) is published quarterly by Elsevier Inc., 360 Park Avenue South, New York, NY 10010-1710. Months of issue are March, June, September, and December. Subscription prices are $259.00 per year for US individuals, $464.00 per year for US institutions, $272.00 per year for Canadian individuals, $524.00 per year for Canadian institutions, $331.00 per year for international individuals, $562.00 per year for international institutions and $100.00 per year for US, Canadian and international students/residents. To receive student/resident rate, orders must be accompanied by name of affiliated institution, date of term, and the signature of program/residency coordinator on institution letterhead. Orders will be billed at individual rate until proof of status is received. Foreign air speed delivery is included in all Clinics subscription prices. All prices are subject to change without notice. **POST-MASTER:** Send address changes to Cardiac Electrophysiology Clinics, Elsevier Health Sciences Division, Subscription Customer Service, 3251 Riverport Lane, Maryland Heights, MO 63043. **Customer Service: 1-800-654-2452 (US and Canada). From outside of the US and Canada, call 314-477-8871. Fax: 314-447-8029. E-mail: JournalsCustomer-Service-usa@elsevier.com (for print support); JournalsOnlineSupport-usa@elsevier.com (for online support).**

Reprints. For copies of 100 or more of articles in this publication, please contact the Commercial Reprints Department, Elsevier Inc., 360 Park Avenue South, New York, NY 10010-1710. Tel.: 212-633-3874; Fax: 212-633-3820; E-mail: reprints@elsevier.com.

Cardiac Electrophysiology Clinics is covered in *MEDLINE/PubMed (Index Medicus).*

Contributors

CONSULTING EDITORS

LUIGI DI BIASE, MD, PhD, FACC, FESC, FHRS
Albert Einstein College of Medicine at Montefiore Health System, New York, New York, USA

EMILY P. ZEITLER, MD, MHS, FHRS
Dartmouth Health, The Dartmouth Institute, Lebanon, New Hampshire; Dartmouth Geisel School of Medicine, Hanover, New Hampshire, USA

EDITORS

RAFIK TADROS, MD, PhD
Cardiovascular Genetics Centre, Montreal Heart Institute, Faculty of Medicine, Université de Montréal, Montreal, Quebec, Canada

JULIA CADRIN-TOURIGNY, MD, PhD
Cardiovascular Genetics Centre, Montreal Heart Institute, Faculty of Medicine, Université de Montréal, Montreal, Quebec, Canada

JASON D. ROBERTS, MD, MAS
McMaster University, DBCVSRI, Population Health Research Institute, Hamilton Health Sciences, Hamilton, Ontario, Canada

AUTHORS

MICHAEL J. ACKERMAN, MD, PhD
Department of Cardiovascular Medicine, Division of Heart Rhythm Services, Windland Smith Rice Genetic Heart Rhythm Clinic, Department of Pediatric and Adolescent Medicine, Division of Pediatric Cardiology, Department of Molecular Pharmacology and Experimental Therapeutics, Windland Smith Rice Sudden Death Genomics Laboratory, Mayo Clinic, Rochester, Minnesota, USA

AHMAD AL SAMARRAIE, MD
Cardiovascular Genetics Centre, Montreal Heart Institute, Faculty of Medicine, University of Montreal, Montreal, Quebec, Canada

WAEL ALQARAWI, MD, MSc
Department of Cardiac Sciences, College of Medicine, King Saud University, Riyadh, Saudi Arabia; University of Ottawa Heart Institute, University of Ottawa, Ottawa, Canada

ABDULELAH H. ALSAEED, MBBS
Department of Cardiac Sciences, College of Medicine, King Saud University, Riyadh, Saudi Arabia

AHMAD S. AMIN, MD, PhD
Department of Clinical Cardiology, Amsterdam UMC, Location University of Amsterdam, Amsterdam Cardiovascular Sciences, Amsterdam, the Netherlands

IGNASI ANGUERA, MD, PhD
Department of Cardiology, Hospital Universitari de Bellvitge, L'Hospitalet de Llobregat, Bioheart-Cardiovascular Diseases Group, Cardiovascular, Respiratory and Systemic Diseases and Cellular Aging Program, Institut d'Investigació Biomèdica de Bellvitge–IDIBELL, L'Hospitalet de Llobregat, Barcelona, Spain

AUKE T. BERGEMAN, MD
Department of Cardiology, Heart Centre, Amsterdam UMC Location Academic Medical Centre, University of Amsterdam, Amsterdam Cardiovascular Sciences, Heart Failure and Arrhythmias, Amsterdam, the Netherlands

CONNIE R. BEZZINA, PhD
Department of Experimental Cardiology, Amsterdam UMC, Location University of Amsterdam, Amsterdam Cardiovascular Sciences, Amsterdam, the Netherlands

EMILY E. BROWN, MGC
Certified Genetic Counselor, Division of Cardiology, Johns Hopkins University, Baltimore, Maryland, USA

HENNING BUNDGAARD, MD, DMSc
The Unit for Inherited Cardiac Diseases, Department of Cardiology, The Heart Centre, Copenhagen University Hospital - Rigshospitalet, Copenhagen OE, Denmark; Department of Clinical Medicine, University of Copenhagen, Copenhagen, Denmark

JULIA CADRIN-TOURIGNY, MD, PhD
Cardiovascular Genetics Centre, Montreal Heart Institute, Faculty of Medicine, Université de Montréal, Montreal, Quebec, Canada

ALEX HØRBY CHRISTENSEN, MD, PhD
The Unit for Inherited Cardiac Diseases, Department of Cardiology, The Heart Centre, Copenhagen University Hospital - Rigshospitalet, Copenhagen OE, Denmark; Department of Cardiology, Copenhagen University Hospital - Herlev-Gentofte Hospital, Herlev, Denmark; Department of Clinical Medicine, University of Copenhagen, Copenhagen, Denmark

SUSAN CHRISTIAN, MSc, PhD, CGC
Assistant Clinical Professor, Department of Medical Genetics, University of Alberta, Edmonton, Alberta, Canada

EDUARD CLAVER, MD
Department of Cardiology, Hospital Universitari de Bellvitge, L'Hospitalet de Llobregat, Bioheart-Cardiovascular Diseases Group, Cardiovascular, Respiratory and Systemic Diseases and Cellular Aging Program, Institut d'Investigació Biomèdica de Bellvitge–IDIBELL, L'Hospitalet de Llobregat, Barcelona, Spain

YAANIK B. DESAI, MD
Department of Medicine, Division of Cardiovascular Medicine, Stanford University School of Medicine, Falk CRVC, Stanford, California, USA

ANDREA DI MARCO, MD, PhD
Department of Cardiology, Hospital Universitari de Bellvitge, L'Hospitalet de Llobregat, Bioheart-Cardiovascular Diseases Group, Cardiovascular, Respiratory and Systemic Diseases and Cellular Aging Program, Institut d'Investigació Biomèdica de Bellvitge–IDIBELL, L'Hospitalet de Llobregat, Barcelona, Spain; Division of Cardiovascular Sciences, School of Medical Sciences, Faculty of Biology, Medicine and Health, University of Manchester, Manchester Academic Health Science Centre, Manchester, United Kingdom

TARA DZWINIEL, MSc, CCGC
Assistant Clinical Professor, Department of Medical Genetics, University of Alberta, Edmonton, Alberta, Canada

SIMON HANSOM, BSc(Hons), MBBS, MRCP(UK)
Assistant Professor and Staff Electrophysiologist, Arrhythmia Service, Division of Cardiology, University of Ottawa Heart Institute, Ottawa, Ontario, Canada

WIERT F. HOEKSEMA, MD
Department of Clinical Cardiology, Amsterdam UMC, Location University of Amsterdam, Amsterdam Cardiovascular Sciences, Amsterdam, the Netherlands

DANIA KALLAS, MS
Department of Pediatrics, Division of Cardiology, BC Children's Hospital, Heart Center, Vancouver, British Columbia, Canada

ANDREW D. KRAHN, MD, FHRS
Professor of Medicine, Division of Cardiology, University of British Columbia, Vancouver Canada

DENI KUKAVICA, MD, PhD
Department of Molecular Medicine, University of Pavia, Molecular Cardiology, IRCCS Istituti Clinici Scientifici Maugeri, Pavia, Italy; Molecular Cardiology, Centro Nacional de Investigaciones Cardiovasculares (CNIC), Madrid, Spain

ZACHARY LAKSMAN, MD, MSc, FRCPC
Assistant Professor, Department of Medicine, School of Biomedical Engineering, Vancouver, British Columbia, Canada

CIORSTI J. MACINTYRE, MD
Department of Cardiovascular Medicine, Division of Heart Rhythm Services, Windland Smith Rice Genetic Heart Rhythm Clinic, Mayo Clinic, Rochester, Minnesota, USA

ANDREA MAZZANTI, MD, PhD
Department of Molecular Medicine, University of Pavia, Molecular Cardiology, IRCCS Istituti Clinici Scientifici Maugeri, Pavia, Italy; Molecular Cardiology, Centro Nacional de Investigaciones Cardiovasculares (CNIC), Madrid, Spain

BRITTNEY MURRAY, MS
Certified Genetic Counselor, Division of Cardiology, Johns Hopkins University, Baltimore, Maryland, USA

VICTORIA N. PARIKH, MD
Department of Medicine, Division of Cardiovascular Medicine, Stanford Center for Inherited Cardiovascular Disease, Stanford University School of Medicine, Falk CRVC, Stanford, California, USA

ADRIAN PETZL, MD
Cardiovascular Genetics Centre, Montreal Heart Institute, Faculty of Medicine, University of Montreal, Montreal, Quebec, Canada

PIETER G. POSTEMA, MD, PhD
Department of Clinical Cardiology, Amsterdam UMC, Location University of Amsterdam, Amsterdam Cardiovascular Sciences, Amsterdam, the Netherlands

SILVIA G. PRIORI, MD, PhD
Department of Molecular Medicine, University of Pavia, Molecular Cardiology, IRCCS Istituti Clinici Scientifici Maugeri, Pavia, Italy; Molecular Cardiology, Centro Nacional de Investigaciones Cardiovasculares (CNIC), Madrid, Spain

JASON D. ROBERTS, MD, MAS
McMaster University, DBCVSRI, Population Health Research Institute, Hamilton Health Sciences, Hamilton, Ontario, Canada

THOMAS M. ROSTON, MD, PhD
Division of Cardiology, Centre for Cardiovascular Innovation, The University of British Columbia, Vancouver, British Columbia, Canada

TAMMY RYAN, MD, PhD
McMaster University, Department of Medicine, Division of Cardiology, Hamilton General Hospital, DBCVSRI, Hamilton, Ontario, Canada

SHUBHAYAN SANATANI, MD
Department of Pediatrics, Division of Cardiology, BC Children's Hospital, Heart Center, Vancouver, British Columbia, Canada

CHRISTIAN STEINBERG, MD
Institut universitaire de cardiologie et pneumologie de Québec (IUCPQ-UL), Laval University, Quebec, Quebec, Canada

ANDREA SUGAMIELE, BS
Department of Molecular Medicine, University of Pavia, Pavia, Italy

RAFIK TADROS, MD, PhD
Cardiovascular Genetics Centre, Montreal Heart Institute, Faculty of Medicine, Université de Montréal, Montreal, Quebec, Canada

ALESSANDRO TRANCUCCIO, MD
Department of Molecular Medicine, University of Pavia, Molecular Cardiology, IRCCS Istituti Clinici Scientifici Maugeri, Pavia, Italy; Molecular Cardiology, Centro Nacional de Investigaciones Cardiovasculares (CNIC), Madrid, Spain

CHRISTIAN VAN DER WERF, MD, PhD
Department of Cardiology, Heart Centre, Amsterdam UMC Location Academic Medical Centre, University of Amsterdam, Amsterdam Cardiovascular Sciences, Heart Failure and Arrhythmias, Amsterdam, the Netherlands

ARTHUR A.M. WILDE, MD, PhD
Department of Cardiology, Heart Centre, Amsterdam UMC Location Academic Medical Centre, University of Amsterdam, Amsterdam Cardiovascular Sciences, Heart Failure and Arrhythmias, Amsterdam, the Netherlands

Contents

Cardiac genetic counseling is the process of helping individuals adapt to a personal diagnosis or family history of an inherited heart condition. The process is shown to benefit patients and includes specialized skills, such as counseling children and interpreting complex genetic results. Emerging areas include: evolving service delivery models for caring for patients and communicating risk to relatives, new areas of need including postmortem molecular autopsy, and new populations of individuals found to carry a likely pathogenic/pathogenic cardiac variant identified through genomic screening. This article provides an overview of the cardiac genetic counseling process and evolving areas in the field.

Genetic testing has increasingly been shown to provide critical information regarding the treatment and management of patients with hereditary cardiomyopathies and arrhythmias and is available for a wide variety of conditions. It can provide information regarding arrhythmia risk, lifestyle recommendations, such as exercise avoidance, pharmaceutical therapies, and prognosis. Beyond the proband, genetic testing can be a valuable tool for cascade screening in the family. Genetic testing should be accompanied with genetic counseling, as genetic tests should be accompanied by expert interpretation, support in cascade family evaluation, and psychosocial considerations. Overall, it should be routinely implemented in arrhythmia and cardiomyopathy clinics.

Diagnosis and risk stratification of rare genetic heart diseases remains clinically challenging. In many cases, there are few data and insufficient numbers to support randomized controlled trials. While implantable cardioverter defibrillator (ICD) use is vital to protect higher-risk individuals from life-threatening ventricular arrhythmias, low-risk individuals also require protection from unnecessary ICDs and their associated complications. Once an ICD has been implanted, appropriate device programming is essential to ensure maximal protection while balancing the risks of inappropriate therapy.

Inherited cardiomyopathy and arrhythmia syndromes are associated with significant morbidity and mortality, particularly in young people. Medical management of these conditions has primarily been limited to agents previously developed for more common forms of heart disease and not tailored to their distinct pathophysiology. As our understanding of their underlying genetics and disease mechanisms has improved, an era of targeted therapies for these rare conditions has begun to emerge. In recent years, several novel agents have been developed and tested in preclinical models and, in some cases, have advanced to both the clinical trial and clinical approval stages with exciting results. These new treatments are derived from multiple classes of therapeutics, including small molecules, antisense oligonucleotides, small interfering RNAs, adeno-associated virus–mediated gene therapies, and in vivo gene editing. Collectively, they carry the promise of revolutionizing management of affected patients and their families.

Brugada syndrome (BrS) is an inherited arrhythmia syndrome with distinctive electrocardiographic abnormalities in the right precordial leads and predisposes to ventricular arrhythmias and sudden cardiac death in otherwise healthy patients. Its complex genetic architecture and pathophysiological mechanism are not yet completely understood, and risk stratification remains challenging, particularly in patients at intermediate risk of arrhythmic events. Further understanding of its complex genetic architecture may help improving future risk stratification, and advances in management may contribute to alternatives to implantable cardioverter-defibrillators. Here, the authors review the latest insights and developments in BrS.

Long QT Syndrome (LQTS) is a potentially life-threatening yet highly treatable inherited cardiac channelopathy. When evaluating these patients, it is important to consider patient-specific as well as genotype-specific factors in order to adequately encompass the many nuances to care that exist in its management. The tendency to follow a "one-size-fits-all" approach needs to be replaced by treatment strategies that embrace the unique considerations of the individual patient in the context of their genotype. Herein, the authors aim to review the spectrum of LQTS, including the considerations when tailoring a personalized, genotype-tailored treatment program for a patient's LQTS.

Catecholaminergic polymorphic ventricular tachycardia (CPVT) is an inherited arrhythmia syndrome characterized by bidirectional or polymorphic ventricular arrhythmia provoked by exercise or emotion. Most cases are caused by pathogenic variants in the gene encoding the cardiac ryanodine receptor (RYR2). The options for treating patients with CPVT have increased during the years, and evidence suggests that these have led to lower arrhythmic event rates. In addition, numerous potential new therapies are being investigated. In this review, we summarize the state of knowledge on both established and potential future treatment strategies for patients with CPVT and describe our approach to their management.

Unexplained cardiac arrest (UCA) is a working diagnosis that should be replaced by a final diagnosis once evaluation is completed. Complete evaluation of UCA should include high-yield tests like cardiac magnetic resonance imaging, exercise treadmill test, and sodium-channel blocker challenge to identify latent causes of UCA. If no clear etiology is revealed after complete evaluation, idiopathic ventricular fibrillation may be diagnosed, and the strength of its diagnosis can be divided into definitive, probable, and possible based on the number of high-yield tests performed. Care should be provided by a multidisciplinary team with expertise in this area.

Calcium release deficiency syndrome (CRDS) is a newly described form of inherited arrhythmia caused by damaging loss-of-function variants in the cardiac ryanodine receptor (RyR2). Unlike the prototypical RyR2 gain-of-function channelopathy, known as catecholaminergic polymorphic ventricular tachycardia, patients with CRDS are predisposed to sudden death usually in the absence of any electrical abnormalities at rest or during stress electrocardiography. This makes diagnosis incredibly challenging, however, an invasive electrophysiologic test appears to be effective in unmasking the phenotype, called the long-burst, long-pause, short-coupled ventricular extra-stimulus protocol. Optimal therapies for patients with CRDS remain unestablished, although flecainide appears to be a promising candidate drug.

Short-coupled ventricular fibrillation (SCVF) is a distinct phenotype among individuals with unexplained cardiac arrest accounting for 7% to 14% of cases of idiopathic ventricular fibrillation (IVF). IVF is typically initiated by a trigger premature ventricular contraction with a short-coupling interval of less than 350 milliseconds. In the absence of specific electrocardiographic features or provocative tests, the diagnosis remains challenging and requires documentation of IVF onset. Most cases are diagnosed during follow-up at the time of IVF recurrence. SCVF is characterized by a high risk of IVF recurrence. Insertion of an implantable cardioverter-defibrillator and quinidine are the keystones of SCVF management.

Familial ST-depression syndrome represents a novel inherited disease characterized by nonischemic ST-segment depressions in multiple leads. The ECG phenotype appears to debut around puberty, while the typical onset of arrhythmias occurs around 50 years of age. Clinical manifestations include supraventricular arrhythmias, fast polymorphic ventricular tachycardia, sudden cardiac death, and left ventricular systolic dysfunction. The optimal treatment is unknown but asymptomatic individuals without red flags may not need treatment. In contrast, ICD implantation should be considered in patients with probable arrhythmic syncope and in those fulfilling general criteria for ICD treatment. Future research should focus on establishing the disease prevalence, optimizing risk stratification and treatment, and elucidating the underlying genetic etiology.

Arrhythmogenic cardiomyopathy is an umbrella term for a group of inherited diseases of the cardiac muscle characterized by progressive fibro-fatty replacement of the myocardium. As suggested by the name, the disease confers electrical instability to the heart and increases the risk of the development of life-threatening arrhythmias, representing one of the leading causes of sudden cardiac death (SCD), especially in young athletes. In this review, the authors review the current knowledge of the disease, highlighting the state-of-the-art approaches to the prevention of the occurrence of SCD.

Hypertrophic cardiomyopathy (HCM) is the most prevalent inherited cardiac disease. Since the modern description of HCM more than seven decades ago, great focus has been placed on preventing its most catastrophic complication: sudden cardiac death (SCD). Implantable cardioverter-defibrillators (ICD) have been recognized to provide effective prophylactic therapy. Over the years, two leading societies, the European Society of Cardiology (ESC) and the American Heart Association/American College of Cardiology (AHA/ACC), have proposed risk stratification models to assess SCD in adults. European guidelines rely on a risk calculator, the HCM Risk-SCD, while American guidelines propose a stand-alone risk factor approach. Recently, risk prediction models were also developed in the pediatric population. This article reviews the latest recommendations on the risk stratification of SCD in HCM and summarises current indications for ICD use.

Left ventricular ejection fraction-based arrhythmic risk stratification in nonischemic cardiomyopathy (NICM) is insufficient and has led to the failure of primary prevention implantable cardioverter defibrillator trials, mainly due to the inability of selecting patients at high risk for sudden cardiac death (SCD). Cardiac magnetic resonance offers unique opportunities for tissue characterization and has gained a central role in arrhythmic risk stratification in NICM. The presence of myocardial scar, denoted by late gadolinium enhancement, is a significant, independent, and strong predictor of ventricular arrhythmias and SCD with high negative predictive value. T1 maps and extracellular volume fraction, which are able to quantify diffuse fibrosis, hold promise as complementary tools but need confirmatory results from large studies.

Arrhythmogenic left ventricular cardiomyopathy is characterized by early malignant ventricular arrhythmia associated with varying degrees and times of onset of left ventricular dysfunction. Variants in numerous genes have been associated with this phenotype. Here, the authors review the literature on recent cohort studies of patients with variants in desmoplakin, lamin A/C, filamin-C, phospholamban, RBM20, TMEM43, and selected channelopathy genes also associated with structural disease. Unlike traditional sudden cardiac death risk assessment in nonischemic cardiomyopathy, left ventricular systolic function is an insensitive predictor of risk in patients with these genetic diagnoses.

CARDIAC ELECTROPHYSIOLOGY CLINICS

SERIES OF RELATED INTEREST

Cardiology Clinics
https://www.cardiology.theclinics.com/
Interventional Cardiology Clinics
https://www.interventional.theclinics.com/
Heart Failure Clinics
https://www.heartfailure.theclinics.com/

THE CLINICS ARE AVAILABLE ONLINE!
Access your subscription at:
www.theclinics.com

Foreword
Progress and Promise

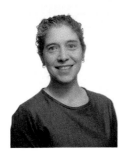
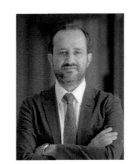

Emily P. Zeitler, MD, MHS, FHRS   Luigi Di Biase, MD, PhD, FACC, FESC, FHRS
Consulting Editors

It has been nearly 10 years since the *Cardiac Electrophysiology Clinics* published reviews on inherited cardiac arrhythmia syndromes. We hope you agree with us after reading this issue that it was worth the wait. There has been tremendous progress in this space over the past 10+ years reflecting stunning advancement in a variety of fields including (but not limited to) genetics, epidemiology, and imaging, which has resulted in remarkable improvements in clinical care. These advancements have culminated in more accurate risk-stratification techniques to help direct care to those who most need it without unnecessarily treating those who don't.

Drs Tadros, Cadrin-Tourigny, and Roberts have compiled a terrific cast of contributors to this issue of the *Cardiac Electrophysiology Clinics* to highlight this advancement, which journeys all the way from the genetic bases of disease to genetic counseling, and from mechanisms of ventricular arrhythmia to patient selection for an ICD, just to name two arcs. You will be amazed to learn (or be reminded) of all of the extraordinary progress that has been made. Indeed, the developments in the field—among other factors—have led to heterogeneity in the application of scientific discoveries at the point of care and in the compiling of recommendations from professional societies. Several of the articles in this issue explore aspects of these differences in interpretation and application of scientific findings. It is these areas of debate that are ripe for future investigation, and we look forward to following that ongoing inquiry. Hopefully, we won't have to wait another 10 years to highlight the next period of advancement.

We believe that the most remarkable aspect of this issue is the obvious and direct potential for application at the point of care for interested readers. We envision that this issue will occupy an easy-to-reach spot on the shelf (be it physical or digital) for repeated reference. While many of us treat patients with inherited cardiac disease on a regular basis, the dramatic heterogeneity of that patient group can make each interaction challenging. So, updated and well-researched reviews on specific scenarios from authoritative sources will be valuable to so many.

As always, we are indebted to the talented group of authors and investigators who have contributed to this issue of the *Cardiac Electrophysiology Clinics*. We are reminded once again of the collaborative spirit and zest for scientific engagement and discovery that so pervades clinical cardiac electrophysiology.

Emily P. Zeitler, MD, MHS, FHRS
Dartmouth Health and
The Dartmouth Institute
1 Medical Center Drive
Lebanon, NH 03756, USA

Luigi Di Biase, MD, PhD, FACC, FESC, FHRS
Albert Einstein College of Medicine
at Montefiore Health System
New York, NY 10467, USA

E-mail addresses:
emily.p.zeitler@hitchcock.org (E.P. Zeitler)
dibbia@gmail.com (L. Di Biase)

Card Electrophysiol Clin 15 (2023) xiii
https://doi.org/10.1016/j.ccep.2023.07.001
1877-9182/23/© 2023 Published by Elsevier Inc.

cardiacEP.theclinics.com

Preface
A Primer on Inherited Cardiac Arrhythmias and Cardiomyopathies

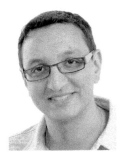 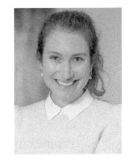 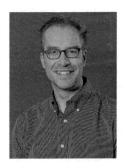

Rafik Tadros, MD, PhD   Julia Cadrin-Tourigny, MD, PhD   Jason D. Roberts, MD, MAS

Editors

The field of cardiogenetics is at a crossroads. Three decades have passed since the identification of the first genes underlying inherited cardiac diseases predisposing to sudden death. Over time, a diverse array of genes has been implicated in cardiac conditions with variable levels of robust evidence, and we now better appreciate the complex genetic architectures of inherited arrhythmias and cardiomyopathies. Our improved understanding of genetics has resulted in better diagnostic and screening strategies for patients and their relatives. This better understanding of human genetics has concomitantly improved our knowledge of disease mechanisms resulting in enhanced and personalized therapy, oftentimes decreasing the requirement for implantable cardiac defibrillators. The future of cardiogenetics is now, with the rapid development of targeted therapies, including gene therapies. It is expected that clinical trials of gene therapy in humans will be initiated in the next few months, with the hope of finding a definitive cure in some of the inherited cardiac diseases predisposing to sudden death.

This issue of *Cardiac Electrophysiology Clinics* provides a comprehensive and practical update of heritable cardiac diseases causing sudden death and is intended for cardiologists, cardiac electrophysiologists, and other health care professionals involved in caring for patients and families with such conditions.

The first part of the issue consists of reviews of general principles in cardiogenetics, including principles of genetic counseling ("Principles of Genetic Counseling in Inherited Heart Conditions") and testing ("A Practical Guide to Genetic Testing in Inherited Heart Disease"), as well as practical aspects of implantable device programming ("Implantable Devices in Genetic Heart Disease: Disease-Specific Device Selection and Programming") and the emerging role of targeted therapies ("Emerging Targeted Therapies for Inherited Cardiomyopathies and Arrhythmias").

The second part consists of practical reviews of heritable arrhythmia syndromes that occur in the absence of overt structural heart disease. Novelties in traditional primary arrhythmia syndromes are reviewed: Brugada in "Novelties in Brugada Syndrome: Complex Genetics, Risk Stratification, and Catheter Ablation," long QT in "Personalized Care in Long QT Syndrome: Better Management, More Sports, and Fewer Devices," and catecholaminergic polymorphic ventricular tachycardia in "Catecholaminergic Polymorphic Ventricular Tachycardia: A Review of Therapeutic Strategies." "Investigation of Unexplained Cardiac Arrest: Phenotyping and Genetic Testing" summarizes the investigation of unexplained cardiac arrest, highlighting the mounting role of genetic testing. Newly recognized phenotypes are also discussed: calcium release deficiency syndrome in "Calcium Release

Card Electrophysiol Clin 15 (2023) xv–xvi
https://doi.org/10.1016/j.ccep.2023.06.006
1877-9182/23/© 2023 Published by Elsevier Inc.

cardiacEP.theclinics.com

Deficiency Syndrome: A New Inherited Arrhythmia Syndrome," short-coupled ventricular fibrillation in "Short-Coupled Ventricular Fibrillation," and familial ST depression syndrome in "The Novel Familial ST-Depression Syndrome—Current Knowledge and Perspectives."

The third part reviews risk stratification of sudden death in heritable cardiomyopathies, including arrhythmogenic right ventricular cardiomyopathy ("Prevention of Sudden Death and Management of Ventricular Arrhythmias in Arrhythmogenic Cardiomyopathy"), hypertrophic cardiomyopathy ("Sudden Death Risk Assessment in Hypertrophic Cardiomyopathy Across the Lifespan: Reconciling the American and European Approaches"), and the emerging role of cardiac magnetic resonance and genetics in risk stratification in left ventricular (arrhythmogenic) cardiomyopathy ("Impact of Cardiac Magnetic Resonance to Arrhythmic Risk Stratification in Nonischemic Cardiomyopathy" and "Genetic Risk Stratification in Arrhythmogenic Left Ventricular Cardiomyopathy").

We are grateful both to the editors-in-chief for the trust placed in us to develop and review the content of this issue and for the contributions of all the immensely talented expert authors. We hope that this issue of *Cardiac Electrophysiology Clinics* will be useful to clinicians and scientists interested in and caring for patients with heritable heart diseases predisposing to sudden cardiac death and their families.

Rafik Tadros, MD, PhD
Montreal Heart Institute and
Université de Montréal
Montreal, Quebec H1T 1C8, Canada

Julia Cadrin-Tourigny, MD, PhD
Montreal Heart Institute and
Université de Montréal
Montreal, Quebec H1T 1C8, Canada

Jason D. Roberts, MD, MAS
Population Health Research Institute and
McMaster University
Hamilton, Ontario L8L 2X2, Canada

E-mail addresses:
rafik.tadros@umontreal.ca (R. Tadros)
julia.cadrin-tourigny@umontreal.ca (J. Cadrin-Tourigny)
Jason.Roberts@phri.ca (J.D. Roberts)

Introduction

Inherited Cardiac Diseases Predisposing to Sudden Death

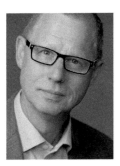

Andrew D. Krahn, MD, FHRS

It is not uncommon to hear the expression "heart disease runs in my family" in both medical and social settings, and indeed, we have virtually all been affected by heart disease in some form or another. The genetic revolution is moving at a staggering pace as we unravel the genetic contribution to cardiomyopathy and sudden death. Indeed, the relatively recently coined term "Arrhythmogenic Cardiomyopathy" speaks to the concept that cardiac conditions that pose a risk of sudden death have a variable "dose" of myopathic and arrhythmogenic elements, which must be considered when approaching patients and families in counseling risk and its resultant management. As a clinical teacher in our inherited arrhythmia clinic (www.heartsinrhythm.ca), I often tell trainees that half the time, the diagnosis is fairly clear and the management is straightforward, but the other half is fraught with uncertainty, both in phenotype and in genetic data and its interpretation and resultant clinical decision making. As you will see when you read on, we are definitely making progress in unraveling that difficult half.

In this issue of *Cardiac Electrophysiology Clinics*, the focus is on the intersection of clinical phenotype with our mechanistic and genetic understanding of familiar foes, such as Long QT syndrome and Brugada, to novel syndromes such as Calcium Release Deficiency Syndrome and Short-Coupled Ventricular Fibrillation. Topics in this series were chosen to be clinically relevant to all practicing Cardiologists, Electrophysiologists, and their partners in Medical Genetics.

Most compelling to me as a senior member of this community, is the author intersection of a founder group of leaders in the field, and a remarkable new generation of clinician scientists who are rapidly advancing our field, including the three editors of this issue. From bench to bedside to policy, and monogenic to oligogenic to polygenic, it is obvious that the field is becoming more complex, and much more precise, in its understanding of individual patients. Most exciting is the rapid progress to highly effective and even curative solutions.

I encourage you to dig into this compendium of state-of-the-art reviews, to gain or strengthen your understanding of this compelling field, the nuances of the individual syndromes, and the opportunity to bring said expertise to your patients and their families.

Andrew D. Krahn, MD, FHRS
Division of Cardiology
University of British Columbia
Vancouver, Canada

E-mail address:
akrahn@mail.ubc.ca

Card Electrophysiol Clin 15 (2023) xvii
https://doi.org/10.1016/j.ccep.2023.07.002
1877-9182/23/© 2023 Published by Elsevier Inc.

Principles of Genetic Counseling in Inherited Heart Conditions

Susan Christian, MSc, PhD, CGC*, Tara Dzwiniel, MSc, CCGC

KEYWORDS

- Genetic counseling • Arrhythmia • Cardiomyopathy • Inherited heart condition

KEY POINTS

- Genetic counseling is a key process to ensure optimal use of cardiac genetic testing and appropriate interpretation of cardiac genetic test results.
- Models of care for genetic counseling are evolving with expanding technologies and demand.
- New patient populations are being identified with unique characteristics and needs.

INTRODUCTION

Cardiac genetic counseling is the process of helping individuals with a personal or family history of an inherited heart condition understand the benefits and limitations of genetic testing/test results and adapt to the diagnosis. It integrates an educational and psychosocial component and involves families as a unit rather than individuals. Historically, there has been significant focus on pretest counseling; however, more recently a greater appreciation of the importance of genetic counseling in the posttest setting has become clear with regard to interpretation of results and communication of risk within a family. The field is quickly evolving with the introduction of new service delivery models of care, new areas of need, and new patient populations. This review article provides an overview of the cardiac genetic counseling process and evolving areas in the field.

DISCUSSION

Introduction of Cardiac Genetic Counseling

Genetic counseling was first introduced in the cardiac setting with the discovery of genes associated with inherited arrhythmias and cardiomyopathies in the 1990s and early 2000s.[1-5] It was quickly appreciated that heart conditions, such as long QT syndrome, catecholaminergic polymorphic ventricular tachycardia (CPVT), Brugada syndrome, hypertrophic cardiomyopathy (HCM), dilated cardiomyopathy, and arrhythmogenic right ventricular cardiomyopathy (ARVC) are genetically heterogeneous, making genetic testing time consuming and expensive. The development of next-generation sequencing technology, allowing multiple genes to be sequenced at the same time, led to a reduction in the turnaround time and the cost of testing. Genetic testing can provide helpful information in diagnosis and management for an individual with an inherited heart condition, and offer an opportunity for early diagnosis and treatment of their relatives (cascade genetic testing). As a result, cardiac genetic counseling emerged.

The key components of cardiac genetic counseling have been nicely described by Cirino and colleagues[6] and include pretest actions, such as gathering a cardiac-focused family history, selecting the most appropriate test and most appropriate person to test, and managing patient expectations with regard to genetic testing (Fig. 1). In the context of cascade genetic testing, it is also important to include a discussion about genetic discrimination and potential concerns regarding genetic testing leading to altered treatment by employers and insurance companies. Although Canada and the United States have national genetic nondiscrimination laws in place,

Department of Medical Genetics, University of Alberta, Edmonton, Alberta, Canada
* Corresponding author. Department of Medical Genetics, University of Alberta, 826 Medical Sciences Building, Edmonton, Alberta T6H 2H7.
E-mail address: smc12@ualberta.ca

Card Electrophysiol Clin 15 (2023) 229–239
https://doi.org/10.1016/j.ccep.2023.05.001

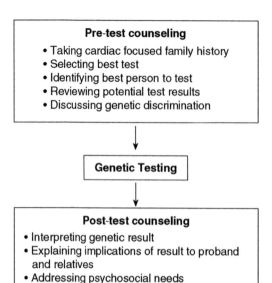

Pre-test counseling
- Taking cardiac focused family history
- Selecting best test
- Identifying best person to test
- Reviewing potential test results
- Discussing genetic discrimination

↓

Genetic Testing

↓

Post-test counseling
- Interpreting genetic result
- Explaining implications of result to proband and relatives
- Addressing psychosocial needs
- Providing resources on support and research

Fig. 1. Overview of the genetic counseling process.

these laws have limitations.[7] Posttest actions include interpreting the patient's genetic result in the context of their clinical presentation and family history, discussing the importance of communicating results with at-risk relatives to guide cardiac screening, and sharing information on support groups and research opportunities. Additional psychosocial counseling is based on patient-specific circumstances, such as how the heart condition presented and impacted the patient and/or their relatives. The process of genetic counseling is typically performed by a health care professional with expertise in genetics and counseling, such as a genetic counselor. However, it may be performed by other health care professionals that have additional training in these areas.

Several published guidelines recommend genetic counseling for patients with or at risk of an inherited heart condition.[8–10] In spite of these recommendations, uptake of genetic counseling is variable for probands ranging from 37% to 68%, and 38% to 84% for at-risk relatives.[11] Helio and colleagues[12] found that patients diagnosed with cardiomyopathy who received genetic counseling tended to be younger at age of diagnosis, were more likely to have familial disease, and presented with less comorbidities compared with those that did not receive genetic counseling.

Utility of Cardiac Genetic Counseling

Genetic counseling is tightly intertwined with genetic testing and as such it is challenging to tease

out the value of genetic counseling independently. Patient empowerment and knowledge of cardiac screening recommendations for relatives have been identified as key outcomes of genetic counseling.[13] Ison and colleagues[13] measured patient empowerment using the genetic counseling outcome scale for patients with a personal or family history of heart disease including inherited arrhythmia or cardiomyopathy. Significantly higher genetic counseling outcome scale scores (greater empowerment) were reported postgenetic counseling. In addition, the proportion of patients aware of screening recommendations for relatives increased from 40% before meeting with a genetic counselor to 76% after the appointment. Patients with a diagnosis of ARVC or at risk of ARVC were also found to have greater patient empowerment and less cardiac fear after one genetic counseling appointment.[14]

High levels of satisfaction with genetic counseling have been reported by several groups.[11] Specifically, Nieuwhof and colleagues[15] found that patients who received genetic counseling from a genetic counselor/genetic nurse had significantly greater satisfaction compared with those that received genetic counseling from a cardiologist.

Genetic Counseling Involving Children

Although inherited heart conditions often present during adulthood, onset during childhood is not uncommon. Engagement with children and adolescents about the pros and cons of cascade genetic testing is therefore an important area of cardiac genetic counseling. Clinical guidelines recommend that children participate to some degree in discussion around the option of genetic testing and potential implications of testing.[16] Genetic counseling with children should start with an assessment of the child's developmental age and maturity and a conversation about the child's understanding of the heart condition in their family. The language used and the depth of discussion vary based on maturity level. In line with recommendations by the American Academy of Pediatrics,[17] obtaining assent from a minor about genetic testing should include:

1. Discussion of the condition
2. Review of potential results and next steps based on the different type of results
3. Assessment of the child's understanding of the information and factors influencing their response
4. Clarification of the child's interest in testing

A systematic review of children and adolescents' understanding of inherited conditions found that for autosomal-dominant conditions, children generally appreciate that disease predisposition runs in families, and most were able to later accurately describe their genetic status.[18] They also describe that a child's understanding of heritability is highly influenced by the experience in their family, highlighting the value of using this as a starting point for discussion.

Decision aids have been created using the International Patient Decision Aid Standards to help guide discussion with families regarding cascade genetic testing for several different inherited heart conditions (https://decisionaid.ohri.ca/Azinvent.php/). The cardiac genetic decision aids review the pros and cons of choosing ongoing cardiac screening versus cascade genetic testing followed by cardiac screening for children that test positive for a familial variant.[19] Most (93%) families interviewed about the cardiac decision aids reported that they would be useful in making a decision about predictive genetic testing for their children.

Role of the Cardiac Genetic Counselor in Variant Interpretation

The ability to offer cascade genetic testing hinges on the correct interpretation of genetic results for the proband. Genetic testing for a proband can yield several types of results, with their own unique impact on family screening recommendations. An informative result (likely pathogenic or pathogenic [LP/P] variant) allows for cascade genetic testing to be offered to relatives. For a proband with a noninformative (negative) result, cardiac screening for their first-degree relatives is still recommended because a negative result cannot exclude the possibility of an inherited condition. When variants of uncertain significance (VUS) are identified, assessing the value of testing other relatives with similar or related disease to help with variant reclassification is within the genetic counselor role.[20]

Variant interpretation is an important part of the cardiac genetic counselor's role. In an online survey of 46 cardiac genetic counselors, Reuter and colleagues[20] showed that nearly all genetic counselors (95.7%) obtain additional information on the variants reported in genetic reports, and that most (81%) critically assess the variant classification. Indeed, correct interpretation of genetic results has been suggested by others as one of the primary roles of cardiac genetic counselors.[21,22]

Importance of ongoing variant evaluation

Genetic results are probabilistic in nature, and variant classification relies on the strength of evidence that a specific variant is disease-causing.[23] Variant classification is seen as a continuum of probability from benign to pathogenic. It follows that the interpretation of genetic variants may differ between clinical genetic laboratories applying modified classification criteria, and may change over time with new data, including genetic variant frequency data obtained from larger and more ethnically diverse cohorts, and functional studies.[24]

Variant reclassifications are not infrequent, and occur in the cardiac genetic realm as in other areas of genetics.[25] Several recent studies in patients with inherited arrhythmia and cardiomyopathy have reported clinically significant variant reclassifications, with reclassification rates ranging from 10% to 41% (Table 1).[26,27] Contributing factors include when the initial genetic testing was done, number of genes per panel, condition tested for, and variant type (eg, missense), although many studies are limited by small sample size.

Variants downgraded from LP/P to VUS have important implications for cascade screening, because relatives who tested negative may have been prematurely discharged from clinical screening. A variant reclassification emphasizes the need for further genetic counseling and ongoing clinical screening of these individuals. Variants that are upgraded from VUS to LP/P, allow for cascade genetic testing for the family. Sarquella-Brugada and coworkers[28] found that nearly 20% of rare arrhythmia variants were reclassified in a 5-year time period. These findings suggest that variant review should be no longer than 5 years from the last classification.

The need for ongoing variant evaluation is further supported by current guidelines.[10,24] Although the psychological impact of variant reclassification on patients has not been extensively studied, one study suggests that variant reclassifications are frequently misunderstood by the patient in terms of implications for themselves and family screening.[29]

Gene curation

Although it is important to consider variant classification, equally important is the notion of whether the gene itself is strongly associated with a given phenotype (gene-disease associations).[30] Over time, genetic testing panels for inherited arrhythmias and cardiomyopathies have increased in size, often with the addition of preliminary evidence genes with limited gene-disease association. This can lead to a higher number of VUS results, which may complicate genetic counseling, potentially increasing uncertainty and the risk of misinterpretation.

To increase the clinical utility and mitigate potential harms of genetic testing, there are ongoing collaborative efforts led by the Clinical Genome

Table 1
Variant reclassification rates in inherited arrhythmia and cardiomyopathy genes

First Author (y)	Population (Study Timeframe)	Reclassification Rate
Das et al,[26] 2014	Hypertrophic cardiomyopathy patients (not indicated)	10% (5/54 unique variants) of variant were reclassified. Two VUS results were upgraded to pathogenic, 1 VUS and 1 pathogenic variant were downgraded to benign, and 1 pathogenic variant was downgraded to VUS.
Bennett et al,[73] 2019	Pediatric inherited arrhythmia patients (2009–2017)	52% (12/23) of unique VUS results were reclassified using 2015 criteria. Of these, 35% (8) were upgraded to pathogenic, and 17% (4) downgraded to benign. 48% (11/23) of VUS results were unable to be reclassified. The year of testing was not a significant factor for reclassification. Those who met clinical diagnostic criteria were more likely to have their variant upgraded to LP/P.
Westphal et al,[74] 2020	Pediatric long QT patients (2001–2018)	14.3% (12/84) of variants were downgraded from LP to VUS.
Cherny et al,[75] 2021	Pediatric arrhythmia and cardiomyopathy patients (2006–2017)	21.5% (71/330) of variants were reclassified, of which 10% were clinically relevant. Of these, most variants were downgraded from LP/P to VUS (7.6%; 25/330), and 2.7% (9/330) were upgraded from VUS to LP/P.
Costa et al,[27] 2021	ARVC patients (1998–2019)	58.8% (47/80 variants) of variants were reclassified, of which 41.3% (n = 33) of reclassifications were clinically relevant. PKP2 variants were less likely to be reclassified. Missense variants were more likely to be reclassified compared with other variant types. 10.1% of patient diagnoses (n = 8) were downgraded from definite ARVC to borderline/possible ARVC because of impact of variant reclassification on major task force criteria. Variants reported before 2015 were more likely to be reclassified than variants reported after 2015.
Davies et al,[76] 2021	CASPER registry (cardiac arrest survivor, sudden death victim, or first-degree relative) (2006–2017)	31% (40/131) of variants had a clinically significant reclassification. VUS results were more likely to be downgraded (73%) to benign than upgraded to pathogenic (27%; P = .03). Variants reported before 2015 were more likely to be reclassified than variants reported after 2015.
Westphal et al,[77] 2022	Pediatric cardiomyopathy patients (2009–2019)	29% (13/45) of variants were reclassified, all of which were downgraded (9/13 went from VUS to likely benign, and 3/13 from LP to VUS).

Abbreviations: LP, likely pathogenic; P, pathogenic.

(ClinGen) gene curation working group to assess the strength of evidence linking a gene to a particular disease.[31] Curated gene lists are published for several cardiogenetic conditions including long QT syndrome, HCM, dilated cardiomyopathy, ARVC, Brugada syndrome, and CPVTa.[32–37]

Genetic counselors have an important role in helping families understand the benefits, limitations, and evolving nature of genetic test information. Variant interpretation and gene curation should be an ongoing, dynamic process that can change over time and with new knowledge. Further research is needed into the psychological impact of variant reclassifications on families.

FUTURE DIRECTIONS

Although cardiac genetic counseling is a new area of genetic counseling, the subspeciality is quickly evolving. Emerging areas include new service delivery models for caring for patients; communicating screening options to at-risk relatives; and new areas of need, such as postmortem molecular autopsy. In addition, new patient populations are arising with increased uptake of genome-wide sequencing leading to the identification of individuals with a secondary finding of an LP/P cardiac variant.

New Service Delivery Models

With the expanding demand for cardiac genetic testing, the genetic counselor workforce is struggling to meet the need. Alternative service delivery models are required to provide patients with the necessary information to make an informed choice about genetic testing. Within the cardiac genetics field, several alternative service delivery models have been piloted and evaluated. Otten and colleagues[38] found that perceived personal control increased and anxiety decreased compared with baseline after patients with HCM attended a group genetic counseling session. Three-quarters of patients indicated that they were satisfied with this format.

A virtual version of group genetic counseling has also been piloted via a live webinar for patients with HCM.[39] This model was compared head-to-head with the traditional genetic counseling model. Comparable improvements between groups were observed in self-perceived knowledge and decisional conflict. Most patients (88%) reported that the webinar was an acceptable replacement for a one-on-one genetic counseling appointment. Furthermore, genetic counseling time was reduced from a traditional 60-minute appointment to on average 24 minutes per patient.

Other service delivery models, such as patient videos and chatbots, may be useful tools to further improve efficiencies in providing pretest counseling. Although these models have been evaluated in other areas of genetic counseling and videos have been developed for cardiac genetic testing, the effectiveness of these models in the setting of inherited heart conditions have yet to be published.

In reality, one service delivery model is unlikely to meet the needs of all patients. The future may involve providing patients with options based on their educational and counseling needs, including viewing a video or reading an information brochure, interacting with a chatbot, attending an in-person or online group genetic counseling session, or meeting with a genetic counselor one-on-one (**Fig. 2**). Information seekers, patients with a complex clinical presentation or family history, and those that have higher counseling needs are more likely to require an individualized genetic counseling appointment. Once genetic testing is complete, new needs may also arise including interpretation of results, and communication of genetic information with relatives. For many cardiac patients, the involvement of a genetic counselor may shift from pretest genetic counseling toward posttest genetic counseling with a focus on positive and unclear test results. This approach requires that cardiologists feel comfortable selecting the most appropriate genetic test and answering patient questions about genetic testing. Ultimately, the assessment of the patient's informational and counseling needs also falls to the cardiologist. Although cardiology providers recognize that genetic testing is an important component to the diagnosis and treatment plan, given the complexity of interpreting results, many feel unprepared to offer genetic testing without the support of a genetic expert (ie, genetic counselor, geneticist, or cardiologist with genetics training).[40,41] This highlights the need for educational supports for ordering providers.

New Strategies for Notifying Relatives

Relatives of an individual with an inherited heart condition have an increased risk of developing the condition regardless of the proband's genetic result. Because of this, cascade screening is recommended for all at-risk relatives. Cascade screening may involve cascade genetic testing when an LP/P variant has been identified in the family, or serial cardiac screening when no genetic cause is found. For cascade screening to be successful, it requires that the proband appreciates the risk to their relatives and communicates this risk to them in a meaningful way.[42] It also requires

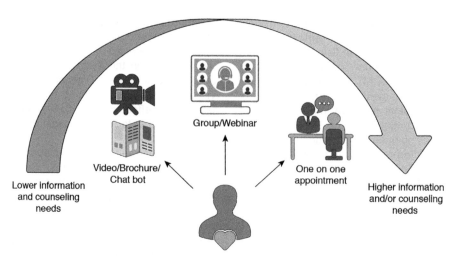

Fig. 2. Models of care based on the informational and counseling needs of a patient. Patient can be offered the option of viewing a video, reading a brochure, interacting with a chatbot, attending a group session/webinar, or meeting one on one with a genetic counselor to best meet their needs.

that the relatives understand the risk and are able and motivated to access the appropriate services. Traditionally, genetic counselors have provided probands with a letter to share with relatives explaining the condition, the risk, and the option of cardiac screening, with or without genetic counseling and genetic testing. Although this approach has been shown to be an effective method to inform relatives of the cardiac genetic risk,[43] approximately 40% of at-risk relatives remain unscreened.[11] As a result, several novel approaches have been introduced to further maximize cascade screening and improve early diagnosis and treatment. These approaches include a personalized family communication aid, patient videos, chatbot, and directly contacting relatives. Studies describing the development and evaluation of these communication tools are described in **Table 2**.

Regardless of the approach, a subset of at-risk relatives remain unscreened. Emphasis has been on the communication of risk information from the proband to their relatives; however, more research is required from the perspective of at-risk relatives regarding their understanding of the information and rationale for not undergoing cascade screening. Development of strategies to overcome barriers to cascade screening is an important next step.

New Areas of Need: Postmortem Genetic Testing

As the availability of genetic testing has increased, so too has the application of next-generation sequencing technologies into new domains, such as postmortem molecular autopsy. A significant proportion of sudden death in the young (<40 years) is caused by inherited arrhythmias and cardiomyopathies.[44] Recent studies suggest the yield of postmortem genetic testing is around 15% to 20%.[45,46] Genetic testing in cases of sudden unexplained death in the young is supported by several guidelines to aid in establishing a cause of death.[47–49] This knowledge can provide closure for the family, and guide clinical screening of relatives when an LP/P variant is identified.

Challenges to this process include inconsistent access to postmortem genetic testing[50,51]; difficulties in obtaining appropriate samples[49]; and a high rate of VUSs, in the range of approximately 47% to 60%.[44,52,53] Postmortem VUS results should be interpreted with caution, because incorrect interpretation leads to incorrect management of the surviving relatives. A collaborative approach between the medical examiner and the health care team managing the first-degree relatives may be helpful to elucidate the more suspicious VUSs from background noise.[54] Genetic counseling should include managing expectations surrounding the diagnostic rate of molecular autopsy, the high likelihood of a VUS result, and the need for periodic re-evaluation of the postmortem genetic findings.

The loss of a family member can have devastating effects on surviving relatives. Studies have shown increased levels of anxiety and depression, poor psychological adaptation and posttraumatic stress, prolonged grieving, and disruption of family dynamics in individuals who have experienced a sudden death of a relative.[55–57] McDonald and colleagues found several unmet needs for parents who experienced a sudden cardiac death in their

Table 2
Models for communicating risk and recommendations for cascade screening to relatives

Communication Approach	First Author (y)	Diagnoses Included	Summary of Findings
Family letters	van der Roest et al,[43] 2009	DCM, HCM, ARVC, LQTS, and Brugada syndrome	88% of probands shared family letter with relatives and of those, 83% had at least 1 relative that received cardiac screening.
Communication aid	Burns et al,[78] 2019	HCM	Outcome pending.
Video	Harris et al,[79] 2019	HCM	93% of probands reported that they had already communicated their diagnosis of HCM to their relatives. Only 1 relative who was not already aware of the diagnosis of HCM in the family received the video.
Chatbot	Schmidlen et al,[80] 2022	Clinically actionable, pathogenic, or likely pathogenic variant result in 1 of 60 ACMG recommended genes	Uptake of cascade screening was significantly greater among relatives of probands who consented to the family screening tool compared with relatives of probands who declined ($P < .001$).
Direct contact	van den Heuvel et al,[81] 2022	Inherited cardiac condition (arrhythmias and cardiomyopathies)	No significant difference was observed in uptake of genetic counseling between the family-mediated (38%) and the direct-contact (37%) group.

Abbreviations: ACMG, American College of Medical Genetics and Genomics; DCM, dilated cardiomyopathy; LQTS, long QT syndrome.

child, particularly in the medical information and psychosocial support domains (**Fig. 3**).[58] Access to support networks may provide a place of emotional safety and comfort to grieving families who are processing their loss.[59]

New Patient Populations: Secondary Findings

The advent of genome-wide sequencing (exome and genome sequencing) has identified a new patient population of individuals with LP/P findings in cardiovascular genes. Currently, the American College of Medical Genetics and Genomics (ACMG) recommends reporting variants in 78 genes, of which approximately half cause cardiovascular disease.[60] Although the ACMG approach has been widely adopted, other groups recommend a more cautious approach to opportunistic screening.[61,62]

In addition to clinical genome-wide sequencing, the return of secondary findings in clinical research and biobanks is becoming more common.[63–65]

Studies suggest that approximately 1% to 2% of those undergoing genome-wide sequencing are found to have a secondary finding.[66,67] This estimate is likely to increase as new genes are added. For example, the recent ACMG secondary findings version 3.1 guideline recommends reporting all LP/P variants in the *TTR* gene, in which the p.Val142Ile (p.V142I) variant alone occurs in 1% to 2.5% of individuals with West African ancestry.[60] Genetic counseling is complicated by the lack of general population penetrance data for most genes,[68] although initial studies suggest that disease penetrance is lower in this population.[69–71] Katz and Webb[17] suggest labeling these findings as a "clinical finding" (phenotypic evidence of

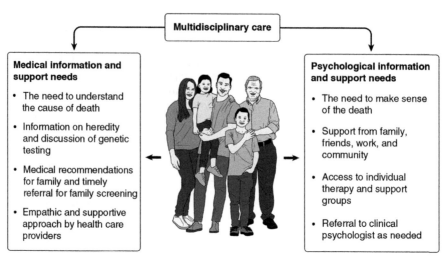

Fig. 3. Informational and psychological needs of families who experience sudden cardiac death in their child.[58] Where possible, care and investigation of the family should be done in a multidisciplinary manner.[49]

disease), "molecular finding" (genetic result), or "clinicomolecular diagnosis" (presence of a clinical and molecular finding) as a way to distinguish between these groups. Genetic counseling will need to be adapted to patients presenting in a genome-first context to help individuals best use this information.[72]

SUMMARY

Cardiac genetic counseling is the process of helping individuals adapt to a personal diagnosis or family history of an inherited heart condition. The process has been shown to benefit patients and includes specialized skills, such as counseling children and interpreting complex genetic results. Emerging areas include: evolving service delivery models for caring for patients and communicating risk to relatives, new areas of need including postmortem molecular autopsy, and new populations of individuals found to carry an LP/P cardiac variant identified through genomic screening.

CLINICS CARE POINTS

- Genetic counseling assists patients in making an informed choice about cardiac genetic testing.

- Decision aids are available to further help families in the choice about predictive genetic testing for children (https://decisionaid.ohri.ca/Azinvent.php/).

- Ongoing, periodic contact with a genetic counselor is important to ensure the most

up-to-date variant classification because this has a critical impact on cascade screening for relatives.

- With increasing demand, novel service delivery models are required.

- Novel patient populations have emerged. Limitations in understanding have led to challenges with interpreting results, making management recommendations, and addressing psychosocial needs.

- More research is needed on the benefit of posttest genetic counseling, the impact of variant reclassification on patients, and barriers to at-risk relatives pursuing cascade screening.

DISCLOSURE

The authors have no conflicts to disclose.

REFERENCES

1. Geisterfer-Lowrance AA, Kass S, Tanigawa G, et al. A molecular basis for familial hypertrophic cardiomyopathy: a beta cardiac myosin heavy chain gene missense mutation. Cell 1990;62(5):999–1006.
2. Curran ME, Splawski I, Timothy KW, et al. A molecular basis for cardiac arrhythmia: HERG mutations cause long QT syndrome. Cell 1995;80(5):795–803.
3. Awad MM, Dalal D, Cho E, et al. DSG2 mutations contribute to arrhythmogenic right ventricular dysplasia/cardiomyopathy. Am J Hum Genet 2006; 79(1):136–42.
4. George CH, Higgs GV, Lai FA. Ryanodine receptor mutations associated with stress-induced ventricular

tachycardia mediate increased calcium release in stimulated cardiomyocytes. Circ Res 2003;93(6):531–40.

5. Antzelevitch C. Molecular biology and cellular mechanisms of Brugada and long QT syndromes in infants and young children. J Electrocardiol 2001;34(Suppl):177–81.

6. Cirino AL, Harris S, Lakdawala NK, et al. Role of genetic testing in inherited cardiovascular disease: a review. JAMA cardiology 2017;2(10):1153–60.

7. Cowan JS, Kagedan BL, Graham GE, et al. Health care implications of the genetic non-discrimination act: protection for Canadians' genetic information. Can Fam Physician 2022;68(9):643–6.

8. Hershberger RE, Givertz M, Ho CY, et al. Genetic evaluation of cardiomyopathy: a Heart Failure Society of America practice guideline. J Card Fail 2018;24(5):281–302.

9. Wilde AAM, Semsarian C, Márquez MF, et al. European Heart Rhythm Association (EHRA)/Heart Rhythm Society (HRS)/Asia Pacific Heart Rhythm Society (APHRS)/Latin American Heart Rhythm Society (LAHRS) expert consensus statement on the state of genetic testing for cardiac diseases. Heart Rhythm 2022;19(7):e1–60.

10. Musunuru K, Hershberger RE, Day SM, et al. Genetic testing for inherited cardiovascular diseases: a scientific statement from the American Heart Association. Circ Genom Precision medicine 2020;13(4):e000067.

11. Cirino AL, Harris SL, Murad AM, et al. The uptake and utility of genetic testing and genetic counseling for hypertrophic cardiomyopathy: a systematic review and meta-analysis. J Genet Counsel 2022. https://doi.org/10.1002/jgc4.1604.

12. Heliö T, Elliott P, Koskenvuo JW, et al. ESC EORP Cardiomyopathy Registry: real-life practice of genetic counselling and testing in adult cardiomyopathy patients. ESC heart failure 2020;7(5):3013–21.

13. Ison HE, Ware SM, Schwantes-An TH, et al. The impact of cardiovascular genetic counseling on patient empowerment. J Genet Counsel 2019;28(3):570–7.

14. Murray B, Tichnell C, Burch AE, et al. Strength of the genetic counselor: patient relationship is associated with extent of increased empowerment in patients with arrhythmogenic cardiomyopathy. J Genet Counsel 2022;31(2):388–97.

15. Nieuwhof K, Birnie E, van den Berg MP, et al. Follow-up care by a genetic counsellor for relatives at risk for cardiomyopathies is cost-saving and well-appreciated: a randomized comparison. Eur J Hum Genet 2017;25(2):169–75.

16. Botkin JR, Belmont JW, Berg JS, et al. Points to consider: ethical, legal, and psychosocial implications of genetic testing in children and adolescents. Am J Hum Genet 2015;97(1):6–21.

17. Katz AL, Webb SA. Informed consent in decision-making in pediatric practice. Pediatrics 2016;138(2). https://doi.org/10.1542/peds.2016-1485.

18. McGill BC, Wakefield CE, Vetsch J, et al. Children and young people's understanding of inherited conditions and their attitudes towards genetic testing: a systematic review. Clin Genet 2019;95(1):10–22.

19. Christian S, Welsh A, Yetman J, et al. Development and evaluation of decision aids to guide families' predictive testing choices for children at risk for arrhythmia or cardiomyopathy. Can J Cardiol 2021;37(10):1586–92.

20. Reuter C, Grove ME, Orland K, et al. Clinical cardiovascular genetic counselors take a leading role in team-based variant classification. J Genet Couns 2018;27(4):751–60.

21. Arscott P, Caleshu C, Kotzer K, et al. A case for inclusion of genetic counselors in cardiac care. Cardiol Rev 2016;24(2):49–55.

22. Ingles J, Yeates L, Semsarian C. The emerging role of the cardiac genetic counselor. Heart Rhythm 2011;8(12):1958–62.

23. Ingles J, Semsarian C. Conveying a probabilistic genetic test result to families with an inherited heart disease. Heart Rhythm 2014;11(6):1073–8.

24. Landstrom AP, Kim JJ, Gelb BD, et al. Genetic testing for heritable cardiovascular diseases in pediatric patients: a scientific statement from the American Heart Association. Circulation Genomic and precision medicine 2021;14(5):e000086.

25. Muir SM, Reagle R. Characterization of variant reclassification and patient re-contact in a cancer genetics clinic. J Genet Counsel 2022. https://doi.org/10.1002/jgc4.1600.

26. Das KJ, Ingles J, Bagnall RD, et al. Determining pathogenicity of genetic variants in hypertrophic cardiomyopathy: importance of periodic reassessment. Genet Med 2014;16(4):286–93.

27. Costa S, Medeiros-Domingo A, Gasperetti A, et al. Impact of genetic variant reassessment on the diagnosis of arrhythmogenic right ventricular cardiomyopathy based on the 2010 task force criteria. Circulation Genomic and precision medicine 2021;14(1):e003047.

28. Sarquella-Brugada G, Fernandez-Falgueras A, Cesar S, et al. Clinical impact of rare variants associated with inherited channelopathies: a 5-year update. Hum Genet 2022;141(10):1579–89.

29. Wong EK, Bartels K, Hathaway J, et al. Perceptions of genetic variant reclassification in patients with inherited cardiac disease. Eur J Hum Genet 2019;27(7):1134–42.

30. Ingles J, Macciocca I, Morales A, et al. Genetic testing in inherited heart diseases. Heart Lung Circ 2020;29(4):505–11.

31. Strande NT, Riggs ER, Buchanan AH, et al. Evaluating the clinical validity of gene-disease associations: an evidence-based framework developed by the clinical genome resource. Am J Hum Genet 2017;100(6):895–906.

32. Ingles J, Goldstein J, Thaxton C, et al. Evaluating the clinical validity of hypertrophic cardiomyopathy genes. Circ Genom Precis Med 2019;12(2):e002460.

33. Jordan E, Peterson L, Ai T, et al. Evidence-based assessment of genes in dilated cardiomyopathy. Circulation 2021;144(1):7–19.

34. James CA, Jongbloed JDH, Hershberger RE, et al. International evidence based reappraisal of genes associated with arrhythmogenic right ventricular cardiomyopathy using the clinical genome resource framework. Circ Genom Precis Med 2021;14(3): e003273.

35. Adler A, Novelli V, Amin AS, et al. An international, multicentered, evidence-based reappraisal of genes reported to cause congenital long QT syndrome. Circulation 2020;141(6):418–28.

36. Hosseini SM, Kim R, Udupa S, et al. Reappraisal of reported genes for sudden arrhythmic death: evidence-based evaluation of gene validity for Brugada syndrome. Circulation 2018;138(12):1195–205.

37. Walsh R, Adler A, Amin AS, et al. Evaluation of gene validity for CPVT and short QT syndrome in sudden arrhythmic death. Eur Heart J 2022; 43(15):1500–10.

38. Otten E, Birnie E, Ranchor AV, et al. A group approach to genetic counselling of cardiomyopathy patients: satisfaction and psychological outcomes sufficient for further implementation. Eur J Hum Genet 2015;23(11):1462–7.

39. Christian S, Tagoe J, Delday L, et al. IMPACT webinars: improving patient access to genetic counselling and testing using webinars-the Alberta experience with hypertrophic cardiomyopathy. Journal of community genetics 2022;13(1):81–9.

40. White S, Jacobs C, Phillips J. Mainstreaming genetics and genomics: a systematic review of the barriers and facilitators for nurses and physicians in secondary and tertiary care. Genet Med 2020; 22(7):1149–55.

41. van Langen IM, Birnie E, Leschot NJ, et al. Genetic knowledge and counselling skills of Dutch cardiologists: sufficient for the genomics era? Eur Heart J 2003;24(6):560–6.

42. Burns C, James C, Ingles J. Communication of genetic information to families with inherited rhythm disorders. Heart Rhythm 2018;15(5):780–6.

43. van der Roest WP, Pennings JM, Bakker M, et al. Family letters are an effective way to inform relatives about inherited cardiac disease. Am J Med Genet 2009;149A(3):357–63.

44. Scheiper-Welling S, Tabunscik M, Gross TE, et al. Variant interpretation in molecular autopsy: a useful dilemma. Int J Leg Med 2022;136(2):475–82.

45. Lahrouchi N, Raju H, Lodder EM, et al. Utility of postmortem genetic testing in cases of sudden arrhythmic death syndrome. J Am Coll Cardiol 2017;69(17):2134–45.

46. Semsarian C, Ingles J. Molecular autopsy in victims of inherited arrhythmias. J Arrhythmia 2016;32(5):359–65.

47. Ackerman MJ, Priori SG, Willems S, et al. HRS/EHRA expert consensus statement on the state of genetic testing for the channelopathies and cardiomyopathies this document was developed as a partnership between the Heart Rhythm Society (HRS) and the European Heart Rhythm Association (EHRA). Heart Rhythm 2011;8(8):1308–39.

48. Gollob MH, Blier L, Brugada R, et al. Recommendations for the use of genetic testing in the clinical evaluation of inherited cardiac arrhythmias associated with sudden cardiac death: Canadian Cardiovascular Society/Canadian Heart Rhythm Society joint position paper. Can J Cardiol 2011;27(2):232–45.

49. Stiles MK, Wilde AAM, Abrams DJ, et al. 2020 APHRS/HRS expert consensus statement on the investigation of decedents with sudden unexplained death and patients with sudden cardiac arrest, and of their families. Heart Rhythm 2021;18(1):e1–50.

50. van den Heuvel LM, Do J, Yeates L, et al. Global approaches to cardiogenetic evaluation after sudden cardiac death in the young: a survey among health care professionals. Heart Rhythm 2021;18(10): 1637–44.

51. Behr ER, Scrocco C, Wilde AAM, et al. Investigation on sudden unexpected death in the young (SUDY) in Europe: results of the European Heart Rhythm Association survey. Europace 2022;24(2):331–9.

52. Iglesias M, Ripoll-Vera T, Perez-Luengo C, et al. Diagnostic yield of genetic testing in sudden cardiac death with autopsy findings of uncertain significance. J Clin Med 2021;10(9). https://doi.org/10.3390/jcm10091806.

53. Williams N, Manderski E, Stewart S, et al. Lessons learned from testing cardiac channelopathy and cardiomyopathy genes in individuals who died suddenly: a two-year prospective study in a large medical examiner's office with an in-house molecular genetics laboratory and genetic counseling services. J Genet Counsel 2020;29(2):293–302.

54. Siskind T, Williams N, Sebastin M, et al. Genetic screening of relatives of decedents experiencing sudden unexpected death: medical examiner's office referrals to a multi-disciplinary cardiogenetics program. Journal of community genetics 2022. https://doi.org/10.1007/s12687-022-00611-1.

55. Yeates L, Hunt L, Saleh M, et al. Poor psychological wellbeing particularly in mothers following sudden cardiac death in the young. Eur J Cardiovasc Nurs 2013;12(5):484–91.

56. Bates K, Sweeting J, Yeates L, et al. Psychological adaptation to molecular autopsy findings following sudden cardiac death in the young. Genet Med 2019;21(6):1452–6.

57. Grubic N, Puskas J, Phelan D, et al. Shock to the heart: psychosocial implications and applications

of sudden cardiac death in the young. Curr Cardiol Rep 2020;22(12):168.

58. McDonald K, Sharpe L, Yeates L, et al. Needs analysis of parents following sudden cardiac death in the young. Open heart 2020;7(2).

59. Steffen EM, Timotijevic L, Coyle A. A qualitative analysis of psychosocial needs and support impacts in families affected by young sudden cardiac death: the role of community and peer support. Eur J Cardiovasc Nurs 2020;19(8):681–90.

60. Miller DT, Lee K, Abul-Husn NS, et al. ACMG SF v3.1 list for reporting of secondary findings in clinical exome and genome sequencing: a policy statement of the American College of Medical Genetics and Genomics (ACMG). Genet Med 2022;24(7):1407–14.

61. de Wert G, Dondorp W, Clarke A, et al. Opportunistic genomic screening. Recommendations of the European Society of Human Genetics. Eur J Hum Genet 2021;29(3):365–77.

62. Boycott K, Hartley T, Adam S, et al. The clinical application of genome-wide sequencing for monogenic diseases in Canada: position Statement of the Canadian College of Medical Geneticists. J Med Genet 2015;52(7):431–7.

63. Schwartz MLB, McCormick CZ, Lazzeri AL, et al. A model for genome-first care: returning secondary genomic findings to participants and their healthcare providers in a large research cohort. Am J Hum Genet 2018;103(3):328–37.

64. Comber DA, Davies B, Roberts JD, et al. Return of results policies for genomic research: current practices and the Hearts in Rhythm Organization (HiRO) approach. Can J Cardiol 2022;38(4):526–35.

65. Soper ER, Suckiel SA, Braganza GT, et al. Genomic screening identifies individuals at high risk for hereditary transthyretin amyloidosis. J Personalized Med 2021;11(1). https://doi.org/10.3390/jpm11010049.

66. Green RC, Berg JS, Grody WW, et al. ACMG recommendations for reporting of incidental findings in clinical exome and genome sequencing. Genet Med 2013;15(7):565–74.

67. Hart MR, Biesecker BB, Blout CL, et al. Secondary findings from clinical genomic sequencing: prevalence, patient perspectives, family history assessment, and health-care costs from a multisite study. Genet Med 2019;21(5):1100–10.

68. Sapp JC, Facio FM, Cooper D, et al. A systematic literature review of disclosure practices and reported outcomes for medically actionable genomic secondary findings. Genet Med 2021;23(12):2260–9.

69. Carruth ED, Young W, Beer D, et al. Prevalence and electronic health record-based phenotype of loss-of-function genetic variants in arrhythmogenic right ventricular cardiomyopathy-associated genes. Circulation Genomic and precision medicine 2019;12(11):e002579.

70. Shah RA, Asatryan B, Sharaf Dabbagh G, et al. Frequency, penetrance, and variable expressivity of dilated cardiomyopathy-associated putative pathogenic gene variants in UK biobank participants. Circulation 2022;146(2):110–24.

71. de Marvao A, McGurk KA, Zheng SL, et al. Phenotypic expression and outcomes in individuals with rare genetic variants of hypertrophic cardiomyopathy. J Am Coll Cardiol 2021;78(11):1097–110.

72. Schwartz MLB, Buchanan AH, Hallquist MLG, et al. Genetic counseling for patients with positive genomic screening results: considerations for when the genetic test comes first. J Genet Counsel 2021;30(3):634–44.

73. Bennett JS, Bernhardt M, McBride KL, et al. Reclassification of variants of uncertain significance in children with inherited arrhythmia syndromes is predicted by clinical factors. Pediatr Cardiol 2019;40(8):1679–87.

74. Westphal DS, Burkard T, Moscu-Gregor A, et al. Reclassification of genetic variants in children with long QT syndrome. Mol Genet Genom Med 2020;8(9):e1300.

75. Cherny S, Olson R, Chiodo K, et al. Changes in genetic variant results over time in pediatric cardiomyopathy and electrophysiology. J Genet Counsel 2021;30(1):229–36.

76. Davies B, Bartels K, Hathaway J, et al. Variant reinterpretation in Survivors of cardiac arrest with preserved ejection fraction (the Cardiac Arrest Survivors With Preserved Ejection Fraction Registry) by clinicians and clinical commercial laboratories. Circulation Genomic and precision medicine 2021;14(3):e003235.

77. Westphal DS, Pollmann K, Marschall C, et al. It is not carved in stone-the need for a genetic reevaluation of variants in pediatric cardiomyopathies. J Cardiovasc Dev Disease 2022;9(2). https://doi.org/10.3390/jcdd9020041.

78. Burns C, Yeates L, Semsarian C, Ingles J. Evaluating a custom-designed aid to improve communication of genetic results in families with hypertrophic cardiomyopathy: study protocol for a randomised controlled trial. BMJ Open 2019;9(1):e026627.

79. Harris S, Cirino AL, Carr CW, et al. The uptake of family screening in hypertrophic cardiomyopathy and an online video intervention to facilitate family communication. Mol Genet Genom Med 2019;7(11):e940.

80. Schmidlen T, Jones CL, Campbell-Salome G, et al. Use of a chatbot to increase uptake of cascade genetic testing. J Genet Counsel 2022;31(5):1219–30.

81. van den Heuvel LM, Hoedemaekers YM, Baas AF, et al. A tailored approach to informing relatives at risk of inherited cardiac conditions: results of a randomised controlled trial. Eur J Hum Genet 2022;30(2):203–10.

A Practical Guide to Genetic Testing in Inherited Heart Disease

Emily E. Brown, MGC*, Brittney Murray, MS

KEYWORDS

• Genetic testing • Cardiomyopathy • Arrhythmia • Inherited heart disease

KEY POINTS

- Genetic testing for inherited cardiomyopathies and arrhythmias can provide important information regarding an individual's medical management, such as arrhythmic risk, lifestyle recommendations, and in some cases, medical therapy.
- Genetic testing allows for targeted cascade screening for all at-risk family members eliminating the need for cardiac screening for those who test negative and guiding tailored screening for genotype-positive individuals.
- Genetic testing should occur in the context of genetic counseling.

INTRODUCTION

Genetic testing is now known to provide critical information regarding the treatment, diagnosis, prognosis, and management of patients with hereditary cardiomyopathies and arrhythmias and is available for a wide variety of conditions, including hypertrophic cardiomyopathy (HCM), dilated cardiomyopathy, left ventricular noncompaction (LVNC), arrhythmogenic cardiomyopathy (ACM), long QT syndrome (LQTS), Brugada syndrome (BrS), and catecholaminergic polymorphic ventricular tachycardia, among others.[1] Consequently, within the past few years, multiple national guidelines and scientific statements recommend incorporating genetic testing into the diagnosis and management of cardiovascular patients.[1–6] However, many physicians feel inadequately prepared to incorporate genetics into their clinical practice.[7,8] Although ideally a patient has access to a genetic counselor and cardiologist trained in cardiovascular genetics,[9] this is not always the case owing to the highly specialized nature of this subspecialty. Therefore, increasing providers' understanding of genetic testing in cardiovascular disease is an efficacious way to increase access to this important management information. This review not only discusses the utility of genetic testing for patients and families with inherited cardiomyopathies and arrhythmias but also provides direction to the correct approach and logistics of incorporating genetic testing in the clinic setting.

DISCUSSION
Utility of Genetic Testing

Diagnostic testing

Genetic testing for cardiomyopathies and arrhythmias can provide a definitive molecular cause for an individual's disease.[1] This can be helpful in differentiating between phenocopies, such as drug-induced LQTS and congenital LQTS, or HCM and hypertensive disease. As such, a molecular diagnosis provides critical information regarding medical management, prognosis, and family screening.[10]

The yield of genetic testing depends on the specific condition along with the age of presentation, severity of disease, and presence of a positive family history (**Fig. 1**).[1] Some conditions, such as

Division of Cardiology, Johns Hopkins University, 600 North Wolfe Street, Blalock 572, Baltimore, MD 21287, USA
* Corresponding author.
E-mail address: ebrow102@jhmi.edu

Card Electrophysiol Clin 15 (2023) 241–247
https://doi.org/10.1016/j.ccep.2023.05.005
1877-9182/23/© 2023 Elsevier Inc. All rights reserved.

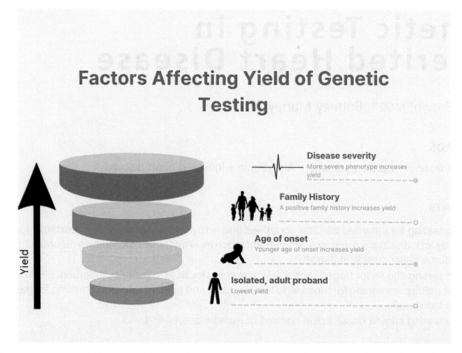

Fig. 1. Genetic testing yield is affected by multiple factors. The lowest yield is typically seen in adult patients with isolated, mild disease. The more factors an individual has, such as a positive family history and severe disease, the higher the yield.

LQTS, have well-characterized genetic causes, and the yield of genetic testing is quite high (~75%), whereas in other conditions, such as LVNC or BrS, the genetic basis is more complex, leading to a low likelihood of a positive result (~10%–20%).[11–14] Nevertheless, a positive result for those patients and families can provide important information, and a low yield alone should not be a reason to defer offering genetic testing.

Risk stratification and medical management

Beyond confirming a diagnosis, genetic testing in cardiomyopathies and arrhythmias can provide valuable insights into an individual's or family's arrhythmia risk allowing for medical intervention and more targeted care. For example, because of the arrhythmic nature and reduced penetrance of LQTS, a positive genetic test result indicates starting beta-blocker therapy even in the setting of a normal QT interval.[9] Without genetic testing, it would be challenging to know who in the family should start this treatment if their electrocardiograms are unremarkable. Genetic testing also allows identification of highly arrhythmic nonischemic cardiomyopathies whereby a patient would benefit from an internal cardiac defibrillator (ICD) at an earlier threshold. In recent guidelines and consensus statements, heart rhythm and cardiology societies now recommend a genotype-based ICD indication, whereby an ICD may be considered in certain genotype carriers (eg, *LMNA*, *FLNC*, *PLN*) with only mildly reduced systolic function.[4,15] Therefore, genetic testing may provide life-saving guidance regarding early risk stratification.

Identifying a genetic cause can also guide specific lifestyle recommendations in these conditions. For example, in LQTS, identifying the specific subtype aids in recognizing specific triggers. Exercise, especially swimming, is a typical trigger of ventricular arrhythmia in LQTS type 1, whereas loud, sudden auditory triggers can be associated with events in LQTS type 2.[12] In addition, for patients with arrhythmogenic right ventricular cardiomyopathy owing to a pathogenic desmosomal variant, frequent endurance exercise increased the risk for life-threatening arrhythmias and heart failure.[16] Consequently, exercise modification is typically recommended for these patients, whereas it may not be required in individuals with other types of ACM.

In a select subset of conditions, identifying the genetic cause will guide pharmacologic therapies. In LQTS type 3 (secondary to a gain of function *SCN5A* pathogenic variant), sodium channel blockers are a potential treatment option.[12] Differentiating phenocopies of HCM, such as transthyretin amyloidosis and Fabry disease, is vital due to gene-specific management.[17,18] Furthermore, although gene-specific therapies have not yet been approved for sarcomeric cardiomyopathies, there are ongoing clinical trials in this space. In the future, it may be even more critical to know the genetic cause for this very reason.[19]

In other cases, although identifying the genetic cause may not change medical therapies, it provides valuable anticipatory guidance for patients and families. The Sarcomeric Human Cardiomyopathy Registry found that patients with HCM owing to a sarcomeric mutation had a 2-fold increased risk of an adverse outcome compared with patients with a negative genetic test result.[20] Furthermore, patients with cardiomyopathy secondary to multiple pathogenic variants are more likely to develop severe disease.[21,22] Thus, genetic test results can help provide guidance for families regarding the likelihood of heart failure, atrial fibrillation, or other arrhythmias, although variable expressivity is important to keep in mind. Building on this concept, the risk to develop left ventricular systolic dysfunction was higher for patients with LVNC owing to an identifiable genetic cause compared with individuals whose genetic test results were negative.[21] This suggests the need for closer follow-up for patients with LVNC owing to an identifiable pathogenic variant and that they should not be released from cardiac screening. Research has also suggested that in patients hospitalized with acute heart failure attributed to "myocarditis," a positive genetic test result correlated with a lower

recovery and survival rate.[23] Beyond the heart, genetic testing may also identify syndromic forms, whereby subsequent features may develop later, prompting the evaluation of other specialists, such as neurologists.[17] In these cases, genetic testing can help families better understand the course of the condition and anticipate what is to come.

Cascade screening

Another key benefit of genetic testing is being able to use a positive result for cascade screening in relatives. Most hereditary cardiomyopathies and arrhythmias are autosomal dominant, indicating that all first-degree relatives have a 50% chance of also carrying the pathogenic/likely pathogenic variant and potentially developing the condition.[1,2] Without genetic testing, all first-degree relatives will need periodic cardiac screening, which can lead to significant expense, stress, and time for patients and families. However, if a relative tests negative for the familial variant, in most cases, they are released from continued cardiac screenings.[1–4,6] Therefore, genetic testing is a helpful tool to cardiac screening in the family (**Fig. 2**).

In family members with positive genetic test results, ongoing cardiac screening can identify latent disease or cardiac disease at an earlier stage, allowing for intervention.[24] This is increasing in importance as gene-specific therapies are developed. For example, in transthyretin amyloidosis, small molecule therapies stabilize the transthyretin

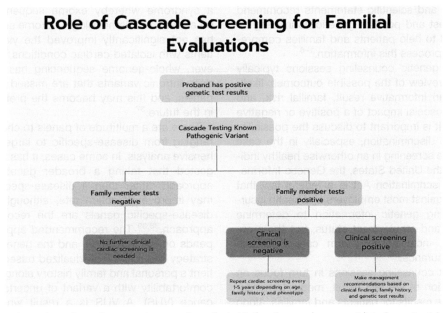

Role of Cascade Screening for Familial Evaluations

Proband has positive genetic test results

Cascade Testing Known Pathogenic Variant

Family member tests negative

No further clinical cardiac screening is needed

Family member tests positive

Clinical screening is negative

Repeat cardiac screening every 1-5 years depending on age, family history, and phenotype

Clinical screening positive

Make management recommendations based on clinical findings, family history, and genetic test results

Fig. 2. Genetic testing allows for cascade screening of at-risk family members providing important information regarding risk and need for ongoing management/assessment.

protein and therefore prevent further progression of the condition. Early identification before large amounts of amyloid fibrils have deposited is critical.[18] In overall family screening, a positive genetic test result has also been associated with increased uptake of cardiac screening compared with individuals who declined predictive genetic testing.[25]

The ability to offer cascade screening can be especially powerful in cases of sudden cardiac death. The tragic sudden loss of a family member owing to a sudden cardiac death has far-reaching effects on a family, including concern for similar outcomes for other relatives. Although the autopsy may reveal signs of a cardiomyopathy allowing for cascade screening, in around half of cases of sudden death in the young (under 35 years old), the cause remains unexplained after autopsy.[26] Genetic testing provides a molecular diagnosis for families in around 20% of cases, allowing for cascade screening and medical follow-up for at-risk family members.[26]

Role of Genetic Counseling

The role of the genetic counselor is described in detail in another article in this issue,[27] but the authors would be remiss to not briefly highlight the importance of this piece in the genetic testing process. The National Society of Genetic Counselors defines genetic counseling as "the process of helping people understand and adapt to the medical, psychological and familial implications of genetic contributions to disease."[28] Multiple guidelines and scientific statements recommend both pretest and posttest genetic counseling be performed to help patients and families comprehend and process this information.[1–6]

Pretest genetic counseling sessions typically include a review of the possible outcomes, likelihood of an informative result, familial risk, and the psychosocial impact of a positive or negative result.[6,29] It is important to discuss the possibility of genetic discrimination, especially in the case of cascade screening in an otherwise healthy individual. In the United States, the Genetic Information Nondiscrimination Act is a federal law that defends against most employers and health insurances using genetic information to determine coverage and employment status, but there are loopholes, including long-term care insurance and life insurance.[30]

Posttest counseling sessions in turn focus on interpretation of the test result, medical implications of the results for patients and families, along with individuals' psychosocial response. There can be a wide variety of reactions to the results ranging from "survivor guilt" in individuals who test negative for a familial variant, relief at finally having a diagnosis, to anxiety regarding the risk to develop a condition. Exploration of these reactions is a critical part of results disclosure and should not be discounted.[29,31,32] The genetic counseling session will also include a discussion of who else in the family is at risk and practical steps on how to best disseminate this information, such as a family letter.[31,32]

Logistics

Genetic testing can be performed on a variety of sample types, including blood and saliva. For postmortem testing, blood or frozen tissue is preferred. It is recommended to bank some DNA for additional analysis at a later date, if needed.[33] Often buccal kits are available allowing for patients to swab their cheeks and return the kit to the laboratory. In addition, genetic counseling is available increasingly by telemedicine allowing for the process of genetic counseling and testing to be done from the convenience of patients' own homes.

Appropriate genetic test selection is key to providing proficient care. In general, it is best to start genetic testing in the most severely affected individual in the family owing to the possibility of multiple variants leading to a more severe phenotype or the possibility of a nongenetic phenocopy in a less-affected relative.[34] Testing should begin with panel testing unless the individual has multisystemic features suggestive of a syndrome whereby exome sequencing may be a preferred methodology.[1] Exome sequencing has not significantly improved the yield in patients with isolated cardiac conditions.[35,36] However, whole-genome sequencing has identified deep intronic variants that are missed on typical panels, and this may become the preferred test in the future.[37]

There are a multitude of panels to choose from ranging from disease-specific to large comprehensive analysis. In some cases, it has been suggested that taking a broader genetic testing approach rather than a disease-specific panel may improve detection rate, although typically disease-specific panels are the recommended approach.[38,39] The recommended approach depends on the indication, and the genetic testing strategy should be individualized based on a patient's personal and family history along with their comfortability with a variant of uncertain significance (VUS). A VUS is a result whereby the consequence of a genetic variation is unclear. Burns and colleagues[34] previously showed that ordering a comprehensive cardiomyopathy panel for HCM did not improve detection, only increasing the likelihood of a VUS. However, for individuals with a mixed phenotype, such as ACM, a genetic testing approach, which includes a wide array of genes associated with cardiomyopathy and arrhythmia, has been shown to be beneficial.[38] In a cohort of patients with arrhythmogenic right ventricular cardiomyopathy/dysplasia, 10% of patients had pathogenic variants in nondesmosomal genes.[38] There are some groups that have taken a broad approach regardless of the indication. Dellefave-Castillo and colleagues[40] recently published that a combined arrhythmia and cardiomyopathy panel identified 10% more positive results than a disease-specific panel alone, but more than 50% of individuals had a VUS. It should be noted that in some cases these positive results are incidental findings not related to the disease at hand, and as such, the yield is not improved.[40,41]

Genes included on the individual cardiomyopathy and arrhythmia panels can vary slightly by laboratory. In general, genes included have been shown to be associated with that specific phenotype after an in-depth review. The Clinical Genome Resource is a resource funded by the National Institutes of Health aiming to determine the clinical relevance of genes and variants. Their expert curation panels review all associated genes and evaluate the validity of the association.[42-44] Their findings are published to guide laboratories on which genes to include on panels. The international consensus statement led by Wilde[1] recommends only testing for genes that are classified with at least a "moderate" association.

Identification of the pathogenic variant in the family allows for cascade screening of at-risk relatives.[1-6] It is important relatives are tested only for the known pathogenic variant rather than a full panel (see **Fig. 2**).[6] Testing with a full panel can lead to unnecessary confusion if VUS are identified.[6]

SUMMARY

Overall, genetic testing should be offered to patients with inherited arrhythmias and cardiomyopathies. Testing results can provide important information in regards to an individual's medical management and also allow for cascade screening throughout the family. Genetic testing should begin in an affected individual and be accompanied by pretest and posttest genetic counseling to review and explore the medical and psychosocial implications of the results.

CLINICS CARE POINTS

- Genetic testing can confirm a diagnosis.
- Genetic testing for inherited cardiomyopathies and arrhythmias can provide important information regarding an individual's medical management, such as arrhythmic risk, lifestyle recommendations, and in some cases, medical therapy.
- Genetic testing allows for targeted cascade screening for all at-risk family members, eliminating the need for cardiac screening for those who test negative and guiding tailored screening for genotype-positive individuals.
- Genetic testing should be performed with proper genetic counseling by health care professionals with expertise in cardiac genetics.

DISCLOSURE

Ms E.E. Brown and Ms B. Murray are consultants for My Gene Counsel.

REFERENCES

1. Wilde AAM, Semsarian C, Marquez MF, et al. European Heart Rhythm Association (EHRA)/Heart Rhythm Society (HRS)/Asia Pacific Heart Rhythm Society (APHRS)/Latin American Heart Rhythm Society (LAHRS) expert consensus statement on the state of genetic testing for cardiac diseases. Heart Rhythm 2022;19(7):e1–60.
2. Hershberger RE, Givertz MM, Ho CY, et al. Genetic evaluation of cardiomyopathy-a heart failure society of America practice guideline. J Card Fail 2018;24(5):281–302.
3. Ommen SR, Mital S, Burke MA, et al. 2020 AHA/ACC guideline for the diagnosis and treatment of patients with hypertrophic cardiomyopathy: a report of the American College of Cardiology/American Heart Association joint committee on clinical practice guidelines. Circulation 2020;142(25):e558–631.
4. Towbin JA, McKenna WJ, Abrams DJ, et al. 2019 HRS expert consensus statement on evaluation, risk stratification, and management of arrhythmogenic cardiomyopathy: executive summary. Heart Rhythm 2019;16(11):e373–407.
5. Stiles MK, Wilde AAM, Abrams DJ, et al. 2020 APHRS/HRS expert consensus statement on the investigation of decedents with sudden unexplained death and patients with sudden cardiac arrest, and of their families. Heart Rhythm 2021;18(1):e1–50.
6. Musunuru K, Hershberger RE, Day SM, et al. Genetic testing for inherited cardiovascular diseases:

a scientific statement from the American Heart Association. Circ Genom Precis Med 2020;13(4): e000067.

7. Schaibley VM, Ramos IN, Woosley RL, et al. Limited genomics training among physicians remains a barrier to genomics-based implementation of precision medicine. Front Med 2022;9:757212.

8. White S, Jacobs C, Phillips J. Mainstreaming genetics and genomics: a systematic review of the barriers and facilitators for nurses and physicians in secondary and tertiary care. Genet Med 2020; 22(7):1149–55.

9. Priori SG, Wilde AA, Horie M, et al. HRS/EHRA/APHRS expert consensus statement on the diagnosis and management of patients with inherited primary arrhythmia syndromes: document endorsed by HRS, EHRA, and APHRS in May 2013 and by ACCF, AHA, PACES, and AEPC in June 2013. Heart Rhythm 2013;10(12):1932–63.

10. Cirino AL, Harris S, Lakdawala NK, et al. Role of genetic testing in inherited cardiovascular disease: a review. JAMA Cardiol 2017;2(10):1153–60.

11. Shimizu W, Horie M. Phenotypic manifestations of mutations in genes encoding subunits of cardiac potassium channels. Circ Res 2011;109(1):97–109.

12. Schwartz PJ, Ackerman MJ, Antzelevitch C, et al. Inherited cardiac arrhythmias. Nat Rev Dis Primers 2020;6(1):58.

13. Miller EM, Hinton RB, Czosek R, et al. Genetic testing in pediatric left ventricular noncompaction. Circ Cardiovasc Genet 2017;10(6). https://doi.org/10.1161/circgenetics.117.001735.

14. Ross SB, Singer ES, Driscoll E, et al. Genetic architecture of left ventricular noncompaction in adults. Hum Genome Var 2020;7:33.

15. Zeppenfeld K, Tfelt-Hansen J, de Riva M, et al. 2022 ESC Guidelines for the management of patients with ventricular arrhythmias and the prevention of sudden cardiac death: developed by the task force for the management of patients with ventricular arrhythmias and the prevention of sudden cardiac death of the European Society of Cardiology (ESC) Endorsed by the Association for European Paediatric and Congenital Cardiology (AEPC). Eur Heart J 2022; 43(40):3997–4126.

16. James CA, Bhonsale A, Tichnell C, et al. Exercise increases age-related penetrance and arrhythmic risk in arrhythmogenic right ventricular dysplasia/cardiomyopathy-associated desmosomal mutation carriers. J Am Coll Cardiol 2013;62(14):1290–7.

17. Pieroni M, Ciabatti M, Saletti E, et al. Beyond sarcomeric hypertrophic cardiomyopathy: how to diagnose and manage phenocopies. Curr Cardiol Rep 2022. https://doi.org/10.1007/s11886-022-01778-2.

18. Ruberg FL, Grogan M, Hanna M, et al. Transthyretin amyloid cardiomyopathy: JACC state-of-the-art review. J Am Coll Cardiol 2019;73(22):2872–91.

19. Helms AS, Thompson AD, Day SM. Translation of new and emerging therapies for genetic cardiomyopathies. JACC Basic Transl Sci 2022;7(1):70–83.

20. Ho CY, Day SM, Ashley EA, et al. Genotype and lifetime burden of disease in hypertrophic cardiomyopathy: insights from the sarcomeric human cardiomyopathy registry (SHaRe). Circulation 2018;138(14):1387–98.

21. van Waning JI, Caliskan K, Hoedemaekers YM, et al. Genetics, clinical features, and long-term outcome of noncompaction cardiomyopathy. J Am Coll Cardiol 2018;71(7):711–22.

22. Kelly M, Semsarian C. Multiple mutations in genetic cardiovascular disease: a marker of disease severity? Circ Cardiovasc Genet 2009;2(2):182–90.

23. Brown EE, McMilllan KN, Halushka MK, et al. Genetic aetiologies should be considered in paediatric cases of acute heart failure presumed to be myocarditis. Cardiol Young 2019;29(7):917–21.

24. van Velzen HG, Schinkel AFL, Baart SJ, et al. Outcomes of contemporary family screening in hypertrophic cardiomyopathy. Circ Genom Precis Med 2018;11(4):e001896.

25. Christian S, Atallah J, Clegg R, et al. Uptake of predictive genetic testing and cardiac evaluation for children at risk for an inherited arrhythmia or cardiomyopathy. J Genet Couns 2018;27(1):124–30.

26. Napolitano C, Bloise R, Monteforte N, et al. Sudden cardiac death and genetic ion channelopathies: long QT, Brugada, short QT, catecholaminergic polymorphic ventricular tachycardia, and idiopathic ventricular fibrillation. Circulation 2012;125(16):2027–34.

27. Dzwiniel T., Christian S., Principles of Genetic Counseling in Inherited Heart Conditions. (In press)

28. Resta R, Biesecker BB, Bennett RL, et al. A new definition of genetic counseling: National Society of Genetic Counselors' task force report. J Genet Couns 2006;15(2):77–83.

29. Ahmad F, McNally EM, Ackerman MJ, et al. Establishment of specialized clinical cardiovascular genetics programs: recognizing the need and meeting standards: a scientific statement from the American Heart Association. Circ Genom Precis Med 2019;12(6):e000054.

30. Prince AE, Roche MI. Genetic information, nondiscrimination, and privacy protections in genetic counseling practice. J Genet Couns 2014;23(6): 891–902.

31. Arscott P, Caleshu C, Kotzer K, et al. A case for inclusion of genetic counselors in cardiac care. Cardiol Rev 2016;24(2):49–55.

32. Ingles J, Yeates L, Semsarian C. The emerging role of the cardiac genetic counselor. Heart Rhythm 2011;8(12):1958–62.

33. Middleton O, Baxter S, Demo E, et al. National Association of Medical Examiners position paper: retaining postmortem samples for genetic testing. Academic Forensic Pathology 2013;3(2):191–4.

34. Burns C, Bagnall RD, Lam L, et al. Multiple gene variants in hypertrophic cardiomyopathy in the era of next-generation sequencing. Circ Cardiovasc Genet 2017;10(4). https://doi.org/10.1161/circgenetics.116.001666.

35. Seidelmann SB, Smith E, Subrahmanyan L, et al. Application of whole exome sequencing in the clinical diagnosis and management of inherited cardiovascular diseases in adults. Circ Cardiovasc Genet 2017;10(1). https://doi.org/10.1161/circgenetics.116.001573.

36. Retterer K, Juusola J, Cho MT, et al. Clinical application of whole-exome sequencing across clinical indications. Genet Med 2016;18(7):696–704.

37. Bagnall RD, Ingles J, Dinger ME, et al. Whole genome sequencing improves outcomes of genetic testing in patients with hypertrophic cardiomyopathy. J Am Coll Cardiol 2018;72(4):419–29.

38. Murray B, Tichnell C, Tandri H, et al. Influence of panel selection on yield of clinically useful variants in arrhythmogenic right ventricular cardiomyopathy families. Circ Genom Precis Med 2020;13(5):548–50.

39. Grondin S, Davies B, Cadrin-Tourigny J, et al. Importance of genetic testing in unexplained cardiac arrest. Eur Heart J 2022;43(32):3071–81.

40. Dellefave-Castillo LM, Cirino AL, Callis TE, et al. Assessment of the diagnostic yield of combined cardiomyopathy and arrhythmia genetic testing. JAMA Cardiol 2022;7(9):966–74.

41. Smith E, Care M, Burke-Martindale C, et al. Secondary findings using broad pan cardiomyopathy and arrhythmia panels in patients with a personal or family history of inherited cardiomyopathy or arrhythmia syndrome. Am J Cardiol 2022;178:137–41.

42. Morales A, Kinnamon DD, Jordan E, et al. Variant interpretation for dilated cardiomyopathy: refinement of the American College of Medical Genetics and Genomics/ClinGen guidelines for the DCM precision medicine study. Circ Genom Precis Med 2020;13(2):e002480.

43. Adler A, Novelli V, Amin AS, et al. An international, multicentered, evidence-based reappraisal of genes reported to cause congenital long QT syndrome. Circulation 2020;141(6):418–28.

44. Morales A, Ing A, Antolik C, et al. Harmonizing the collection of clinical data on genetic testing requisition forms to enhance variant interpretation in hypertrophic cardiomyopathy (HCM): a study from the ClinGen cardiomyopathy variant curation expert panel. J Mol Diagn 2021;23(5):589–98.

Implantable Devices in Genetic Heart Disease
Disease-Specific Device Selection and Programming

Simon Hansom, MBBS, MRCP(UK)[a], Zachary Laksman, MD, MSc, FRCPC[b],*

KEYWORDS

- Genetic • Inherited • Arrhythmia • Defibrillator • Programming

KEY POINTS

- Diagnosis of genetic heart diseases can be challenging and appropriate risk stratification is a critical next step.
- Shared decision making is vital when making decisions related to ICD implantation.
- ICDs are associated with significant rates of morbidity and mortality.
- Appropriate device programming is critical to adequately protect patients from both life threatening ventricular arrhythmia and inappropriate therapy.

INTRODUCTION

The genetic diseases discussed in this article encompass an array of primary arrhythmia syndromes, channelopathies, and cardiomyopathies. Typically these patients are young, and in the case of primary arrhythmia syndromes and channelopathies, have preserved ventricular function often without a clearly defined arrhythmic substrate. For those with associated structural disease, namely hypertrophic cardiomyopathy (HCM) or arrhythmogenic right ventricular cardiomyopathy (ARVC), the disease process and the arrhythmic substrate remain dynamic throughout life. Diagnosis can be difficult, hampered by complex diagnostic criteria that are challenging to apply, and often open to varying interpretations. Following correct diagnosis, risk stratification is critical, but particularly nuanced, lacking well-defined thresholds for device implantation and the support of large randomized controlled trials (RCTs).

Faced with such uncertainty, and the fear of sudden cardiac death (SCD) in a young patient, physicians may have a low threshold for ICD implantation. However, ICD implantation in these patients is fraught with potential problems, ranging from inappropriate therapy to device related complications. The potential for psychological harm and repeated surgical interventions throughout their lifetime is significant. On that basis, while it is vital to adequately protect those at high risk of life-threatening ventricular arrhythmia (LTVA), it is equally important to protect those truly low-risk individuals from the potential complications of a lifelong ICD. Since the advent of the subcutaneous ICD (S-ICD) an alternative system is now available that spares the vasculature of these young individuals. However, there are clear differences in the functionality and complications associated with S-ICDs that may preclude its use in some situations. Ultimately, in all cases, the decision for ICD implantation should

[a] Division of Cardiology, Arrhythmia Service, University of Ottawa Heart Institute, 40 Ruskin Street, Ottawa, Ontario K1Y 4W7, Canada; [b] Department of Medicine and the School of Biomedical Engineering, Room 211 – 1033 Davie Street, Vancouver, British Columbia V6E 1M7, Canada
* Corresponding author.
E-mail address: zlaksman@mail.ubc.ca

Card Electrophysiol Clin 15 (2023) 249–260
https://doi.org/10.1016/j.ccep.2023.04.001
1877-9182/23/© 2023 Elsevier Inc. All rights reserved.

be a shared decision between the physician and patient.

Following device implantation, careful consideration should be given to its programming, not only to ensure patients are protected from LTVA, but also to minimize the possibility of inappropriate device therapy. Unfortunately, as opposed to the ischemic population, device programming considerations are neither well established, nor well supported by randomized data in these rare diseases.

This article assumes a prior understanding of device programming and familiarity with discriminators employed by the various manufacturers. It seeks to provide an overview of each condition, its pathophysiological basis, and the key considerations regarding appropriate device selection and subsequent programming.

CATECHOLAMINERGIC POLYMORPHIC VENTRICULAR TACHYCARDIA

Catecholaminergic polymorphic ventricular tachycardia (CPVT) is an ion channelopathy associated with adrenergically mediated ventricular arrhythmia (VA), syncope, and SCD. Typical triggers involve emotional or physical stress resulting in bidirectional VT (BDVT), polymorphic VT (PMVT) and ventricular fibrillation (VF).

The role of beta-blockade and flecainide in the reduction of arrhythmic events is recognized, and management of CPVT primarily focuses on aggressive pharmacologic management and the use of sympathetic denervation in select cases. Consequently, consensus recommendations reserve ICDs for those who experience recurrent syncope, cardiac arrest, or polymorphic/bidirectional VT despite these measures.[1] Standalone ICD implantation is not recommended and is potentially harmful.

ICD implantation in this group is nuanced and remains controversial. Given the critical role of catecholamines in the genesis of arrhythmia, ICD therapy may itself induce arrhythmia (**Fig. 1**), at times with a fatal outcome.[2] Furthermore, there appears to be a high failure rate of defibrillator therapy in CPVT patients. A retrospective review of 13 CPVT patients who had undergone ICD implantation demonstrated that just 32% of appropriate shocks were effective. Shocks delivered during VF appeared most effective (83%), whereas those delivered during PMVT/BDVT or monomorphic ventricular tachycardia (MMVT) were largely ineffective, with a 98% failure rate. Seventeen ATP therapies were also delivered, of which only 2 appeared effective.[3]

A recent systematic review of 503 CPVT patients, all of whom had an ICD, demonstrated a 40% incidence of at least 1 appropriate shock during follow-up. Electrical storm was seen in 19.6% of patients, nearly equaling the 20.8% incidence of receiving at least 1 inappropriate shock. Device complication rates including lead failure, infection, or surgical revision, occurred in 32% of cases.[4]

The classical CPVT patient is usually an adolescent/young adult at the time of diagnosis with a normal resting 12-lead electrocardiogram (ECG). The relative merits of an endocardial versus subcutaneous system should therefore be carefully considered given the predilection to PMVT/VF, and the largely ineffective role of ATP.[3] Associated conduction disease is also extremely rare such that pacing is unlikely to be required. Conversely, complex atrial arrhythmias are frequently seen in CPVT, accounting for 45% of inappropriate shocks. The lack of robust data supporting improved discrimination with a dual-chamber system and the inherent risk of endocardial leads in such a young population may ultimately favor S-ICD implantation.

Approaches to device programming include the use of a single, high-rate VF zone plus or minus a monitor zone, while others have utilized dual (VT and VF) zones.[3] Ultimately, optimal programming should focus on minimizing inappropriate therapy utilizing available discriminators. As advocated by some authors, the use of a single, high-rate zone with prolonged detection would seem optimal.[4]

In the case of redetection, shocks should be programmed to noncommitted where possible and maximally delayed to prevent incessant high-voltage therapy and avoiding 'death by ICD'.

The failure of therapy during episodes of PMVT/BDVT is challenging to address with currently available device algorithms. Theoretically, prolonged detection may facilitate degeneration to VF alongside permitting additional time for spontaneous termination. Ideally, an optimal device would recognize bidirectional VT, distinguish it from VF, and allow tailored programming to optimize device effectiveness.

In the case of S-ICD programming, improved SVT discrimination with conditional zone use has been demonstrated.[5,6] Based on current guideline recommendations, the conditional zone should be programmed at greater than or equal to 200 bpm with the shock zone at greater than or equal to 230 bpm.[5] Use of the smart pass filter to minimize inappropriate therapy is also encouraged.[6]

ARRHYTHMOGENIC CARDIOMYOPATHY

Understanding of arrhythmogenic right ventricular cardiomyopathy (ARVC) has advanced considerably since its initial identification over 40 years

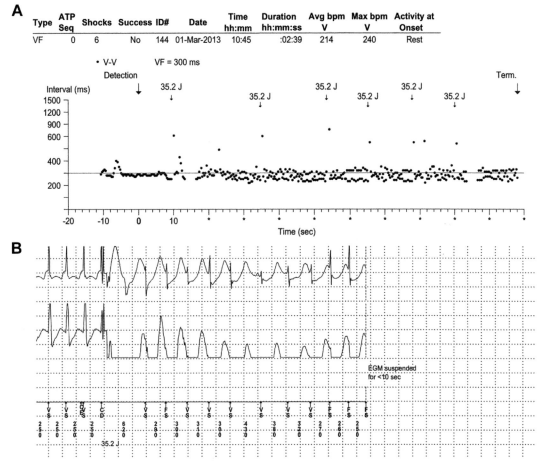

Fig. 1. (*A*) Ventricular interval dot plot obtained from a single-chamber ICD in a patient with CPVT. Initial tachycardia, cycle length 280 milliseconds, falls in the VF zone. Following detection, a 35J shock is delivered with degeneration of the tachycardia into VF/polymorphic ventricular tachycardia, following which a further 5 unsuccessful shocks are delivered followed by spontaneous termination. (*B*) Demonstrates the corresponding intracardiac electrograms (EGMs) displaying the RV tip-ring and can-coil EGMs. Initial tachycardia suggestive of possible SVT given identical appearance to presenting EGM (not shown) and relative timing of tip-ring and can-coil electrograms.

ago. The pathophysiological finding of patchy myocyte loss and fibrofatty replacement are well described. Aside from classical RV disease, biventricular and even isolated left-sided subtypes are increasingly identified.[7]

ARVC passes through a continuum of progressive electrical and structural changes as it develops, influencing not only the clinical presentation but also the substrate and burden of consequent arrhythmia, although increased risk is present at all stages.[8]

ARVC indiscriminately affects the young, with a peak onset between the second and forth decades of life.[7] Although some individuals may initially present with syncope or palpitations, for some the first episode may be SCD. Indeed, ARVC is felt to account for approximately 10% of unexplained cardiac arrests and 4% of SCD.[9]

For those individuals who suffer and survive a sudden cardiac arrest, the decision for ICD therapy is largely straightforward. However, the spectrum of disease identified through cascade screening poses additional challenges to the clinician, hampered by the highly variable penetrance and expressivity. Following diagnosis, risk stratification is a critical step given that 27.7% of patients in 1 cohort experienced their first VA within 4 years of initial diagnosis.[10]

Given the progressive structural changes and the potential for monomorphic VT, the benefit of antitachycardia pacing (ATP) likely increases as the disease advances (**Fig. 2**). Indeed, of 108 patients from the North American Multidisciplinary study of ARVC, 48 experienced 489 episodes of monomorphic VT, 92% of which were successfully terminated with ATP.[11] Given the proximity of the

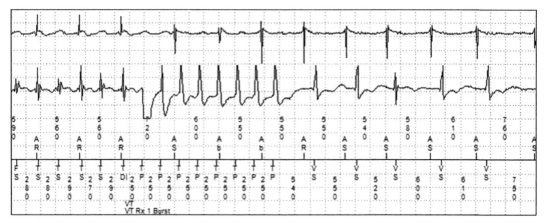

Fig. 2. Intracardiac electrograms from a dual-chamber ICD in a patient with arrhythmogenic right ventricular cardiomyopathy. Atrial and ventricular (tip to ring) bipolar EGMs are shown. Ventricular tachycardia noted with appropriate detection and delivery of an 8-beat burst of ATP with successful termination.

RV lead to the VT circuit, this is not of surprise and lends weight to the decision to implant a transvenous ICD (TV-ICD), rather than an S-ICD. Furthermore, S-ICD shock and conditional zones are limited to minimum ventricular rates of 170 bpm. This, coupled with the potential for slower VTs with advanced disease and the potential for further slowing VT circuits with escalating antiarrhythmic therapy, may limit their use.

Endocardial leads, however, are not without their issues. With increasingly advanced disease, involvement of RV apical regions is frequently seen with potential implications for the sensing and threshold of apically positioned leads.[12] The resulting reduction in the sensed R wave and its relative ratio to the T wave may create issues with R wave sensing and T wave oversensing (TWOS). Careful review of these parameters at each interrogation is therefore recommended.

ARVC patients have an increased incidence of atrial arrhythmias. On this basis, diligent use of SVT discriminators is critical in reducing the risk of inappropriate therapy. Additional consideration should also be given to disabling the high-rate time-out feature for this reason.

Avoidance of therapy, including potentially unnecessary ATP, is important given the possibility for acceleration and distressing high-voltage therapies. Extrapolating from previous studies how many treated VTs may have self-terminated with prolonged detection times is challenging, but allowing adequate time for spontaneous termination is critical in minimizing therapies.

ATP, particularly in the case of secondary prevention, should be programmed 10 to 20 bpm below the clinical VT (particularly where further escalation of medical therapy may occur).[5]

Therefore, programming of multiple bursts of ATP at slower VT rates is likely advantageous, and in such slow zones, an absence of shock therapy is reasonable. However, in these cases, additional higher rate VT zones must be included in case of acceleration. Further ATP may be programmed in these zones, including more aggressive ATP therapies; however, shock therapy should be placed at the end of the zone to effectively treat potentially rapid, poorly tolerated VT. Furthermore, care should be taken to avoid unnecessarily delaying effective therapy at higher ventricular rates. ATP, even at rapid VT cycle lengths of 200 to 250 milliseconds has been shown to successfully terminate episodes, supporting the role of ATP during charging in the VF zone.[11]

Finally, in experienced centers, radiofrequency catheter ablation is increasingly employed to treat recurrent VA.[13] A potential future could be envisaged, whereby catheter ablation of scar-mediated VT, in combination with S-ICD implantation, provides protection from LTVA, and in doing so spares the vasculature of these young patients.

HYPERTROPHIC CARDIOMYOPATHY

Hypertrophic cardiomyopathy is a heterogenous sarcomere disorder characterized by myocyte disarray and scar formation and is associated with an increased risk of VA and SCD. Although the advent of ICDs has resulted in a significant reduction in mortality to below 1% per annum, VAs still account for 51% of deaths in these individuals.[14]

Although HCM is primarily an obstructive disease, with some 70% of cases having mechanical outflow obstruction,[15] the underlying cellular disarray, microvascular ischemia, and myocardial fibrosis are all implicated in the increased arrhythmia burden. A recent study of 217 patients with primary prevention ICDs demonstrated an annual appropriate rate of therapy of 3.4%.[16]

There are several important considerations prior to placement of an ICD in cases of HCM. ICDs are associated with an overall complication rate of 4% to 6% per year, including the risks associated with the initial device implant,[17] and sparing the vasculature in these young patients is an important consideration.

For those HCM patients requiring an ICD, relevant guidelines give a class 1 recommendation for the implantation of either a single-chamber TV-ICD or S-ICD with a similar recommendation for the use of a single, over a dual coil ICD lead.[18] Dual-chamber ICDs are given a 2a recommendation where additional atrial pacing or relief of outflow obstruction is required.

The incidence of monomorphic ventricular tachycardia (MMVT) in the HCM population appears high. From a recent study of 56 HCM patients presenting with VA, 68% had MMVT; 14% had MMVT and VF, and 18% had isolated VF.[19] A 78% of those initially resuscitated for sudden death or VF had further VF, and 94% of those implanted following MMVT had further MMVT.[19] Unadjusted ATP effectiveness was 77.7%.

Rowin and colleagues reported rates of inappropriate therapy of 9.7% within the first 5 years after implant.[16] Common causes include TWOS, deviation from the stored electrogram template given progressive hypertrophy, and the prevalence of atrial arrhythmias. Indeed, atrial fibrillation (AF) is frequently seen in patients with HCM. A cohort of over 1500 HCM patients demonstrated an incidence of 20%.[20] Inappropriate therapy secondary to AF was ultimately seen in 39% of cases, with TWOS occurring in 24%.[17]

The role of the S-ICD has continued to gain momentum in the HCM population despite concerns regarding rates of inappropriate therapy, particularly TWOS. Two recent studies[21,22] demonstrated the ability of the S-ICD to effectively terminate LTVA, with similar numbers of successful defibrillation tests in both groups, 98.9% in HCM and 98.5% for non-HCM indications.[22] In the same study, SVT accounted for 86% of inappropriate therapies in TV-ICDs, while in S-ICD recipients, TWOS accounted for 83%, with the remainder secondary to atrial arrhythmia.[22]

A recent publication using data from the ALTITUDE registry examined 2673 patients implanted with an ICD for HCM including 2047 with a TV-ICD and 626 with an S-ICD.[23] ICD therapy per 100 patient years was considerably higher in the TV-ICD group versus the S-ICD group at 14.18 versus 5.25, driven primarily by ATP delivery. The number of appropriate shocks was not significantly different between the 2 groups at 5.87 versus 5.25 respectively. Inappropriate therapy rates were also higher in the TV-ICD group, at 18.55 versus 7.25. Given the additional time taken for charging of the S-ICD compared to the time to deliver ATP with a TV-ICD, episodes otherwise destined for ATP may have spontaneously terminated.

Given the progressive nature of HCM, the potential for increased defibrillation thresholds exists. There appears to be an adequate safety margin for left-sided single coil ICD leads,[18] however, for right-sided implants, consideration should be given as to the use of a dual coil ICD lead and defibrillation threshold testing, particularly in the presence of massive hypertrophy.[24]

Ultimately, device programming with adherence to the published HRS recommendations is encouraged.[5] Accordingly, VT and VF zones should be programmed at 185 bpm and 250 bpm respectively with delayed detection of 5 and 12 seconds with additional SVT discriminators to minimize inappropriate therapy. Given the incidence of MMVT, programming of ATP with delayed detection, particularly in the case of secondary prevention for VT, is suggested. In S-ICD recipients, the role of dual-zone programming is emphasized given its ability to mitigate inappropriate therapy for SVT.[22]

BRUGADA SYNDROME

Despite frequently being referred to as an inherited channelopathy, a single causative mutation in Brugada syndrome (BrS) is only identified in approximately 20% of individuals, with most having no clearly defined genetic basis.[25] BrS is associated with cardiogenic syncope and SCD secondary to polymorphic VT and VF, with a predilection for periods of rest or sleep.[26] Its prevalence is estimated at 1 case per 2000 population worldwide, although this figure is as much as 14 times higher within parts of southeast Asia.[27]

Although the classical ECG features are well described, they are often dynamic, with some individuals requiring provocation to manifest the classical ECG appearance whether by intentional or accidental pharmacologic means or by fever.

Although the mean age of SCD is 39.5 years, SCD occurs throughout life[28] The only therapy with proven efficacy in the treatment of LTVA is the ICD. In patients with confirmed BrS who have survived an out-of-hospital cardiac arrest or had documented sustained VT (with or without syncope), guidelines give a class 1 recommendation for the implantation of an ICD.[1]

A meta-analysis of 1539 patients with BrS and a mean follow-up of 4.9 years demonstrated an 18% incidence of appropriate ICD intervention with a further 18% experiencing inappropriate therapy.[29] Atrial arrhythmias were also commonly seen, with 10% of patients experiencing AF.

Inappropriate therapy, and in particular TWOS, remains a significant issue. A study of 480 Brugada ICD recipients revealed TWOS in 5.8% of patients. This was resolved in 75% of cases by altering the sensing vector from a true tip to ring bipolar configuration to an integrated tip to coil one.[30]

Given the young age and minimal role for ATP, there is justification for an S-ICD. However, given the dynamic potential of the ECG during fever, changes in sympathetic tone or following exposure to provoking medications, the potential for inappropriate therapy exists. The fixed programmed vector in the S-ICD makes it particularly sensitive to changes in the amplitude of the R wave, T wave, or both.[31] Ultimately S-ICD screening failure is seen in approximately 18% of cases of BrS.[32]

In the hope of improving screening success, Conte and colleagues utilized the SMART pass filter during Ajmaline infusion to potentially reduce such failures.[31] Ultimately, this failed to make any statistically significant improvement in success rates, with 30% of candidates failing, which is notable given that 85% of BrS patients' resting electrograms would typically pass.[31]

Considering the potential for dynamic ST segment changes during exercise, exercise testing during screening has also been proposed to reduce rates of inappropriate therapy. In one study, this resulted in ineligibility rates of 24%.[33] Overall, given the high incidence of inappropriate therapy, both exercise testing and potential provocation testing would be reasonable during screening, although supporting data are limited.

In view of the typically high ventricular rates during events, potential for TWOS, and increased burden of AF, careful consideration should be given to the type of ICD and its subsequent programming. Furthermore, SCN5A variant carriers appear prone to atrial arrhythmia and may harbor or go on to develop significant conduction disease. In such cases, a dual-chamber ICD should be considered to facilitate pacing and to assist discrimination.

Regarding programming decisions, the use of a single VF zone at 222 beats per minute appears safe and has been associated with a 2.07% yearly incidence of inappropriate therapy.[34] Furthermore, programming high-rate zones with long detection intervals of 30/40 beats and a high cut-off rate to reduce inappropriate therapy (**Fig. 3**) has been proposed.[28] In cases of secondary prevention, the use of a monitor zone greater than 150 bpm and a fast VT zone at 180 to 200 bpm with appropriate use of discriminators and ATP in all cases is recommended.[28]

CONGENITAL LONG QT SYNDROME

Congenital long QT syndrome (LQTS) is an inherited disorder of cardiac repolarization that predisposes individuals to arrhythmia, syncope, and SCD with the appearance of afterdepolarizations and the potential for triggering torsade de pointes (TdP).[35]

Recurrent syncope is a classical, albeit concerning symptom in LQTS and in the absence of treatment, the frequency of syncopal events is approximately 5% per year, with SCD rates of 0.9% per year.[36]

Beta blockers have become the cornerstone of treatment and are first-line therapy in LQTS.[35] Coupled with avoidance of QT prolonging medications, this approach has significantly impacted event rates in LQTS patients. Although further syncope despite this approach may often represent compliance issues, it is important to recognize those individuals who are truly high risk.

There is abundant literature supporting the role of ICDs in high-risk cases. However, these have primarily focused on survivors of cardiac arrests, where guidelines give a class 1 recommendation for ICD implantation.[37] Beyond this indication, a careful discussion regarding the risks and benefits of device implantation with an LQT expert is strongly recommended. Indeed, some authors advocate the use of left cardiac sympathetic denervation as an alternative to ICD implantation.[38] To this point, during a median follow-up of 54 months, 16 patients from a cohort of 55 patients with LQTS received appropriate therapy. Of those, 15 were initially implanted for secondary prevention.[39]

It is apparent that the risk of cardiac events and SCD is highest in childhood and reduces in later life.[40] Consequently, device implantation decisions are commonly faced in younger patients, and careful consideration needs to be given regarding the lifetime risks of an ICD. A multicenter study of ICD therapies in LQTS followed 67 patients over a median of 47.8 months.[40] Twenty-one percent of patients experienced inappropriate therapy secondary to AF, sinus tachycardia, TWOS, lead failure, or myopotential sensing. In addition, 13% of patients suffered device-related complications.[40]

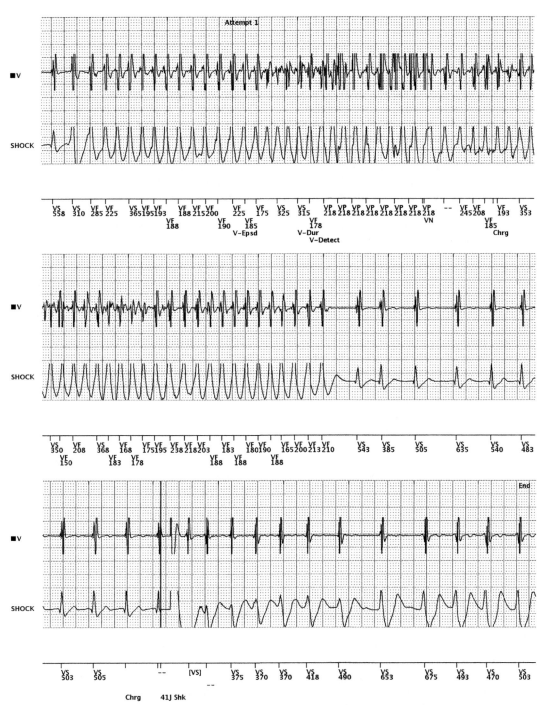

Fig. 3. Electrograms from a single-chamber ICD in a patient with BrS. Ventricular bipolar tip-ring and shock EGMs are shown. Ventricular fibrillation noted with intermittent undersensing. Appropriate detection in the VF zone is followed by satisfaction of the duration discriminator and delivery of an 8-beat burst of ATP with failure of termination. The device subsequently charges. 5.5 seconds later the tachycardia spontaneously terminates. Because of the committed nature of the shock, it is subsequently delivered despite termination.

The argument for an S-ICD in this cohort is clear. In total, 12% of patients from the EFFORT-LESS study had a diagnosis of LQT and subsequently underwent S-ICD implantation;[6] 99.4% successfully cardioverted at less than or equal to 80J and required no significant change in vector programming compared with non-channelopathy patients. However, LQTS patients had higher rates of appropriate and inappropriate therapy, at 33% and 12.5%, respectively, with a combined complication rate of 13%. Screening failure rates of 5% have previously been demonstrated in other case series.[32] Given the typical T wave changes in LQTS, screening should include both right and left parasternal areas during rest and exercise.[6]

The potential for short-long-short sequences initiating TdP is a significant caveat to the S-ICD given the inability to pace, particularly where bradycardia events may be expected. This has a direct impact on the potential utility of S-ICD devices.[6] Furthermore, prevention of bradycardia or pause-dependent events may justify the use of a pacemaker alone in some cases.[41] Consequently, the role of dual-chamber devices to permit atrial pacing, suppress heart rate variability, and prevent relative bradycardia should be carefully considered.

Although pacing alone is not invariably associated with a reduction in appropriate shock rates,[42] other studies have demonstrated both a significant reduction in QTc and cardiac events with this approach, particularly in LQT-2 patients.[42] Additional programming features such as AV hysteresis, given its promotion of intrinsic conduction below the lower rate limit and the potential for bradycardia mediated events, should be avoided.

Additional ICD programming decisions include prolonged detection times to allow for spontaneous termination of TdP and programming of a single VF zone with high rates to minimize inappropriate therapy. Finally, the impact of catecholamine release following device therapy and the potential for electrical storm warrant delayed redetection.

IDIOPATHIC VENTRICULAR FIBRILLATION

Idiopathic ventricular fibrillation (IVF) remains poorly defined as a clinical entity yet accounts for 5% to 7% of cases of aborted cardiac arrests.[43] Diagnosis remains largely one of exclusion given the broad etiologies to PMVT and VF. Diagnostic testing, including consideration of provocation testing, should therefore be carefully considered.

The 2013 HRS/EHRA/APHRS expert consensus statement on the diagnosis and management of patients with inherited primary arrhythmia syndromes gives a class 1 recommendation for ICD implantation in all cases of IVF.[1]

Conte and colleagues reported on the outcome of 245 registry patients with suspected IVF.[44] Ninety-two percent of patients were implanted with an ICD. Over 63 months of follow-up, 3 patients died of a cardiac event, (2 receiving medical therapy and 1 with an ICD). Twenty-one percent of patients experienced arrhythmia recurrence. Seventeen percent received appropriate ICD shocks, and 3% received successful ATP; 4.5% received inappropriate therapy.

Awareness of the critical role of short-coupled PVCs as a trigger in IVF is established.[1,43,44] More recently, publications have also implicated PVCs with longer coupling intervals.[43] In both cases, it is important to appreciate that VF initiation is neither bradycardia- nor pause-dependent, which has implications when selecting not only the type of ICD, but also its subsequent programming.

In addition, arrhythmia suppression with quinidine has been used in the management of short-coupled VF since the late 1980s with impressive results, so much so that it has led some authors to raise the possibility of a multicenter randomized controlled trial against ICD implantation.[45]

Given the rarity of IVF, data are lacking as to the role of S-ICDs. Given the young age, normal 12-lead ECG and absence of conduction disease, such patients appear to be good potential candidates for S-ICD implantation (**Fig. 4**). Frommeyer and colleagues reported the performance of S-ICDs in 24 patients with IVF and electrical heart disease.[46] During follow-up over 29 months, 4 patients had appropriate detection of VA, while 3 cases of oversensing resulted in inappropriate shocks in 2 patients.[46]

Therefore, in the case of S-ICD implants, careful attention should be paid to the screening process. Conte and colleagues demonstrated a 7% failure rate of patients with IVF.[32] Furthermore, where few suitable vectors are identified, the role of exercise testing should be considered. Programming of 2 zones, with the shock zone rate of greater than or equal to 230 bpm and the conditional zone greater than 200 bpm in addition to activation of the Smartpass filter is recommended.

Where a conventional left sided ICD is planned, a single coil lead with a single high-rate VF zone with delayed detection is likely to reduce rates of inappropriate therapy. Additional programming of ATP during charging is reasonable based on the data from Conte.[44]

Although coexisting atrial arrhythmias are uncommon, given the typically young age of the recipients and potential for rapid AV conduction, SVT discriminators should be programmed where possible.

SHORT QT SYNDROME

The short QT syndrome (SQTS) is a rare inheritable channelopathy associated with SCD and AF.[47] Although first recognized over 20 years ago, understanding remains limited, and formulating diagnostic criteria, including appropriate QT cut-offs, has proved challenging.

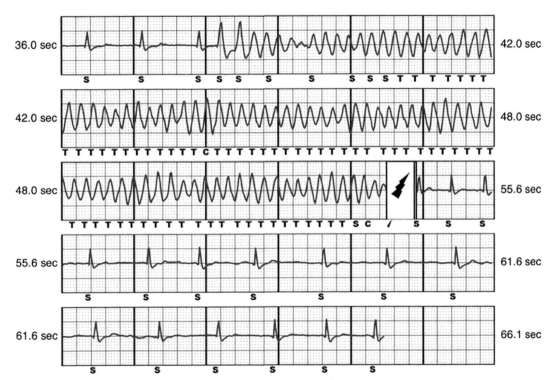

Fig. 4. Boston Emblem S-ICD tracing from a patient with IVF demonstrating a short-coupled PVC initiating polymorphic VT. Following initial undersensing, subsequent appropriate detection and delivery of an 80J shock is seen with successful termination.

Early attempts to form diagnostic and screening criteria demonstrated broad ranges of QTc intervals from the short, to the not so short (248–381 ms).[47] Potential overlap into normal QTc ranges was considerable, and it was apparent that some individuals with short QT intervals went on to a benign outcome.[48] Despite efforts by some authors, in addition to consensus statements, criteria remain unclear or disputed.[1,47,49]

The 2013 HRS/EHRA/APHRS expert consensus statement gave a Class 1 recommendation for ICD implantation in symptomatic patients who survived a cardiac arrest and/or had documented sustained VT, while a class IIb recommendation was given to asymptomatic patients with SQTS and a family history of SCD.[1]

Based on data from the European Short QT registry, SCD is highly prevalent within affected families, with 89% having experienced such an event. Indeed, one-third of patients presented with cardiac arrest as their first clinical manifestation.[50] The incidence of VA during follow-up was 4.9%; however, those on hydroquinidine experienced no events.[50] Complications were seen in 58% of ICD recipients, with one-third receiving inappropriate therapy, divided equally between TWOS and atrial arrhythmia.[50] Indeed, AF rates of 15% to 41% are seen in affected families.[50,51]

TWOS is a particular challenge with SQTS given the shortened QT interval and classically prominent T waves. Reducing the sensitivity of the RV lead may resolve the issue; however, this is dependent on the relative size and ratio of the R and T waves and carries a risk of undersensing VF. Devices that facilitate the programming of the ventricular sensitivity decay allow specific optimization to minimize potential oversensing.[52] Furthermore, a change in the RV sensing vector, where possible, will impact the relative amplitudes of the R and T waves and could be evaluated in such cases.

Where S-ICD implantation is being considered, given the potential for TWOS, exercise testing during screening is recommended. Programming of 2 zones with the shock zone rate greater than or equal to 230 bpm and the conditional zone greater than 200 bpm with activation of the Smartpass filter is recommended.

Regarding conventional TV device selection, a single-chamber ICD programmed with delayed detection and a single, high-rate zone, would minimize inappropriate therapy. Implant parameters are particularly important and maximal sensed R waves are beneficial when attempting to manage TWOS at a later stage. Given the high incidence of atrial arrhythmia, it is understandable to consider the role of a dual-chamber system, however, the evidence to support this approach from a discriminator perspective is lacking. Furthermore, justifying the significant incremental risk of an additional lead is difficult. In all cases, optimal use of SVT discriminators is critical alongside potential deactivation of the SVT timeout.

SUMMARY

These rare genetic heart diseases carry a significant risk of SCD. Yet, following appropriate medical management, risk stratification and ICD implantation, this can be minimized. Caution should, however, be exercised at all stages. Despite the desired and understandable focus on preventing arrhythmic death, ICD implantation in a young patient is a trade-off, exposing him or her to device-related complications, repeated interventions, and the pain and distress of inappropriate therapy. It is vital, therefore, that where ICD implantation is warranted, careful consideration is given not only to the selection of the device. but also its programming.

It is hoped this article has provided a useful insight into these rare diseases and the avoidance of some of the inherent pitfalls related to ICD selection and programming.

CLINICS CARE POINTS

- When considering ICD implantation, shared decision making is critical given the lack of robust data and tools for risk stratification. The emphasis should be to protect high risk individuals from life threatening arrhythmia but also protect truly low risk individuals from the risks of an ICD.
- ICD implantation in patients with CPVT should be approached with abundant caution given ICD shocks may precipitate further life-threatening ventricular arrhythmia.
- Appropriate risk stratification of patients with arrhythmogenic cardiomyopathy is critical remembering that for some patients the first presentation is sudden cardiac death.
- When reviewing patients with hypertrophic cardiomyopathy in the device clinic, the stored template should be frequently updated given deviation with disease progression may increase the risk of inappropriate therapy.
- Given the potential for dynamic ECG changes in Brugada syndrome, particularly in response to fever, the risk of T wave over-sensing should be considering when programming the device.
- Beta blockers remain the cornerstone of treatment in patients with Long QT syndrome with significant reduction in the rates of life-threatening ventricular arrhythmia. Where ICD implantation is being considered, involvement of an inherited arrhythmia specialist is strongly encouraged.

DISCLOSURE

S. Hansom: None. Z. Laksman: Advisory Committee for Boston Scientific, Consulting for Medtronic and Abbott.

REFERENCES

1. Priori SG, Wilde AA, Horie M, et al. HRS/EHRA/APHRS expert consensus statement on the diagnosis and management of patients with inherited primary arrhythmia syndromes: document endorsed by HRS, EHRA, and APHRS in May 2013 and by ACCF, AHA, PACES, and AEPC in June 2013. Heart Rhythm 2013;10(12):1932–63.
2. Sy RW, Gollob MH, Klein GJ, et al. Arrhythmia characterization and long-term outcomes in catecholaminergic polymorphic ventricular tachycardia. Heart Rhythm 2011;8(6):864–71.
3. Roses-Noguer F, Jarman JW, Clague JR, et al. Outcomes of defibrillator therapy in catecholaminergic polymorphic ventricular tachycardia. Heart Rhythm 2014;11(1):58–66.
4. Roston TM, Jones K, Hawkins NM, et al. Implantable cardioverter-defibrillator use in catecholaminergic polymorphic ventricular tachycardia: a systematic review. Heart Rhythm 2018;15(12):1791–9.
5. Stiles MK, Fauchier L, Morillo CA, et al. HRS/EHRA/APHRS/LAHRS focused update to 2015 expert consensus statement on optimal implantable cardioverter-defibrillator programming and testing. EP Europace 2019;21(9):1442–3.
6. Lambiase PD, Eckardt L, Theuns DA, et al. Evaluation of subcutaneous implantable cardioverter-defibrillator performance in patients with ion channelopathies from the EFFORTLESS cohort and comparison with a meta-analysis of transvenous ICD outcomes. Heart rhythm O2 2020;1(5):326–35.
7. Krahn AD, Wilde AA, Calkins H, et al. Arrhythmogenic right ventricular cardiomyopathy. Clinical Electrophysiology 2022;8(4):533–53.
8. Bosman LP, Te Riele AS. Arrhythmogenic right ventricular cardiomyopathy: a focused update on diagnosis and risk stratification. Heart 2022;108(2):90–7.

9. Miles C, Finocchiaro G, Papadakis M, et al. Sudden death and left ventricular involvement in arrhythmogenic cardiomyopathy. Circulation 2019;139(15):1786–97.

10. Cadrin-Tourigny J, Bosman LP, Nozza A, et al. A new prediction model for ventricular arrhythmias in arrhythmogenic right ventricular cardiomyopathy. Eur Heart J 2019;40:1850–8.

11. Link MS, Laidlaw D, Polonsky B, et al. Ventricular arrhythmias in the North American multidisciplinary study of ARVC: predictors, characteristics, and treatment. J Am Coll Cardiol 2014;64(2):119–25.

12. Corrado D, Leoni L, Link MS, et al. Implantable cardioverter-defibrillator therapy for prevention of sudden death in patients with arrhythmogenic right ventricular cardiomyopathy/dysplasia. Circulation 2003;108(25):3084–91.

13. Daimee UA, Assis FR, Murray B, et al. Clinical outcomes of catheter ablation of ventricular tachycardia in patients with arrhythmogenic right ventricular cardiomyopathy: insights from the Johns Hopkins ARVC Program. Heart Rhythm 2021;18(8):1369–76.

14. Trivedi A, Knight BP. ICD therapy for primary prevention in hypertrophic cardiomyopathy. Arrhythmia Electrophysiol Rev 2016;5(3):188.

15. Maron BJ. Clinical course and management of hypertrophic cardiomyopathy. N Engl J Med 2018; 379(7):655–68.

16. Rowin EJ, Burrows A, Madias C, et al. Long-term outcome in high-risk patients with hypertrophic cardiomyopathy after primary prevention defibrillator implants. Circulation 2020;13(10):e008123.

17. Thavikulwat AC, Tomson TT, Knight BP, et al. Appropriate implantable defibrillator therapy in adults with hypertrophic cardiomyopathy. J Cardiovasc Electrophysiol 2016;27(8):953–60.

18. Ommen SR, Mital S, Burke MA, et al. AHA/ACC guideline for the diagnosis and treatment of patients with hypertrophic cardiomyopathy: a report of the American College of Cardiology/American Heart Association Joint Committee on Clinical Practice Guidelines. J Am Coll Cardiol 2020;76(25): e159–240.

19. Dallaglio PD, di Marco A, Weidmann ZM, et al. Anti-tachycardia pacing for shock prevention in patients with hypertrophic cardiomyopathy and ventricular tachycardia. Heart Rhythm 2020;17(7):1084–91.

20. Rowin EJ, Hausvater A, Link MS, et al. Clinical profile and consequences of atrial fibrillation in hypertrophic cardiomyopathy. Circulation 2017;136(25):2420–36.

21. Weinstock J, Bader YH, Maron MS, et al. Subcutaneous implantable cardioverter defibrillator in patients with hypertrophic cardiomyopathy: an initial experience. J Am Heart Assoc 2016;5(2):e002488.

22. Lambiase PD, Gold MR, Hood M, et al. Evaluation of subcutaneous ICD early performance in hypertrophic cardiomyopathy from the pooled EFFORTLESS and IDE cohorts. Heart Rhythm 2016;13(5):1066–74.

23. Jankelson L, Garber L, Sherrid M, et al. Subcutaneous versus transvenous implantable defibrillator in patients with hypertrophic cardiomyopathy. Heart Rhythm 2022;19(5):759–67.

24. Adduci C, Semprini L, Palano F, et al. Safety and efficacy of anti-tachycardia pacing in patients with hypertrophic cardiomyopathy implanted with an ICD. Pacing Clin Electrophysiol 2019;42:610–6.

25. Probst V, Wilde AA, Barc J, et al. SCN5A mutations and the role of genetic background in the pathophysiology of Brugada syndrome. Circ Cardiovasc Genet 2009;2:552–7.

26. Benito B, Brugada R, Brugada J, et al. Brugada syndrome. Prog Cardiovasc Dis 2008;51(1):1–22.

27. Vutthikraivit W, Rattanawong P, Putthapiban P, et al. Worldwide prevalence of Brugada syndrome: a systematic review and meta-analysis. Acta Cardiol Sin 2018;34(3):267.

28. Conte G, Sieira J, Ciconte G, et al. Implantable cardioverter-defibrillator therapy in Brugada syndrome: a 20-year single-center experience. J Am Coll Cardiol 2015;65(9):879–88.

29. Dereci A, Yap SC, Schinkel AF. Meta-analysis of clinical outcome after implantable cardioverter-defibrillator implantation in patients with Brugada syndrome. JACC (J Am Coll Cardiol): Clinical Electrophysiology 2019;5(2):141–8.

30. Rodríguez-Mañero M, de Asmundis C, Sacher F, et al. T-wave oversensing in patients with Brugada syndrome: true bipolar versus integrated bipolar implantable cardioverter defibrillator leads: multicenter retrospective study. Circulation 2015;8(4):792–8.

31. Conte G, Cattaneo F, de Asmundis C, et al. Impact of SMART Pass filter in patients with ajmaline-induced Brugada syndrome and subcutaneous implantable cardioverter-defibrillator eligibility failure: results from a prospective multicentre study. EP Europace 2022;24(5):845–54.

32. Conte G, Kawabata M, de Asmundis C, et al. High rate of subcutaneous implantable cardioverter-defibrillator sensing screening failure in patients with Brugada syndrome: a comparison with other inherited primary arrhythmia syndromes. Europace 2018;20:1188–93.

33. Tachibana M, Nishii N, Morita H, et al. Exercise stress test reveals ineligibility for subcutaneous implantable cardioverter defibrillator in patients with Brugada syndrome. J Cardiovasc Electrophysiol 2017;28(12):1454–9.

34. Veltmann C, Kuschyk J, Schimpf R, et al. Prevention of inappropriate ICD shocks in patients with Brugada syndrome. Clin Res Cardiol 2010 Jan;99(1):37–44.

35. Abrams DJ, MacRae CA. Long QT syndrome. Circulation 2014;129(14):1524–9.

36. Moss AJ, Schwartz PJ, Crampton RS, et al. The long QT syndrome. Prospective longitudinal study of 328 families. Circulation 1991;84(3):1136–44.

37. Al-Khatib SM, Stevenson WG, Ackerman MJ, et al. 2017 AHA/ACC/HRS guideline for management of patients with ventricular arrhythmias and the prevention of sudden cardiac death: a report of the American College of Cardiology/American Heart Association Task Force on Clinical Practice Guidelines and the Heart Rhythm Society. J Am Coll Cardiol 2018;72(14):e91–220.

38. Krahn AD, Laksman Z, Sy RW, et al. Congenital long QT syndrome. Clinical Electrophysiology 2022;8(5):687–706.

39. Olde Nordkamp LR, Wilde AA, Tijssen JG, et al. The ICD for primary prevention in patients with inherited cardiac diseases: indications, use, and outcome: a comparison with secondary prevention. Circulation 2013;6(1):91–100.

40. Nannenberg EA, Sijbrands EJ, Dijksman LM, et al. Mortality of inherited arrhythmia syndromes: insight into their natural history. Circulation 2012;5(2):183–9.

41. Viskin S. Cardiac pacing in the long QT syndrome: review of available data and practical recommendations. J Cardiovasc Electrophysiol 2000;11(5):593–9.

42. Kowlgi GN, Giudicessi JR, Barake W, et al. Efficacy of intentional permanent atrial pacing in the long-term management of congenital long QT syndrome. J Cardiovasc Electrophysiol 2021;32(3):782–9.

43. Belhassen B, Tovia-Brodie O. Short-coupled idiopathic ventricular fibrillation-a literature review with extended follow-up. JACC (J Am Coll Cardiol) 2022;8(7):918–36.

44. Conte G, Belhassen B, Lambiase P, et al. Out-of-hospital cardiac arrest due to idiopathic ventricular fibrillation in patients with normal electrocardiograms: results from a multicentre long-term registry. EP Europace 2019;21(11):1670–7.

45. Steinberg C, Krahn AD. Quinidine vs. ICD therapy in short-coupled ventricular fibrillation—is a randomized trial the next logical step? Eur Heart J 2021;42(38):3993–4.

46. Frommeyer G, Dechering DG, Kochhäuser S, et al. Long-time "real-life" performance of the subcutaneous ICD in patients with electrical heart disease or idiopathic ventricular fibrillation. J Intervent Card Electrophysiol 2016;47(2):185–8.

47. Gollob MH, Redpath CJ, Roberts JD. The short QT syndrome: proposed diagnostic criteria. J Am Coll Cardiol 2011;57(7):802–12.

48. Anttonen O, Junttila MJ, Rissanen H, et al. Prevalence and prognostic significance of short QT interval in a middle-aged Finnish population. Circulation 2007;116(7):714–20.

49. Bjerregaard P. Proposed diagnostic criteria for short QT syndrome are badly founded. J Am Coll Cardiol 2011;58(5):549–50.

50. Giustetto C, Schimpf R, Mazzanti A, et al. Long-term follow-up of patients with short QT syndrome. J Am Coll Cardiol 2011;58(6):587–95.

51. El-Battrawy I, Schlentrich K, Besler J, et al. Sex-differences in short QT syndrome: a systematic literature review and pooled analysis. Eur J Prev Cardiol 2020;27(12):1335–8.

52. Schimpf R, Wolpert C, Bianchi F, et al. Congenital short QT syndrome and implantable cardioverter defibrillator treatment: inherent risk for inappropriate shock delivery. J Cardiovasc Electrophysiol 2003;14(12):1273–7.

Emerging Targeted Therapies for Inherited Cardiomyopathies and Arrhythmias

Tammy Ryan, MD, PhD[a,b], Jason D. Roberts, MD, MAS[a,c,d],*

KEYWORDS

- Genetics • Cardiomyopathy • Arrhythmia • Antisense oligonucleotide • Small interfering RNA
- Gene therapy • Gene editing

KEY POINTS

- Medical therapies for inherited cardiomyopathy and arrhythmia syndromes have historically been limited to agents previously developed for more common forms of heart disease.
- Our improved understanding of their genetics and disease mechanisms, coupled with the development of novel classes of therapeutics, has led to an emerging era of targeted therapies.
- The classes of novel therapies for inherited arrhythmia and cardiomyopathy syndromes include small molecules, antisense oligonucleotides, small interfering RNAs, adeno-associated virus–mediated gene therapies, and in vivo gene editing.
- The first agent in this new era to receive approval for clinical use is mavacamten, a myosin ATPase inhibitor for hypertrophic cardiomyopathy.

INTRODUCTION

Inherited cardiomyopathy and arrhythmia syndromes, although relatively rare, have a proclivity to cause significant morbidity and mortality, particularly in young people. The medical management of these conditions has primarily been limited to agents previously developed for more common forms of heart disease and not tailored to their distinct pathophysiology. As our understanding of their underlying genetics and disease mechanisms has improved, an era of targeted therapies for these rare conditions has begun to emerge. In recent years, several novel agents have been developed and tested in preclinical models and, in some cases, have advanced to both the clinical trial and clinical approval stages with exciting results. These are a diverse group, including small molecules, antisense oligonucleotides (ASOs), small interfering RNAs (siRNAs), adeno-associated virus (AAV)-mediated gene therapies, and in vivo gene-editing therapeutics (**Fig. 1**).

Here, we review the progress that has been made to date with emerging forms of targeted therapies for inherited cardiomyopathies and arrhythmias. We highlight the progress through stages of transition from bench to bedside and discuss the challenges involved in clinical translation.

HYPERTROPHIC CARDIOMYOPATHY

Hypertrophic cardiomyopathy (HCM) is the most common inherited cardiomyopathy with a prevalence approximating 1 in 500. The disease is characterized by thickening of the myocardium, which can result in left ventricular outflow tract (LVOT) obstruction, as well as a predisposition to malignant arrhythmias and sudden cardiac death. The

[a] McMaster University, Hamilton, Ontario, Canada; [b] Department of Medicine, Division of Cardiology, DBCVSRI, Hamilton General Hospital, Room C3-121, 237 Barton Street East, Hamilton, Ontario L8L2X2, Canada; [c] DBCVSRI, Room C3-111, 237 Barton Street East, Hamilton, Ontario L8L2X2, Canada; [d] Population Health Research Institute and Hamilton Health Sciences, Hamilton, Ontario, Canada
* Corresponding author. DBCVSRI, Room C3-111, 237 Barton Street East, Hamilton, Ontario L8L2X2, Canada.
E-mail address: jason.roberts@phri.ca

Card Electrophysiol Clin 15 (2023) 261–271
https://doi.org/10.1016/j.ccep.2023.04.006
1877-9182/23/© 2023 Elsevier Inc. All rights reserved.

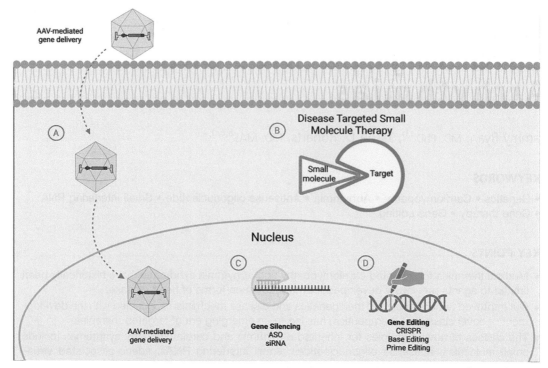

Fig. 1. Classes of emerging targeted treatment strategies for inherited arrhythmia and cardiomyopathy syndromes. (A) Adeno-associated virus (AAV)-mediated gene delivery. (B) Disease-targeted small molecule therapy. (C) Gene silencing through antisense oligonucleotides (ASOs) and small interfering RNAs (siRNA). (D) Gene editing through clustered regularly interspaced short palindromic repeats (CRISPR) nuclease, base editing, and prime editing approaches.

aberrant contractile activity is also associated with diastolic dysfunction, which can manifest with marked shortness of breath and functional limitation. Medical therapy has traditionally been limited to the use of β-blockers, calcium channel blockers, and disopyramide. Surgical myectomy and alcohol septal ablation are options for those with obstructive phenotypes that remain symptomatic despite optimal medical therapy. Although effective, many patients suffer from ongoing dyspnea, chest pain, and heart failure.

HCM is an autosomal dominant condition that has been linked to pathogenic variants in components of the sarcomere, including myosin. A portion of these myosin variants exhibit increased ATPase activity in biochemical assays, which may contribute to increased power output and the hyperdynamic contractile function in HCM. In 2016, Green and colleagues performed a chemical screen to identify small molecules with the ability to reduce the ATPase activity of myosin and identified the small molecule MYK-461, now known as mavacamten **(Fig. 2A).**[1] Treatment of mice harboring pathogenic variants in myosin with mavacamten resulted in reduced contractility, ventricular hypertrophy, and myocardial fibrosis, and its exposure to engineered

heart tissue from human induced pluripotent stem cells (hiPSCs) resulted in reduced contractility and diastolic stiffness.[1,2] Mavacamten also relieved LVOT obstruction in a feline model of HCM.[3]

These preclinical studies were shortly followed by the phase II clinical trials PIONEER-HCM[4] and MAVERICK-HCM,[5] which evaluated the efficacy of mavacamten in obstructive and nonobstructive HCM, respectively. PIONEER-HCM was a nonrandomized study evaluating 2 different mavacamten dosing regimens in 21 patients with obstructive HCM and found that treatment led to reduced dyspnea and improved LVOT gradients. These encouraging results in obstructive HCM were subsequently followed by the phase III EXPLORER-HCM[6] and VALOR-HCM[7] trials.

The EXPLORER-HCM trial was a randomized, double-blind, placebo-controlled trial involving 251 adults with obstructive HCM (LVOT gradient of at least 50 mm Hg) and New York Heart Association (NYHA) class II-III symptoms.[6] Patients treated with mavacamten showed greater improvement in the composite primary endpoint (1.5 mL/kg/min or greater increase in pVO₂ and at least one NYHA class reduction; or a 3.0-mL/kg/min or greater improvement in pVO₂ and no worsening of NYHA

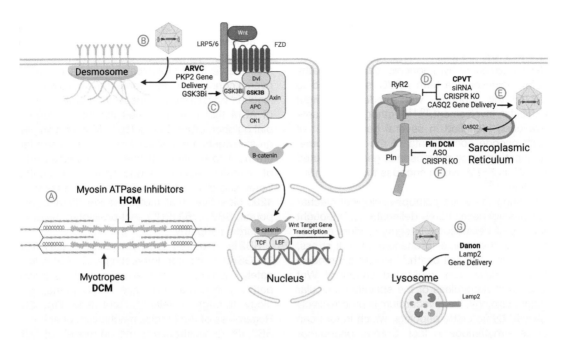

Fig. 2. Cellular targets for novel therapies in inherited arrhythmia and cardiomyopathy syndromes. (A) Small molecule sarcomere-targeted therapies for hypertrophic (HCM) and dilated cardiomyopathies (DCM). (B) Adeno-associated virus (AAV)-mediated *PKP2* gene delivery for arrhythmogenic right ventricular cardiomyopathy (ARVC). (C) Small molecule-based glycogen synthase kinase 3β inhibition (GSK3β) for ARVC. (D) CRISPR nuclease and small interfering RNA (siRNA)-mediated allele-specific RyR2 knockdown for RyR2-catecholaminergic polymorphic ventricular tachycardia (CPVT). (E) AAV-mediated CASQ2 gene delivery for CASQ2-CPVT. (F) CRISPR nuclease and antisense oligonucleotide (ASO)-mediated allele-specific PLN-p.R14 knockdown for phospholamban (PLN) cardiomyopathy. (G) AAV-mediated LAMP2B gene delivery for Danon disease. APC, adenomatous polyposis coli; LEF, lymphoid enhancer factor; TCF, t-cell factor.

class), as well as in the secondary endpoints, including reduced postexercise LVOT gradient and patient-reported symptom scores. VALOR-HCM[7] randomized 112 obstructive HCM patients that met guideline criteria for septal reduction therapy to mavacamten or placebo. Following a 16-week treatment period, mavacamten dramatically reduced the proportion of individuals that continued to meet guideline criteria for intervention (17.9% vs 76.8%).

In the setting of nonobstructive HCM, the phase II randomized MAVERICK-HCM trial found that 16 weeks of mavacamten treatment resulted in reduced N-terminal pro-brain natriuretic peptide (NT-proBNP) and troponin I relative to placebo.[4] Although no improvement in symptoms or exercise capacity was observed, the primary goal of the trial was to evaluate the safety and tolerability of mavacamten, and hence, it was not powered to evaluate clinical outcomes.

The overall safety and tolerability of mavacamten has been reassuring with no statistically significant differences in adverse clinical outcomes being observed. Decreases in ejection fraction on echocardiography have been observed in association with mavacamten; however, this was not unexpected given its mechanism of action. Furthermore, in cases of hyperdynamic function, this reduction in ejection fraction may perhaps be more appropriately viewed as a normalization. A long-term 5-year safety extension study involving study participants from both the EXPLORER-HCM and MAVERICK-HCM trials is ongoing (NCT03723655) and will further inform the safety of this new class of therapy.

A second myosin ATPase inhibitor, aficamten, is currently in phase II clinical trials. Preclinical studies in rats and dogs have shown reductions in fractional shortening and left ventricular ejection fraction (LVEF).[8] Preliminary results shared from REDWOOD-HCM (NCT04219826) indicate that treatment with aficamten reduces LVOT gradients; however, the full trial results remain to be published.[9]

ARRHYTHMOGENIC RIGHT VENTRICULAR CARDIOMYOPATHY

Arrhythmogenic right ventricular cardiomyopathy (ARVC) is an inherited cardiomyopathy that causes ventricular arrhythmias, heart failure, and sudden cardiac death. Recognition that the disease often extends to the left ventricle has led experts to suggest that the condition more appropriately be referred to as arrhythmogenic cardiomyopathy (ACM); however, the term ARVC is still used to refer to the subgroup with predominant right ventricular involvement.[10,11] Pathogenic variants have been identified in several genes, most of which encode components of the desmosome. The most common desmosomal gene implicated in ARVC is *PKP2*, which encodes the plakophilin-2 protein.[12,13]

Although the exact pathophysiological mechanism has not been entirely delineated, it is thought that loss of desmosome integrity renders cardiomyocytes susceptible to changes in wall stress, detachment, and cell death.[14] Preclinical models of ARVC have also implicated canonical Wnt signaling.[15] Regardless of the specific molecular pathophysiology, the myocardium is progressively replaced by fibrofatty deposits, which in turn can act as arrhythmogenic foci. Current pharmacotherapy is primarily aimed at minimizing arrhythmias and consists of β-blockers, antiarrhythmic drugs, and guideline-directed therapy for heart failure in the presence of ventricular dysfunction.[16] Breakthrough malignant ventricular arrhythmias are common and often necessitate catheter ablation. Given that ARVC pathology most often develops in the epicardium and grows inward, combined endocardial and epicardial ablation approaches are often required to achieve effective arrhythmia suppression. Owing to the limitations of current medical therapies for ARVC, there has been significant interest in developing more efficacious, target-directed agents.

The mechanism of *PKP2*-mediated ARVC is considered to be secondary to haploinsufficiency and, in this context, has been investigated as a potential target for gene therapy (see **Fig. 2**B). Proof-of-principle experiments in a hiPSC model of ARVC showed that AAV-mediated delivery of *PKP2* resulted in improved contractility and desmosome structure.[17] Using a *PKP2* mouse model of ARVC, Bradford and colleagues showed that delivery of wild-type *PKP2* using AAV resulted in rescue of PKP2 protein levels and improved cardiac function and survival.[18] PKP2-based gene therapy using an AAV vector is currently being developed for potential clinical application but has not yet reached human studies.

Although gene replacement therapy for genetic culprits presumed to result in haploinsufficiency offers a clear path to a therapeutic, our otherwise limited insight into ACM pathophysiology leaves a lack of a clearly defined biological target for modulation by a small molecule. In this setting,

identification of a novel therapeutic agent can still be achieved through screening a library of candidate drugs against an assay; however, the assay must serve as a biological recapitulation of the overall condition. In this context, Asimaki and colleagues developed a transgenic zebrafish model of ACM that overexpressed the mutant form of plakoglobin (*JUP* 2057del2).[19] Mutant fish had gross evidence of cardiomyopathy and heart failure by 4 to 6 weeks of age and increased rates of mortality relative to wild type by 3 months. Screening of this ACM model against a library of 4200 bioactive small molecules identified a compound, SB216763 (SB2), that prevented the onset of cardiomyopathy.

SB2 is annotated as a glycogen synthase kinase 3β (GSK3β) inhibitor. Interestingly, GSK3β is intricately involved in the Wnt/β-catenin signaling pathway and may influence ARVC pathophysiology through a related input (see **Fig. 2**C). Regardless of the precise mechanism of action of SB2, its administration to mouse models of ACM secondary to mutations in plakoglobin, desmoglein,[20] desmoplakin,[15] TMEM43,[21] and ANK2[22] have been striking. In each instance, administration of SB2 was able to prevent or markedly slow disease development. Although promising, human trials for GSK3β inhibition in ARVC have yet to be initiated.

CATECHOLAMINERGIC POLYMORPHIC VENTRICULAR TACHYCARDIA

Catecholaminergic polymorphic ventricular tachycardia (CPVT) is a malignant, inherited arrhythmia syndrome characterized by episodes of polymorphic VT in response to adrenergic stimulation. The mechanism is thought to be due to store overload–induced calcium release from the sarcoplasmic reticulum during diastole, leading to delayed after-depolarizations. Current first-line management consists of β-blockers, preferably nadolol, and exercise restriction. Although considered a second-line agent, flecainide has proven efficacious for reducing exercise-induced ventricular ectopy and is frequently added as adjuvant therapy.[23,24] Left cervical sympathetic denervation can be effective when medical therapy is insufficient, whereas the role of an implantable cardioverter-defibrillator (ICD) in high-risk patients remains debated.[25,26]

CPVT is associated with pathogenic variants in the cardiac ryanodine receptor (encoded by *RyR2*) and, less commonly, in calsequestrin-2 (encoded by *CASQ2*). *RYR2*-CPVT is autosomal dominant, whereas *CASQ2*-CPVT is usually autosomal recessive.[27,28] Each of these genetic culprits has been the focus of gene-based therapies in pre-clinical models. Autosomal recessive forms of *CASQ2*-CPVT are considered to potentially arise from inadequate buffering of calcium in the sarcoplasmic reticulum.[29] In this context, gene therapy to replace CASQ2 has shown remarkable efficacy in CASQ2 KO,[30] CASQ2-p.R33Q,[31] and CASQ2-p.D307H mice (see **Fig. 2**E).[32]

Given that pathogenic *RyR2* variants cause CPVT secondary to gain of function, *RyR2*-based gene replacement therapy would not be anticipated to be effective. In this context, multiple alternative strategies have been evaluated (see **Fig. 2**D). Ca^{2+}/calmodulin-dependent protein kinase II is an adrenergic-dependent kinase that activates RyR2 through phosphorylation. Its inhibition through small molecules and AAV-based delivery of autocamtide-2-related inhibitory peptide has been shown to be effective at suppressing arrhythmias in multiple RyR2-CPVT mouse models.[33,34] Prior work has also explored the utility of allele-specific silencing of mutant *RyR2* mRNA through the use of an siRNA. A study involving RyR2-p.R4496C CPVT mice revealed that selective siRNA-mediated knockdown of the mutant allele effectively prevented susceptibility to arrhythmia.[35] Notably, arrhythmia suppression was achieved with a 15% reduction in expression of the mutant *RyR2* allele.

A more recent study targeted RyR2 through a gene-editing approach that disrupted the disease-causing allele using clustered regularly interspaced short palindromic repeats (CRISPR)/CRISPR ASsociated protein 9 (Cas9).[36] Mice harboring the RyR2-p.R176Q mutation underwent AAV9-mediated editing of the mutant allele. While control mice developed VT in response to caffeine and isoproterenol exposure, mice that underwent gene editing were resistant to arrhythmias and exhibited normal calcium handling. The safety of this strategy is predicated on the notion that moderately reduced levels of RyR2 may be well tolerated.[35,37] Importantly, emerging evidence has implicated RyR2 loss of function in a novel pathologic entity termed calcium-release deficiency syndrome.[38] It is clear that there is a limit to the degree that RyR2 can be suppressed before it becomes pathologic; however, it is conceivable that there is an adequate therapeutic window to enable sufficient suppression to prevent arrhythmia while still maintaining normal cardiac physiology.

INHERITED DILATED CARDIOMYOPATHIES

Dilated cardiomyopathy (DCM) is a genetically diverse condition caused by pathogenic variants in several different genes.[39,40] Emerging therapies directed at specific targets are reviewed below, but there has also been some progress with the development of agents to stimulate systolic function. Omecamtiv mecarbil (OM) is a myotrope that activates myosin by stabilizing its actin-bound conformation (see **Fig. 2**A).[41] Initially identified in a chemical screen and subsequently modified to optimize its potency and pharmacokinetics, OM was shown to improve cardiac function in animal models. Initial trials in humans showed improved systolic function, but ischemia was also observed at high doses, and ultimately did not demonstrate an improvement in dyspnea in patients with acute heart failure in the ATOMIC-HF trial.[42–44] OM has also been tested in the setting of chronic heart failure in the GALACTIC-HF trial where it demonstrated a modest 8% relative risk reduction in the composite endpoint of heart failure events and death from cardiovascular causes.[45] There is some evidence that the benefit may be more substantial in patients with severely reduced systolic function.[45,46]

More recently, Perea-Gil and colleagues used phenotypic screening of a hiPSC model of DCM to identify novel therapeutic agents.[47] They identified two small-molecule kinase inhibitors that rescued contractile function in cardiomyocytes harboring a pathogenic mutation in *TNNT2*. These molecules appeared to function by promoting serine biosynthesis, which was hypothesized to exert its beneficial impact through modulation of energy metabolism in cardiomyocytes. The study suggested that augmented serine biosynthesis led to increased ATP production through upregulation of oxidative phosphorylation within mitochondria. They were also able to replicate their initial *TNNT2* findings in cardiomyocytes harboring pathogenic variants in several additional DCM genetic culprits, including *TTN*, *LMNA*, *PLN*, *TPM1*, and *LAMA2*. The authors suggested that targeting serine biosynthesis may provide a "genotype-agnostic" strategy for treating DCM that may be beneficial for a broad spectrum of patients rather than being confined to a single genetic subtype.

Titin Cardiomyopathy

Truncating variants within *TTN*,[48] the largest protein encoded by the human genome, are the most common genetic culprit in DCM. Approximately 25% of familial and 18% of sporadic DCM cases have been attributed to *TTN* truncating variants. *TTN* undergoes alternative splicing, and the pathogenicity of individual variants is partially related to whether they reside in an exon that is spliced out or incorporated into the mature mRNA. In this context, exons that have "proportion spliced-in" rates of greater than 90% exhibit the greatest pathogenicity.[49] Because of its large size, gene delivery of *TTN* would prove extremely challenging, and one alternative approach has focused on the development of ASOs to modulate splicing, promoting exclusion of mutated exons. In a hiPSC model of *TTN* cardiomyopathy that harbored a truncating variant in exon 326, ASO-mediated skipping of exon 326 normalized sarcomere structure, while delivery to *TTN* mice harboring the same variant resulted in rescue of sarcomere assembly and contractile function.[50] Despite these promising results, ASOs have yet to enter clinical trials for DCM.

Most recently, *TTN* truncating variants were targeted in hiPSCs using a pharmacologic approach. Fomin and colleagues showed that truncated titin proteins were not incorporated into sarcomeres in DCM patient hearts but instead were sequestered into intracellular aggregates.[51] They generated hiPSCs with a *TTN* truncating variant and found that pharmacologic inhibition of the ubiquitin-proteasome system resulted in increased levels of both wild-type and truncated titin protein and that this translated to increased contractile force, albeit to a lesser extent than in cells in which the variant was corrected using CRISPR/Cas9. These results offer another potential pathway to modulate titin expression in DCM but will require further exploration.

Cardiolaminopathy

Lamins are intermediate filament proteins that provide mechanical structure to the nucleus and modulate chromatin architecture.[52] A-type lamins, lamin A and C, are both expressed from the *LMNA* gene through alternative splicing. After *TTN*, pathogenic variants in *LMNA* are the most common cause of DCM and have been implicated in approximately 6% of cases.[53] Lamin cardiomyopathy is particularly aggressive, characterized by early-onset conduction system disease, atrial fibrillation, heart failure, malignant ventricular arrhythmias, and sudden cardiac death.[54] Management is currently limited to standard heart failure therapies and ICDs for those considered at high risk of sudden cardiac death (SCD).[55]

Although the pathophysiology is incompletely understood, some studies have implicated abnormal activation of mitogen-activated protein kinase signaling.[56–58] Treatment with the small-molecule PF-07265803 (formerly ARRY-371797), a selective inhibitor of p38α, showed improved LV function in a Lmna$^{H222P/H222P}$ mouse model.[56] A phase II clinical trial with 12 patients showed improved 6-minute walk test and preserved

exercise capacity,[59] but the phase III randomized controlled trial REALM-DCM has recently been discontinued because of anticipated futility.[60]

The ubiquitous expression of lamins makes the specific cause of cardiolaminopathy even more challenging to determine and target. Indeed, recent evidence suggests that endothelial dysfunction may also contribute to the pathophysiology and be a target for therapy. Using endothelial cells derived from LMNA hiPSCs, Sayed and colleagues performed concomitant gene expression and chromatin accessibility profiling, which revealed downregulation of the transcription factor KLF2 and a resultant failure to respond appropriately to shear stress by aligning in the direction of flow and augmenting the expression of endothelial nitric oxide synthase to increase nitric oxide production.[61] In the presence of the KLF2 agonist lovastatin, cocultures of mutant *LMNA* hiPSC-derived cardiomyocytes and endothelial cells exhibited improvements in arrhythmic calcium transients and diastolic function. To date, this study has not been followed up with trials in patients.

Phospholamban Cardiomyopathy

Phospholamban (PLN) is a sarcoplasmic reticulum protein that is integral in the regulation of SERCA2a (sarcoplasmic/endoplasmic reticulum Ca^{2+} ATPase 2a)-mediated calcium reuptake. In its unphosphorylated state, PLN binds to SERCA2a, inhibiting its ability to traffic cytoplasmic calcium back to the sarcoplasmic reticulum. When phosphorylated, PLN releases SERCA2a, allowing it to move calcium into the sarcoplasmic reticulum and thereby promoting lusitropy.[62] Pathogenic variants in PLN cause an ACM characterized by malignant arrhythmias and heart failure.[63] Among the most prevalent variants in PLN is R14Del, which is thought to result in "superinhibition" of SERCA2a.[64]

PLN-p.R14del has been targeted for genome editing, first in an hiPSC model of PLN cardiomyopathy using transcription activator-like effector nucleases,[65] then subsequently in mice, using AAV9-CRISPR/Cas9 (see **Fig. 2**F).[66] The humanized mouse model exhibited biventricular dilatation, and hearts were more vulnerable to arrhythmia (although this could only be demonstrated in an explant model). These defects were both ameliorated in animals that underwent gene editing. In a similar manner, ASOs targeting *PLN* were shown to improve cardiac dysfunction and survival (see **Fig. 2**F).[67] Interestingly, in this study, the *PLN*-ASO also had a positive impact in an unrelated mouse model of DCM, as well as in a rat model of ischemic cardiomyopathy. These findings suggest that targeting PLN may be of more general clinical benefit in various forms of cardiomyopathy. While targeting of the SERCA2a/PLN interaction through a gene therapy approach has previously failed to improve outcomes in heart failure patients,[68] the concept is biologically plausible, and it may be that novel methods of genetic or protein modulation, such as those discussed here, may prove more effective.

DANON DISEASE

Danon disease is an autophagic vacuolar myopathy caused by pathogenic variants in lysosome-associated membrane protein 2 (LAMP2). It is an X-linked disorder, and penetrance in male patients is nearly 100%. Affected individuals may develop cardiac hypertrophy and ventricular pre-excitation.[69] Prognosis is poor, and affected males rarely survive beyond 30 years of age without a heart transplant.

Studies in hiPSCs derived from patients with Danon disease have shown that replacement of LAMP2 restores some cellular functions, including mitochondrial bioenergetics and mitophagy.[70] Based on this, Manso and colleagues assessed the impact of systemic AAV-mediated delivery of LAMP2B in a mouse model of Danon disease and found some improvement in autophagic flux, cardiac contractile function (although this mouse model does not exhibit the cardiac hypertrophy typically seen in Danon disease), and survival (see **Fig. 2**G).[71] AAV9:LAMP2B has since entered phase I clinical trials, and preliminary results indicate that replacement of LAMP2B is associated with improved exercise tolerance, reduced natriuretic peptide levels, and normalized myocardial morphology on electron microscopy.[72] There were significant adverse events, including acute kidney injury requiring dialysis, exacerbations of skeletal myopathy, and thrombocytopenia; however, they were generally manageable with transient immunosuppression.

GENE EDITING

The advent of CRISPR/Cas9 for gene editing[73,74] has led to a surge in the use of this technology in the last decade, and multiple programs have recently begun to advance to clinical-stage investigations. CRISPR involves an endonuclease, termed a Cas, and a single guide RNA (sgRNA) (see **Fig.** 1D). The sgRNA is configured to be complementary to the targeted genomic sequence to be modified.[73] The Cas endonuclease in the initial iteration of CRISPR induces a DNA double-stranded break. Although the location of the break is precise, the subsequent edit is dependent on the cell's own repair processes (either nonhomologous end joining or homology-directed repair). Nonhomologous end joining is the dominant repair process and often results in insertions and deletions, with the potential to cause frameshifts. In this context, the initial iteration of CRISPR can effectively disrupt or knockout a gene; however, it has limited ability to revert a damaging variant to the wild type. Given that gene knockout is pathogenic for most genes involved in inherited arrhythmias and cardiomyopathies, this form of CRISPR is unlikely to be able to provide therapeutic benefit in isolation. In addition, there has been concern that the double-stranded DNA breaks may lead to harmful chromosomal rearrangements.[75]

These limitations prompted the development of base editing technology, which can directly alter targeted base pairs without inducing double-stranded breaks or relying on innate cellular repair processes.[76] Two types of base editors have been developed, namely adenine and cytosine base editors.[77] Each contains a catalytically inactive Cas9 (that does not make double-stranded DNA breaks) and a DNA-modifying enzyme. Base editors can currently perform transition edits (A > G and C > T), but not transversions, which require converting a purine base to a pyrimidine or vice versa. Shortly following the advent of base editing, a third iteration of CRISPR was introduced, termed prime editing. Prime editing enables the full array of genomic modifications, including base pair substitutions (both transitions and transversions), along with insertions and deletions without requiring double-strand DNA breaks.[78] Although promising, prime editing is at an earlier stage of development relative to base editing, and its efficacy in nonhuman primates has yet to be established.

Although base editing and prime editing techniques carry the potential to provide cures for monogenic inherited arrhythmias and cardiomyopathies, there are multiple obstacles that need to first be overcome. Delivery of CRISPR machinery to the liver through lipid nanoparticles has been optimized and performed effectively in humans; however, efficient vehicles for delivery to the heart have yet to be established.[79] In addition, most forms of inherited arrhythmias and cardiomyopathies develop secondary to a broad array of variants within culprit genes. It is unlikely to be feasible to develop a different CRISPR therapeutic for each individual disease-causing variant, and in this context, it is not immediately clear how CRISPR-based approaches will be able to provide treatments for the diverse array of disease-causing variants in patients when gene knockout is not therapeutic.

Regardless of these current uncertainties, the advent of gene editing technology holds tremendous potential for these genetic conditions with the possibility of providing definitive cures. The first base editor to enter clinical trials in humans is within the cardiovascular domain and aims to silence liver-based PCSK9 expression with the goal of providing life-long low-density lipoprotein cholesterol lowering and protection against coronary artery disease following a single treatment.[80]

SUMMARY

Recent years have been associated with the emergence of several novel forms of therapy for inherited cardiomyopathies and arrhythmias that include small molecules, ASOs, siRNAs, AAV-based gene therapy, and various gene-editing approaches. The myosin ATPase inhibitor mavacamten is currently the furthest along, having been approved for use in obstructive HCM by the Food and Drug Administration this year. CRISPR-based tools have ushered in a genome editing revolution in the last 10 years and are now rapidly entering the clinical realm. We have now reached a precipice whereby the ability to edit genes is no longer in question, although rigorous scrutiny and long-term follow-up data will be necessary to ensure its safety. The potential of this emerging era of therapies precisely targeted toward underlying disease pathophysiology hopefully represents a pivotal turning point in the management of inherited cardiac diseases.

DISCLOSURES

Dr T. Ryan receives research funding from Pfizer Inc. Dr J.D. Roberts has received consulting fees from Bristol Myers Squibb and Ionis Pharmaceuticals.

REFERENCES

1. Green EM, Wakimoto H, Anderson RL, et al. A small-molecule inhibitor of sarcomere contractility suppresses hypertrophic cardiomyopathy in mice. Science 2016;351(6273):617–21.
2. Sewanan LR, Shen S, Campbell SG. Mavacamten preserves length-dependent contractility and improves diastolic function in human engineered heart tissue. Am J Physiol Heart Circ Physiol 2021;320(3):H1112–23.
3. Stern JA, Markova S, Ueda Y, et al. A small molecule inhibitor of sarcomere contractility acutely Relieves left ventricular outflow tract obstruction in feline hypertrophic cardiomyopathy. PLoS One 2016;11(12):e0168407.
4. Heitner SB, Jacoby D, Lester SJ, et al. Mavacamten treatment for obstructive hypertrophic cardiomyopathy: a clinical trial. Ann Intern Med 2019;170(11):741–8.
5. Ho CY, Mealiffe ME, Bach RG, et al. Evaluation of Mavacamten in symptomatic patients with Nonobstructive hypertrophic cardiomyopathy. J Am Coll Cardiol 2020;75(21):2649–60.
6. Olivotto I, Oreziak A, Barriales-Villa R, et al. Mavacamten for treatment of symptomatic obstructive hypertrophic cardiomyopathy (EXPLORER-HCM): a randomised, double-blind, placebo-controlled, phase 3 trial. Lancet 2020;396(10253):759–69.
7. Desai MY, Owens A, Geske JB, et al. Myosin inhibition in patients with obstructive hypertrophic cardiomyopathy referred for septal reduction therapy. J Am Coll Cardiol 2022;80(2):95–108.
8. Hwee DT, Hatrman J, Wang J, et al. Pharmacologic Characterization of the cardiac myosin inhibitor, CK-3773274: a potential therapeutic approach for hypertrophic cardiomyopathy. Circ Res 2019;125(S1). https://doi.org/10.1161/res.125.suppl_1.332. Abstract 332.
9. BioSpace. Cytokinetics announces positive topline results from cohort 3 of REDWOOD-HCM. Accessed 2022/09/03, 2022. https://www.biospace.com/article/releases/cytokinetics-announces-positive-topline-results-from-cohort-3-of-redwood-hcm.
10. Bosman LP, Te Riele A. Arrhythmogenic right ventricular cardiomyopathy: a focused update on diagnosis and risk stratification. Heart 2022;108(2):90–7.
11. Krahn AD, Wilde AAM, Calkins H, et al. Arrhythmogenic right ventricular cardiomyopathy. JACC Clin Electrophysiol 2022;8(4):533–53.
12. Dalal D, Molin LH, Piccini J, et al. Clinical features of arrhythmogenic right ventricular dysplasia/cardiomyopathy associated with mutations in plakophilin-2. Circulation 2006;113(13):1641–9.
13. van Tintelen JP, Entius MM, Bhuiyan ZA, et al. Plakophilin-2 mutations are the major determinant of familial arrhythmogenic right ventricular dysplasia/cardiomyopathy. Circulation 2006;113(13):1650–8.
14. Corrado D, Thiene G. Arrhythmogenic right ventricular cardiomyopathy/dysplasia: clinical impact of molecular genetic studies. Circulation 2006;113(13):1634–7.
15. Garcia-Gras E, Lombardi R, Giocondo MJ, et al. Suppression of canonical Wnt/beta-catenin signaling by nuclear plakoglobin recapitulates phenotype of arrhythmogenic right ventricular cardiomyopathy. J Clin Invest 2006;116(7):2012–21.
16. Towbin JA, McKenna WJ, Abrams DJ, et al. HRS expert consensus statement on evaluation, risk stratification, and management of arrhythmogenic cardiomyopathy. Heart Rhythm 2019;16(11):e301–72.
17. Inoue H, Nakamura S, Higo S, et al. Modeling reduced contractility and impaired desmosome assembly due to plakophilin-2 deficiency using isogenic iPS cell-derived cardiomyocytes. Stem Cell Rep 2022;17(2):337–51.

18. Bradford W, Liang Y, Mataaarachchi N, et al. Plako-philin-2 gene therapy prevents arrhythmogenic right ventricular cardiomyopathy development in a novel mouse model harboring patient genetics. Faseb J 2021;35(S1):03193.

19. Asimaki A, Kapoor S, Plovie E, et al. Identification of a new modulator of the intercalated disc in a zebra-fish model of arrhythmogenic cardiomyopathy. Sci Transl Med 2014;6(240):240ra74.

20. Chelko SP, Asimaki A, Andersen P, et al. Central role for GSK3beta in the pathogenesis of arrhythmo-genic cardiomyopathy. JCI Insight 2016;1(5).

21. Padron-Barthe L, Villalba-Orero M, Gomez-Salinero JM, et al. Severe cardiac dysfunction and death caused by arrhythmogenic right ventricular cardiomyopathy type 5 are improved by inhibition of glycogen synthase kinase-3beta. Circulation 2019;140(14):1188–204.

22. Roberts JD, Murphy NP, Hamilton RM, et al. Ankyrin-B dysfunction predisposes to arrhythmogenic car-diomyopathy and is amenable to therapy. J Clin Invest 2019;129(8):3171–84.

23. van der Werf C, Kannankeril PJ, Sacher F, et al. Fle-cainide therapy reduces exercise-induced ventricu-lar arrhythmias in patients with catecholaminergic polymorphic ventricular tachycardia. J Am Coll Car-diol 2011;57(22):2244–54.

24. Kannankeril PJ, Moore JP, Cerrone M, et al. Efficacy of flecainide in the treatment of catecholaminergic polymorphic ventricular tachycardia: a randomized clinical trial. JAMA Cardiol 2017;2(7):759–66.

25. van der Werf C, Lieve KV, Bos JM, et al. Implantable cardioverter-defibrillators in previously undiagnosed patients with catecholaminergic polymorphic ven-tricular tachycardia resuscitated from sudden car-diac arrest. Eur Heart J 2019;40(35):2953–61.

26. Mazzanti A, Kukavica D, Trancuccio A, et al. Outcomes of patients with catecholaminergic polymorphic ven-tricular tachycardia treated with beta-blockers. JAMA Cardiol 2022;7(5):504–12.

27. Lahat H, Pras E, Olender T, et al. A missense mutation in a highly conserved region of CASQ2 is associated with autosomal recessive catecholamine-induced polymorphic ventricular tachycardia in Bedouin families from Israel. Am J Hum Genet 2001;69(6): 1378–84.

28. Ng K, Titus EW, Lieve KV, et al. An International Multicenter evaluation of inheritance Patterns, arrhythmic risks, and underlying mechanisms of CASQ2-catecholaminergic polymorphic ventricular tachycardia. Circulation 2020;142(10):932–47.

29. Titus EW, Deiter FH, Shi C, et al. The structure of a cal-sequestrin filament reveals mechanisms of familial arrhythmia. Nat Struct Mol Biol 2020;27(12):1142–51.

30. Denegri M, Avelino-Cruz JE, Boncompagni S, et al. Viral gene transfer rescues arrhythmogenic pheno-type and ultrastructural abnormalities in adult calsequestrin-null mice with inherited arrhythmias. Circ Res 2012;110(5):663–8.

31. Denegri M, Bongianino R, Lodola F, et al. Single deliv-ery of an adeno-associated viral construct to transfer the CASQ2 gene to knock-in mice affected by cate-cholaminergic polymorphic ventricular tachycardia is able to cure the disease from birth to advanced age. Circulation 2014;129(25):2673–81.

32. Kurtzwald-Josefson E, Yadin D, Harun-Khun S, et al. Viral delivered gene therapy to treat catecholamin-ergic polymorphic ventricular tachycardia (CPVT2) in mouse models. Heart Rhythm 2017;14(7): 1053–60.

33. Liu N, Ruan Y, Denegri M, et al. Calmodulin kinase II inhibition prevents arrhythmias in RyR2(R4496C+/-) mice with catecholaminergic polymorphic ventricular tachycardia. J Mol Cell Cardiol 2011;50(1):214–22.

34. Bezzerides VJ, Caballero A, Wang S, et al. Gene ther-apy for catecholaminergic polymorphic ventricular tachycardia by inhibition of Ca(2+)/calmodulin-dependent kinase II. Circulation 2019;140(5):405–19.

35. Bongianino R, Denegri M, Mazzanti A, et al. Allele-specific silencing of mutant mRNA rescues ultrastruc-tural and arrhythmic phenotype in mice Carriers of the R4496C mutation in the ryanodine receptor gene (RYR2). Circ Res 2017;121(5):525–36.

36. Pan X, Philippen L, Lahiri SK, et al. In Vivo Ryr2 edit-ing corrects catecholaminergic polymorphic ventric-ular tachycardia. Circ Res 2018;123(8):953–63.

37. Bround MJ, Wambolt R, Cen H, et al. Cardiac ryano-dine receptor (Ryr2)-mediated calcium Signals Spe-cifically Promote Glucose oxidation via Pyruvate Dehydrogenase. J Biol Chem 2016;291(45): 23490–505.

38. Sun B, Yao J, Ni M, et al. Cardiac ryanodine receptor calcium release deficiency syndrome. Sci Transl Med 2021;13:579.

39. Repetti GG, Toepfer CN, Seidman JG, et al. Novel therapies for prevention and early treatment of car-diomyopathies. Circ Res 2019;124(11):1536–50.

40. Jordan E, Peterson L, Ai T, et al. Evidence-based Assessment of genes in dilated cardiomyopathy. Circulation 2021;144(1):7–19.

41. Malik FI, Hartman JJ, Elias KA, et al. Cardiac myosin activation: a potential therapeutic approach for sys-tolic heart failure. Science 2011;331(6023):1439–43.

42. Cleland JG, Teerlink JR, Senior R, et al. The effects of the cardiac myosin activator, omecamtiv mecar-bil, on cardiac function in systolic heart failure: a double-blind, placebo-controlled, crossover, dose-ranging phase 2 trial. Lancet 2011;378(9792): 676–83.

43. Teerlink JR, Clarke CP, Saikali KG, et al. Dose-dependent augmentation of cardiac systolic func-tion with the selective cardiac myosin activator, ome-camtiv mecarbil: a first-in-man study. Lancet 2011; 378(9792):667–75.

44. Teerlink JR, Felker GM, McMurray JJV, et al. Acute treatment with omecamtiv mecarbil to increase contractility in acute heart failure: the ATOMIC-AHF study. J Am Coll Cardiol 2016;67(12):1444–55.

45. Teerlink JR, Diaz R, Felker GM, et al. Cardiac myosin activation with omecamtiv mecarbil in systolic heart failure. N Engl J Med 2021;384(2):105–16.

46. Felker GM, Solomon SD, Claggett B, et al. Assessment of omecamtiv mecarbil for the treatment of patients with Severe heart failure: a post Hoc analysis of data from the GALACTIC-HF randomized clinical trial. JAMA Cardiol 2022;7(1):26–34.

47. Perea-Gil I, Seeger T, Bruyneel AAN, et al. Serine biosynthesis as a novel therapeutic target for dilated cardiomyopathy. Eur Heart J 2022;43(36):3477–89.

48. Herman DS, Lam L, Taylor MR, et al. Truncations of titin causing dilated cardiomyopathy. N Engl J Med 2012;366(7):619–28.

49. Roberts AM, Ware JS, Herman DS, et al. Integrated allelic, transcriptional, and phenomic dissection of the cardiac effects of titin truncations in health and disease. Sci Transl Med 2015;7(270):270ra6.

50. Gramlich M, Pane LS, Zhou Q, et al. Antisense-mediated exon skipping: a therapeutic strategy for titin-based dilated cardiomyopathy. EMBO Mol Med 2015;7(5):562–76.

51. Fomin A, Gartner A, Cyganek L, et al. Truncated titin proteins and titin haploinsufficiency are targets for functional recovery in human cardiomyopathy due to TTN mutations. Sci Transl Med 2021;13(618):eabd3079.

52. Gruenbaum Y, Foisner R. Lamins: nuclear intermediate filament proteins with fundamental functions in nuclear mechanics and genome regulation. Annu Rev Biochem 2015;84:131–64.

53. Parks SB, Kushner JD, Nauman D, et al. Lamin A/C mutation analysis in a cohort of 324 unrelated patients with idiopathic or familial dilated cardiomyopathy. Am Heart J 2008;156(1):161–9.

54. Chen SN, Mestroni L, Taylor MRG. Genetics of dilated cardiomyopathy. Curr Opin Cardiol 2021;36(3):288–94.

55. Zeppenfeld K, Tfelt-Hansen J, de Riva M, et al. ESC Guidelines for the management of patients with ventricular arrhythmias and the prevention of sudden cardiac death. Eur Heart J 2022. https://doi.org/10.1093/eurheartj/ehac262.

56. Muchir A, Wu W, Choi JC, et al. Abnormal p38alpha mitogen-activated protein kinase signaling in dilated cardiomyopathy caused by lamin A/C gene mutation. Hum Mol Genet 2012;21(19):4325–33.

57. Muchir A, Reilly SA, Wu W, et al. Treatment with selumetinib preserves cardiac function and improves survival in cardiomyopathy caused by mutation in the lamin A/C gene. Cardiovasc Res 2012;93(2):311–9.

58. Wu W, Muchir A, Shan J, et al. Mitogen-activated protein kinase inhibitors improve heart function and prevent fibrosis in cardiomyopathy caused by mutation in lamin A/C gene. Circulation 2011;123(1):53–61.

59. Judge DP, Lakdawala NK, Taylor MRG, et al. Long-term efficacy and safety of ARRY-371797 (PF-07265803) in patients with lamin A/C-related dilated cardiomyopathy. Am J Cardiol 2022.

60. Pfizer. Pfizer to Discontinue Development Program for PF-07265803 for LMNA-Related Dilated Cardiomyopathy. Accessed 2022/09/25, 2022. https://www.pfizer.com/news/announcements/pfizer-discontinue-development-program-pf-07265803-lmna-related-dilated.

61. Sayed N, Liu C, Ameen M, et al. Clinical trial in a dish using iPSCs shows lovastatin improves endothelial dysfunction and cellular cross-talk in LMNA cardiomyopathy. Sci Transl Med 2020;(554):12. https://doi.org/10.1126/scitranslmed.aax9276.

62. MacLennan DH, Kranias EG. Phospholamban: a crucial regulator of cardiac contractility. Nat Rev Mol Cell Biol 2003;4(7):566–77.

63. Hof IE, van der Heijden JF, Kranias EG, et al. Prevalence and cardiac phenotype of patients with a phospholamban mutation. Neth Heart J 2019;27(2):64–9.

64. Haghighi K, Kolokathis F, Gramolini AO, et al. A mutation in the human phospholamban gene, deleting arginine 14, results in lethal, hereditary cardiomyopathy. Proc Natl Acad Sci U S A 2006;103(5):1388–93.

65. Stillitano F, Turnbull IC, Karakikes I, et al. Genomic correction of familial cardiomyopathy in human engineered cardiac tissues. Eur Heart J 2016;37(43):3282–4.

66. Dave J, Raad N, Mittal N, et al. Gene editing reverses arrhythmia susceptibility in humanized PLN-R14del mice: modeling a European cardiomyopathy with global impact. Cardiovasc Res 2022;22.

67. Grote Beverborg N, Spater D, Knoll R, et al. Phospholamban antisense oligonucleotides improve cardiac function in murine cardiomyopathy. Nat Commun 2021;12(1):5180.

68. Greenberg B, Butler J, Felker GM, et al. Calcium upregulation by percutaneous administration of gene therapy in patients with cardiac disease (CUPID 2): a randomised, multinational, double-blind, placebo-controlled, phase 2b trial. Lancet 2016;387(10024):1178–86.

69. Zhai Y, Miao J, Peng Y, et al. Clinical features of Danon disease and insights gained from LAMP-2 deficiency models. Trends Cardiovasc Med 2021. https://doi.org/10.1016/j.tcm.2021.10.012.

70. Hashem SI, Murphy AN, Divakaruni AS, et al. Impaired mitophagy facilitates mitochondrial damage in Danon disease. J Mol Cell Cardiol 2017;108:86–94.

71. Manso AM, Hashem SI, Nelson BC, et al. Systemic AAV9.LAMP2B injection reverses metabolic and

physiologic multiorgan dysfunction in a murine model of Danon disease. Sci Transl Med 2020; 18(535):12.

72. Greenber g B, Eshraghian E, Battiprolu P, et al. Abstract 10727: results from first-in-human clinical trial of RP-A501 (AAV9:LAMP2B) gene therapy treatment for Danon disease. Circulation 2021;(A10727):144.

73. Jinek M, Chylinski K, Fonfara I, et al. A programmable dual-RNA-guided DNA endonuclease in adaptive bacterial immunity. Science 2012;337(6096):816–21.

74. Cong L, Ran FA, Cox D, et al. Multiplex genome engineering using CRISPR/Cas systems. Science 2013;339(6121):819–23.

75. Kosicki M, Tomberg K, Bradley A. Repair of double-strand breaks induced by CRISPR-Cas9 leads to large deletions and complex rearrangements. Nat Biotechnol 2018;36(8):765–71.

76. Komor AC, Kim YB, Packer MS, et al. Programmable editing of a target base in genomic DNA without double-stranded DNA cleavage. Nature 2016; 533(7603):420–4.

77. Gaudelli NM, Komor AC, Rees HA, et al. Programmable base editing of A*T to G*C in genomic DNA without DNA cleavage. Nature 2017;551(7681): 464–71.

78. Anzalone AV, Randolph PB, Davis JR, et al. Search-and-replace genome editing without double-strand breaks or donor DNA. Nature 2019;576(7785):149–57.

79. Gillmore JD, Gane E, Taubel J, et al. CRISPR-Cas9 in vivo gene editing for Transthyretin Amyloidosis. Reply. N Engl J Med 2021;385(6):493–502.

80. Kingwell K. Base editors hit the clinic. Nat Rev Drug Discov 2022;21(8):545–7.

Novelties in Brugada Syndrome: Complex Genetics, Risk Stratification, and Catheter Ablation

Wiert F. Hoeksema, MD[a], Ahmad S. Amin, MD, PhD[a],
Connie R. Bezzina, PhD[b], Arthur A.M. Wilde, MD, PhD[a],
Pieter G. Postema, MD, PhD[a],*

KEYWORDS

• Brugada syndrome • Ventricular arrhythmias • Ventricular fibrillation • Sudden cardiac death

KEY POINTS

- The genetic architecture of Brugada syndrome (BrS) is complex and seems to be polygenic rather than monogenic, to which combinations of common variants as well as rare variants contribute.
- Progress in genome-wide association studies and the development of polygenic risk scores may contribute to our understanding of BrS.
- Risk stratification in BrS is still imperfect, particularly in patients with intermediate risk of arrhythmic events and sudden cardiac death.
- Catheter ablation may have an important role in the future management of BrS, although it is premature to consider catheter ablation in patients at low-to-intermediate risk for arrhythmic events.

INTRODUCTION

Brugada syndrome (BrS) is an inherited primary arrhythmia syndrome, first described in 1953 by Osher and Wolff,[1] and subsequently by several others including Martini and colleagues in 1989[2] and Pedro and Josep Brugada, after whom it became named, in 1992.[3] Its hallmark electrocardiographic signature is traditionally characterized by a J-point elevation $\geq$0.2 mV with a coved ST elevation and T-wave inversion in the right precordial leads.[4] This distinctive electrocardiogram (ECG) pattern is called the type 1 Brugada ECG pattern. The Brugada ECG pattern may be transient and can occur spontaneously or after provocation (eg, by fever or certain drugs). BrS is associated with a predisposition to ventricular arrhythmias (VAs) and sudden cardiac death (SCD), most often in otherwise healthy and young adults. The first disease expression is usually at the age of 30 to 50 years, although first expression can be during childhood, but many patients will remain asymptomatic throughout their life.

Over the last decades, the criteria to diagnose BrS were changed several times following consensus meetings.[5–7] For example, currently, only a spontaneous type 1 (coved type, **Fig. 1**) Brugada ECG pattern is diagnostic for BrS, whereas formerly a non-spontaneous type 1 Brugada ECG pattern (eg, drug-induced) was by itself considered diagnostic as well.[7] A spontaneous type 1 Brugada ECG pattern has an estimated global prevalence of 0.05%,[8] although there is large variation by geographical location, race, and sex. BrS is much

[a] Department of Clinical Cardiology, Amsterdam UMC, Location University of Amsterdam, Amsterdam Cardiovascular Sciences, Heart Failure & Arrhythmias, Meibergdreef 9, Amsterdam, the Netherlands; [b] Department of Experimental Cardiology, Amsterdam UMC, Location University of Amsterdam, Amsterdam Cardiovascular Sciences, Heart Failure & Arrhythmias, Meibergdreef 9, Amsterdam, the Netherlands
* Corresponding author. Department of Clinical Cardiology, Amsterdam UMC, Location University of Amsterdam, Meibergdreef 9, 1105 AZ, Amsterdam, The Netherlands.
E-mail address: p.g.postema@amsterdamumc.nl

Card Electrophysiol Clin 15 (2023) 273–283
https://doi.org/10.1016/j.ccep.2023.05.002
1877-9182/23/© 2023 Elsevier Inc. All rights reserved.

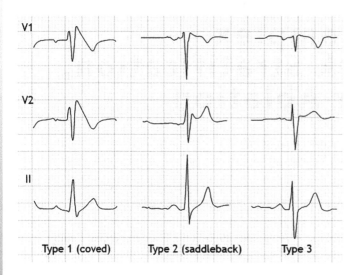

V1

V2

II

Type 1 (coved)   Type 2 (saddleback)   Type 3

Fig. 1. The three Brugada ECG patterns. As described in the most recent expert consensus,[7] a type 1 Brugada ECG pattern is characterized by a J-point elevation and a coved ST segment of ≥2 mm with a subsequent T-wave inversion in ≥ 1 of the right precordial leads. A type 2 Brugada ECG pattern is characterized by a J-point elevation of ≥0.5 mm (usually ≥2 mm in V2) with a "saddleback"-shaped ST segment elevation and positive T wave in ≥ 1 of the right precordial leads. A type 3 Brugada ECG pattern is characterized by a coved or saddleback-shaped ST segment elevation of 1 mm.

more common in Southeast Asia (prevalence 0.37%) than in North America (prevalence 0.005%), as systematically reviewed.[9] BrS is nine times more common in Asians than in Caucasians[9] and 80% of all patients are male.[10] The actual prevalence of BrS is hard to estimate but may be higher as patients can remain asymptomatic their entire life. However, current stricter diagnostic criteria promote less lenient BrS diagnoses.[7]

The most severe symptoms of BrS are VAs and SCD. To date, the most efficient protection against SCD in BrS patients often seems to be the implantation of an implantable cardioverter-defibrillator (ICD) in high-risk patients.[4,11] In low-to-intermediate risk patients, however, inappropriate shocks and complications with risk of fatal outcomes due to ICD implantation outbalance the risks of SCD without an ICD.[12] This underlines the need for refined risk stratification, which is indeed challenging and subject of debate, and management alternatives in the prevention of SCD. Here, the authors review the latest insights on BrS with a focus on its complex genetic architecture, its challenging risk stratification, and recent advances in its management.

GENETICS

Rare genetic variants in the SCN5A gene, which encodes for the α-subunit of the cardiac sodium channel (Na$_v$1.5), were first reported as a cause of BrS in 1998.[13] BrS causing genetic variants in SCN5A result in "loss-of-function" of the channel (ie, less sodium current).[13,14] At first, BrS was thought to follow a relatively simple Mendelian autosomal dominant inheritance, caused by rare large-effect pathogenic variants. However, research conducted

in the past two decades has markedly improved our understanding of the underlying genetic architecture, pointing toward a more complex inheritance pattern.

Several lines of evidence support complex inheritance in BrS. First, when a pathogenic variant in SCN5A is found in a family, only a small proportion of family members with the familial disease-causing variant show clinical signs of the disease (reduced penetrance).[15] Second, pathogenic variants in SCN5A often result in highly variable disease expressivity (eg, in symptom occurrence and/or in symptom severity), even in related individuals carrying the same pathogenic variant. For example, one individual may have a spontaneous type 1 Brugada ECG pattern, whereas others with the same variant only show a type 1 ECG pattern after sodium channel blocker (SCB) provocation. In addition, many cases of BrS are often sporadic, and familial clustering is not often observed. Last, in affected families, a phenotype-genotype mismatch has been described,[16] with genotype-negative–phenotype-positive individuals, which also challenges the concept of a relatively simple, monogenic inheritance pattern.

Besides the fact that pathogenic variants in SCN5A were demonstrated to have a highly variable disease expressivity, pathogenic variants in SCN5A have also been associated with different clinical phenotypes and overlap syndromes.[17] For example, variants in SCN5A have also been linked to long QT syndrome type 3 (LQT3—albeit that this phenotype requires a "gain-of-function" of the altered sodium channel protein), dilated cardiomyopathy, atrial arrhythmias, and/or combination of these phenotypes (**Fig. 2**B).[18] The feature

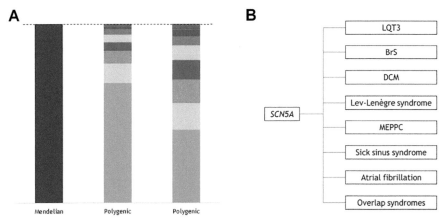

Fig. 2. (*A*) The genetic susceptibility may be composed of multiple susceptibility variants, resulting in polygenic inheritance. In Mendelian disorders, a large-effect genetic variant (dark grey bar) by itself allows the disease threshold to be reached (*dashed line*). In complex inheritance, the disease threshold is presumed to be reached by the aggregate effect of multiple susceptibility variants that have a spectrum of frequency and effect size, ranging from low-frequency variants of moderate to large effect to common variants of small effect. (*B*) Pleiotropy (ie, pathogenic variants in one gene may cause different clinical phenotypes) in *SCN5A*. LQT3, long QT syndrome type 3; DCM, dilated cardiomyopathy; MEPPC, multifocal ectopic Purkinje-related premature contractions.

that variants in one gene may cause different clinical phenotypes is called pleiotropy. This contributes to the assumption that pathogenic variants in one gene do not merely cause one disease, and diseases are not merely caused by one gene.[19]

Candidate gene studies conducted before 2018 proposed 20 additional genes as being associated with BrS. However, the causative role of genetic variants in all of these genes has been disputed, with *SCN5A* remaining as the only gene robustly associated with the disorder.[20] Pathogenic variants in *SCN5A* are only found in ±20% of familial BrS cases.[21] As mentioned above, a more complex inheritance pattern is now assumed, wherein multiple variants likely contribute to disease susceptibility (ie, polygenic inheritance pattern, **Fig. 2**A). The genetic architecture of BrS thus may consist of, for instance, one rare variant and multiple common variants, or in another scenario, multiple common variants. These common variants are frequently seen in the overall population and usually have small effects, in contrast to rare variants which usually have larger effects.[22]

In a genome-wide association study (GWAS) conducted by Bezzina and colleagues[23] on 312 cases and 1115 controls, common variants at two loci (*SCN10A* and near *HEY2*) were associated with BrS. In a subsequent replication, SNPs in *SCN5A* have also been associated with BrS. Although these common variants may not be causative by themselves, the three loci in aggregate were demonstrated to significantly increase disease susceptibility. Variants in the *SCN5A-SCN10A* loci were earlier known to affect cardiac

conduction, whereas the associated variants in *HEY2*, which encodes for a transcription factor, implicated a role of a cardiac transcription factor in the pathophysiology of BrS. Importantly, this GWAS showed that GWAS can associate common variants with rare diseases, which were formerly assumed to be Mendelian.

In subsequent studies, the role of genetic variants in aggregate, in the form of polygenic risk scores (PRSs), was evaluated.[24–26] In such studies, patient-specific PRSs are derived by counting the number of risk variants carried at each locus associated in GWAS, each weighted by their effect size, as was first described for BrS by Tadros and colleagues.[25] In this study composed of 1368 patients, it was demonstrated that a PRS based on the three BrS-associated common SNPs known at the time[23] was an independent risk factor for the development of an SCB-induced type 1 Brugada ECG pattern. This study can be considered a first step in evaluating whether such PRS may have a role in the management of patients with the disorder. In a more recent genome-wide association meta-analysis in 2820 patients with BrS, 12 genetic loci harboring 21 independent SNPs were associated with BrS[26] (**Fig. 3**A), thereby identifying multiple novel loci. The subsequently derived patient-specific PRS for BrS, based on the 21 associating SNPs, was significantly higher in patients with a spontaneous type 1 ECG (**Fig. 3**C), although it was not significantly higher in patients who suffered a life-threatening arrhythmic event. The PRS was higher in patients who did not carry a known (likely) pathogenic variant in *SCN5A* as compared with patients who did (**Fig. 3**B), indicating a higher burden

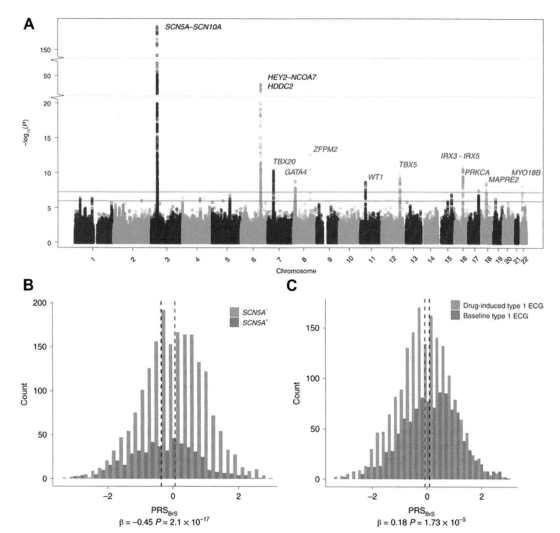

Fig. 3. The results from a GWAS and subsequently derived PRS for BrS, in this case from a recent genome-wide association meta-analysis by Barc and colleagues.[26] (*A*) A Manhattan plot with the closest genes at 12 loci, of which those displayed in red were newly associated. (*B*) Histograms of PRS for BrS distribution demonstrating a significantly lower mean PRS in *SCN5A*-positive compared with *SCN5A*-negative patients. (*C*) Histograms of PRS for BrS distribution demonstrating a significantly higher mean PRS in patients with a spontaneous type 1 Brugada ECG pattern compared with patients with a drug-induced type 1 Brugada ECG pattern. (*Adapted from* Barc J, Tadros R, Glinge C, et al. Genome-wide association analyses identify new Brugada syndrome risk loci and highlight a new mechanism of sodium channel regulation in disease susceptibility. Nat Genet. Mar 2022;54(3):232–239; with permission.)

of BrS-associated common variants in *SCN5A* negative patients. Progress deciphering genetic variants contributing to susceptibility to BrS may thus have a role in the development of our understanding of BrS and its complex inheritance pattern.

Currently, single-gene testing for *SCN5A* is recommended as indicated in the most recent expert consensus on genetic testing for cardiac diseases.[27] Briefly, in index patients besides testing for (likely) pathogenic variants in *SCN5A*, testing for other genes should not be routinely performed.

Subsequently, family members are recommended to be genetically tested in instances where a pathogenic *SCN5A* variant has been identified. For the family members of other patients, that is, those without a pathogenic (or probably pathogenic) *SCN5A* variant, clinical evaluations (SCB provocation testing) are proposed. It is very critical however that the clinical diagnosis of the index patient is correct. Moreover, like genetic testing, SCB provocation testing certainly does not provide 100% sensitivity and specificity, which may result in more difficult diagnostic and treatment dilemmas.

PATHOPHYSIOLOGY

The underlying pathophysiological mechanism is still not completely understood. Since its first description as a distinct clinical entity, there have been two major hypotheses, that is, the repolarization and depolarization theories.[28]

At first, the repolarization theory, based on studies conducted in canine cardiac wedges, was described by Yan and colleagues.[29] In the canine model, differences in I_{TO} (transient outward potassium current) expression and thus in action potential in the different cardiac layers were observed and presumed to be the underlying arrhythmogenic mechanism. After blocking sodium or calcium currents, a prominent notch and a loss of the dome were observed in the action potential in the epicardial layer of the right ventricle (RV), which were not seen in the endocardial layer. Thereby, a transmural dispersion of the action potential in the RV would result in repolarization heterogeneity, ST segment elevation, and consequently in phase 2 reentrant arrhythmia initiating extrasystoles.

Conversely, several years later the depolarization theory was introduced.[30] The depolarization theory centers on a reduced sodium current (predominantly $Na_v1.5$) and hence a conduction delay in the RV and right ventricular outflow tract (RVOT; thus, the distinctive Brugada ECG pattern is observed in the right precordial leads). In this theory, the typical Brugada ECG pattern is a consequence of the conduction delay in the RV. The RVOT remains negative for a relatively long period compared with the RV, causing an electrical current toward the RVOT. During repolarization, this is the other way around. This discontinuous depolarization causes depolarization mismatch border zones where VAs can arise. The depolarization theory is supported by observed minor structural alterations in the RVOT.[31,32] This includes strain abnormalities on echocardiogram,[33] late gadolinium enhancement on cardiac MRI,[34] fibrosis and fibrofatty depositions in histological studies, and the observation of a substrate of late potentials and fragmented electrograms near the RVOT,[35] the clinical relevance of which is underscored by the promising effects of catheter ablation of this substrate (see below). Because of the more evident structural abnormalities, which may be more evident due to advances in cardiac imaging, it has even been theorized that BrS may be categorized with structural heart diseases in the future.[36]

Both hypotheses, that is, the repolarization and depolarization theories, are well supported[28] and may even coexist. On the contrary, there are solid arguments against both separate hypotheses.[37] As recently proposed elsewhere, perhaps the umbrella term for the pathophysiological mechanisms underlying BrS should be an impaired conduction reserve of the RVOT.[37]

DIAGNOSIS

As mentioned before, the criteria to diagnose BrS have not remained the same over the years. Formerly, BrS was diagnosed in patients presenting with either a spontaneous type 1 Brugada ECG pattern or a non-spontaneous type 1 Brugada ECG pattern, that is, only after intravenous provocation testing with SCBs (eg, ajmaline, flecainide, procainamide).[38] In patients presenting with a less characteristic type 2 or 3 Brugada ECG pattern, BrS was diagnosed when this pattern converted to a type 1 Brugada ECG pattern. However, the expert Task Force of 2016 urged for awareness about possibly overdiagnosing BrS,[7] particularly in asymptomatic patients with a type 1 Brugada ECG pattern only after SCB provocation testing. SCB provocation testing presumably has a high sensitivity,[39] which can even be increased by placing precordial leads higher than V1–V3, at the third or second intercostal space.[40] Yet, SCB provocation testing may have a lower than expected specificity.[41–43] Besides, SCB provocation testing results in a type 1 Brugada ECG pattern more frequently in patients with AV nodal reentry tachycardia[44] or an accessory pathway[45] compared with controls. These individuals who may be coincidentally "uncovered" as being affected by BrS are probably at very low risk of arrhythmic events.[46] Still, as the clinical notion of BrS was developed in an era with expanding usage of ICDs,[47] a possible consequence of being labeled as a BrS patient is the apparent urge to promote ICD implantations. To avoid overdiagnosis and presumed unnecessary (and potentially life-threatening) treatment, a scoring system has been proposed to diagnose BrS, the Shanghai scoring system (**Table 1**).[7] In addition to a non-spontaneous type 1 Brugada ECG pattern, patients should have, for instance, a history of aborted SCD, documented VAs or arrhythmic syncope to make BrS diagnosis probable/definite. Importantly, diseases that mimic BrS (phenocopies) should be excluded before diagnosing BrS.[4]

RISK STRATIFICATION

Foremost in BrS management is the patient-specific decision whether a patient is at risk of having arrhythmic events, that is, (polymorphic— rarely monomorphic) ventricular tachycardia (VT) or ventricular fibrillation (VF) and possibly a subsequent cardiac arrest, and thus whether ICD implantation is warranted.

Table 1
Shanghai score system as proposed in the most recent expert consensus[7]

	Points
I. ECG (12-Lead/Ambulatory)**[a]	
A. Spontaneous type 1 Brugada ECG pattern at nominal or high leads	3.5
B. Fever-induced type 1 Brugada ECG pattern at nominal or high leads	3
C. Type 2 or 3 Brugada ECG pattern that converts with provocative drug challenge	2
**One item from this category must apply.	
II. Clinical History[a]	
A. Unexplained cardiac arrest or documented VF/polymorphic VT	3
B. Nocturnal agonal respirations	2
C. Suspected arrhythmic syncope	2
D. Syncope of unclear mechanism/ unclear etiology	1
E. Atrial flutter/fibrillation in patients <30 years without alternative etiology	0.5
III. Family History[a]	
A. First- or second-degree relative with definite BrS	2
B. Suspicious SCD (fever, nocturnal, Brugada aggravating drugs) in a first- or second-degree relative	1
C. Unexplained SCD <45 years in first- or second-degree relative with negative autopsy	0.5
IV. Genetic Test Result	
A. Probable pathogenic mutation in BrS susceptibility gene	0.5
Score (requires at least one ECG finding)	
= 3.5 points: Probable/definite BrS	
2–3 points: Possible BrS	
<2 points: Nondiagnostic	

[a] Only award points once for highest score within this category.

Adapted from Antzelevitch C, Yan G-X, Ackerman MJ, et al. J-Wave syndromes expert consensus conference report: Emerging concepts and gaps in knowledge. Heart Rhythm. 2016/10/01/ 2016;13(10):e295-e324.

In BrS patients at high risk for VAs, that is, those who suffered an aborted SCD or those in whom a sustained VA was previously documented, the evidence is undisputed and an ICD is recommended.[4,11] Patients who are at low risk for VAs, the asymptomatic patients with a Brugada ECG pattern only after SCB provocation, an ICD is not recommended. These asymptomatic patients have an annual arrhythmic event rate of ≤0.5%[46]—which is lower than the severe complication rate of, for example, ICDs. However, particularly in the patients who are at intermediate risk for VAs, risk stratification remains challenging. This group consists mostly of patients with a Shanghai score of 4 to 6.5[48,49] (see **Table 1**). The predictive value of previous clinical presentation (particularly arrhythmic syncope) and the presence of a spontaneous type 1 Brugada ECG pattern, early repolarization ECG pattern, or fragmented QRS complex is generally suggested but not thoroughly tested.[4,50] In a search for strong predictors, it seemed that also the value of programmed electrical stimulation (PES) is not undisputed. Large registries show conflicting results on the predictive value of the inducibility of VAs during PES.[46,51] Besides, the predictive value of PES is hard to assess. An ICD is usually implanted when PES is positive, and because an ICD may register more arrhythmias than would become clinically evident in patients without an ICD, the predictive value is easily overestimated.

In this complicated matter, multiple risk scores have been proposed.[50,52] The Shanghai scoring system has, next to a diagnosis scoring system, also been proposed as a risk score, albeit not by the original authors.[48] Both the Sieira and Shanghai risk scores seem capable of predicting arrhythmic events in patients at low and high risk for arrhythmic events. However, both scores have a moderate area under the curve (AUC Shanghai score 0.73 [0.67–0.79] and AUC Sieira 0.71 [0.61–0.81]), which even decreases when specifically looking at patients at intermediate risks.[53] Of note, including PES in the risk score did not result in a higher predictive accuracy. Another BrS risk score consisting of four variables,[50] that is, a spontaneous type 1 Brugada ECG pattern, probable arrhythmic syncope and a type 1 Brugada ECG pattern and early repolarization in the peripheral leads, may seem promising. This score is developed in a large cohort of 1110 patients but is yet to be externally validated.

In conclusion, currently, there is a large population in whom it is still not yet clear whether they may benefit from an ICD. Studies in larger populations and preferably with a longer follow-up are necessitated to develop risk scores with an improved predictive value. Besides, in the future, other factors may help in risk stratification in this intermediate risk population, including PRS (see "Genetics").

MANAGEMENT

Management considerations in BrS highly depend on risk stratification. In patients at low risk for VAs, where the benefits of protection from SCD by an ICD do not outweigh the risks of an ICD (ie, inappropriate shocks and other potentially severe complications), lifestyle advices are recommended.[4,11] These are composed of measures aiming to avoid developing the type 1 Brugada ECG pattern (and thus VAs and SCD) and include the following. Patients should avoid certain drugs (eg, antiarrhythmic and psychotropic drugs) and anesthetic agents (see www.BrugadaDrugs.org for an up-to-date overview[54]) and are advised against excessive use of alcohol and use of cannabis or cocaine. Fever should be adequately suppressed by antipyretics, and whenever this is unsuccessful, admission may be considered for rhythm monitoring.

In patients at higher risk for VAs, an ICD is recommended,[4,11] whereas in patients at intermediate risk (see "Risk stratification"), an ICD should be considered. Because BrS is generally diagnosed at a relatively young age, a subcutaneous ICD (S-ICD) may be worthwhile.[55] Thus, lead-related complications could be prevented in this relatively active patient population. However, the S-ICD may have sensing issues in patients with dynamic ECGs such as a type 1 Brugada ECG pattern,[56] so patients should be carefully selected. For this selection, screening after exercise testing and SCB provocation testing have recently been proposed,[57] although this needs to be confirmed in clinical studies.

For patients with (recurrent) appropriate ICD shocks, quinidine should certainly be considered. Quinidine is a class 1a anti-arrhythmic drug and works as an outward transient potassium current (I_{TO}) inhibitor which can rescue the decreased depolarization reserve in BrS patients.[58] In the previous century, quinidine was commonly used in the prevention of atrial and VAs. In 2004, it was first reported as possibly effective in the treatment of arrhythmic events secondary to BrS,[59] where other studies followed.[60,61] The QUIDAM study,[62] a randomized double-blind study with 18-month cross-over phases, showed no appropriate shocks in patients who were on quinidine. However, only one appropriate shock was seen in the control group. Although its efficacy results seem promising, quinidine also has a high rate of side effects (incidence 17–58%[59,60,62]). The most reported side effects are gastrointestinal. In the QUIDAM study, side effects led to discontinuation of treatment in 26% of cases.[62] Therefore, the optimal dose should always be determined in accordance with patients' wishes. A lower dose may decrease side effects,[63] but a long-term appreciably sized study of its efficacy at lower doses is currently lacking. Of note, quinidine is unfortunately not (easily) accessible in every country, with all the consequences thereof.[64,65]

Although quinidine was formerly also mentioned in the guidelines to treat BrS patients with electrical storm (class I[11] to IIa[66] recommendation), in the latest ESC guidelines this role is exclusively for isoproterenol (class IIa).[4] This notwithstanding quinidine still has a major role in the treatment of BrS.[67]

CATHETER ABLATION

In therapy-refractory patients, that is, patients with an ICD implanted and recurrent appropriate shocks despite the maximum tolerated quinidine dose (or when quinidine is inaccessible), catheter ablation for BrS may have an important role in the future. Although the first reports on catheter ablation for premature ventricular complexes in BrS are from 2003,[68] considerable progress has been made only more recently over the past decade. Nademanee and colleagues[69] were the first to demonstrate that the epicardial ablation of the arrhythmic substrate located near the RVOT, and anterior right ventricular wall could result in the abolishment of the type 1 Brugada ECG pattern and the prevention of VA recurrences. The arrhythmic substrate was characterized by a typical electrogram pattern, consisting of a low voltage delayed and prolonged ventricular duration with fragmentation near the RVOT and anterior right ventricular wall. This electrogram pattern may be caused by epicardial fibrosis, which is also seen in postmortem and in vivo (during epicardial ablation for BrS) samples from BrS cases.[32] Both epicardial and interstitial fibrosis were seen in the RVOT as well as reduced gap junction expression on the location where abnormal potentials were recorded.

The largest study on catheter ablation for BrS to date is the prospective BRUGADA_I trial published by Pappone and colleagues.[70] In this study, 135 patients were included of whom 72 patients were less symptomatic (ie, no documented arrhythmia during symptoms) or asymptomatic, although VAs were inducible. Only 27 patients had recurrent VAs and ICD shocks. With epi-endocardial mapping, substrate augmentation by ajmaline provocation, and subsequent epicardial radiofrequency ablation, the Brugada ECG pattern abolishment was achieved and maintained in 98.5% (n = 133) for a median follow-up of 10 months. Moreover, no VA recurrences were registered in 98.5% during follow-up. However, median follow-up was only 10 months. Because patients are usually relatively young at the time of diagnosis, the results of a longer term follow-up are necessary. Besides, a large proportion of this study was less symptomatic or asymptomatic and consequently not at high risk for VAs (see "Risk stratification"). Therefore, it is conceivable that the baseline risk of VA occurrence in these patients was already very low.[71] Although not reported in this study, epicardial ablation may come with complications[72] not worth its presumed benefits in less symptomatic and low-risk BrS patients. So it is too early to consider catheter ablation in other patients than therapy-refractory patients, not to speak of considering it as an ICD competitor.

Besides, to declare catheter ablation an ICD competitor may be premature without randomized trials to confirm these results. A first step to this question is the Brugada Syndrome Ablation for the prevention of VF Episodes study (www.ClinicalTrials.gov NCT02704416),[73] a randomized controlled trial with only an ICD in one arm and an epicardial ablation for BrS with an ICD in the other. Hopefully, in the coming years, the role of catheter ablation for BrS will become clearer, whether it remains a last resort in therapy-refractory patients or becomes a worthy alternative to an ICD.

SUMMARY

BrS is an inherited primary arrhythmia syndrome with a distinctive ECG pattern and a predisposition to SCD in otherwise healthy individuals. Although BrS is considered to have a genetic component, there are still many gaps of knowledge about its complex genetic architecture and underlying pathophysiological mechanisms. In the last decade, progress in the understanding of its genetic architecture has been made, which resulted in the hypothesis that its inheritance pattern is polygenic, with more variants yet to be discovered. PRS derived from newly identified variants may in turn help in our understanding of the genetic architecture and pathophysiological mechanism of BrS, and thereby possibly in risk stratification. A very challenging issue is risk stratification indeed as it is still imperfect, especially for patients at intermediate risk for arrhythmic events, necessitating larger studies with a longer follow-up. However, advances in BrS management are encouraging. ICD complication rates may, for example, be reduced by advances in ICD technology. In patients with or without ICD, VA occurrence or recurrence may be effectively prevented with quinidine. Last, the promising results of catheter ablation for BrS certainly promote enthusiasm but should

currently only be exploited in (severely) symptomatic patients.

CLINICS CARE POINTS

- The routine assessment for genetic variants other than those located in *SCN5A* is currently not recommended.
- As Brugada syndrome (BrS) risk stratification remains challenging and the predictive value of programmed electrical stimulation is disputed, one should carefully consider whether implantable cardioverter-defibrillator (ICD) implantation is warranted.
- ICD type should be carefully selected, because not all BrS patients seem suited for subcutaneous ICD implantation.
- Quinidine can be prescribed in BrS patients with a presumed higher risk of arrhythmic events, and isoproterenol can be used in case of an electrical storm.
- Catheter ablation, although promising, remains only recommended as a treatment modality in severely symptomatic BrS patients.

DISCLOSURE

Dr P.G. Postema is supported by the Dutch Heart Foundation, Netherlands grant 03-003-2021-T061. Drs A.A.M. Wilde and C.R. Bezzina are supported by the Dutch Heart Foundation grant 2018-30 PREDICT2 project. Dr C.R. Bezzina acknowledges the support of the EJP-RD project LQTS-NEXT (ZonMW 40–46300–98–19009).

REFERENCES

1. Osher HL, Wolff L. Electrocardiographic pattern simulating acute myocardial injury. Am J Med Sci 1953;226(5):541–5.
2. Martini B, Nava A, Thiene G, et al. Ventricular fibrillation without apparent heart disease: description of six cases. Am Heart J 1989;118(6):1203–9.
3. Brugada P, Brugada J. Right bundle branch block, persistent ST segment elevation and sudden cardiac death: a distinct clinical and electrocardiographic syndrome. A multicenter report. J Am Coll Cardiol 1992;20(6):1391–6.
4. Zeppenfeld K, Tfelt-Hansen J, de Riva M, et al. 2022 ESC Guidelines for the management of patients with ventricular arrhythmias and the prevention of sudden cardiac death: Developed by the task force for the management of patients with ventricular arrhythmias and the prevention of sudden cardiac

death of the European Society of Cardiology (ESC) Endorsed by the Association for European Pediatric and Congenital Cardiology (AEPC). Eur Heart J 2022;43(40):3997–4126.

5. Wilde AA, Antzelevitch C, Borggrefe M, et al. Proposed diagnostic criteria for the Brugada syndrome: consensus report. Circulation 2002;106(19):2514–9.

6. Antzelevitch C, Brugada P, Borggrefe M, et al. Brugada syndrome: report of the second consensus conference: endorsed by the heart rhythm society and the European heart rhythm association. Circulation 2005;111(5):659–70.

7. Antzelevitch C, Yan G-X, Ackerman MJ, et al. J-Wave syndromes expert consensus conference report: emerging concepts and gaps in knowledge. Heart Rhythm 2016;13(10):e295–324.

8. Postema PG. About Brugada syndrome and its prevalence. EP Europace 2012;14(7):925–8.

9. Vutthikraivit W, Rattanawong P, Putthapiban P, et al. Worldwide prevalence of brugada syndrome: a systematic review and meta-analysis. Acta Cardiol Sin 2018;34(3):267–77.

10. Eckardt L. Gender differences in Brugada syndrome. J Cardiovasc Electrophysiol 2007;18(4):422–4.

11. Al-Khatib SM, Stevenson WG, Ackerman MJ, et al. 2017 AHA/ACC/HRS guideline for management of patients with ventricular arrhythmias and the prevention of sudden cardiac death: executive summary: a report of the american college of cardiology/American heart association task force on clinical practice guidelines and the heart rhythm society. Circulation 2018;138(13):e210–71.

12. Sacher F, Probst V, Maury P, et al. Outcome after implantation of a cardioverter-defibrillator in patients with brugada syndrome. Circulation 2013;128(16):1739–47.

13. Chen Q, Kirsch GE, Zhang D, et al. Genetic basis and molecular mechanism for idiopathic ventricular fibrillation. Nature 1998;392(6673):293–6.

14. Rook MB, Bezzina Alshinawi C, Groenewegen WA, et al. Human SCN5A gene mutations alter cardiac sodium channel kinetics and are associated with the Brugada syndrome. Cardiovasc Res 1999;44(3):507–17.

15. Priori SG, Napolitano C, Gasparini M, et al. Clinical and genetic heterogeneity of right bundle branch block and ST-segment elevation syndrome. Circulation 2000;102(20):2509–15.

16. Probst V, Wilde AA, Barc J, et al. SCN5A mutations and the role of genetic background in the pathophysiology of Brugada syndrome. Circ Cardiovasc Genet 2009;2(6):552–7.

17. Remme CA, Wilde AAM, Bezzina CR. Cardiac sodium channel overlap syndromes: different faces of SCN5A mutations. Trends Cardiovasc Med 2008;18(3):78–87.

18. Wilde AAM, Amin AS. Clinical spectrum of SCN5A mutations: long QT Syndrome, Brugada syndrome,

and cardiomyopathy. JACC Clin Electrophysiol 2018;4(5):569–79.

19. Cerrone M, Remme CA, Tadros R, et al. Beyond the one gene–one disease paradigm. Circulation 2019;140(7):595–610.

20. Hosseini SM, Kim R, Udupa S, et al. Reappraisal of reported genes for sudden arrhythmic death. Circulation 2018;138(12):1195–205.

21. Kapplinger JD, Tester DJ, Alders M, et al. An international compendium of mutations in the SCN5A-encoded cardiac sodium channel in patients referred for Brugada syndrome genetic testing. Heart Rhythm 2010;7(1):33–46.

22. Gibson G. Rare and common variants: twenty arguments. Nat Rev Genet 2012;13(2):135–45.

23. Bezzina CR, Barc J, Mizusawa Y, et al. Common variants at SCN5A-SCN10A and HEY2 are associated with Brugada syndrome, a rare disease with high risk of sudden cardiac death. Nat Genet 2013;45(9):1044–9.

24. Juang J-MJ, Liu Y-B, Chen C-YJ, et al. Validation and disease risk assessment of previously reported genome-wide genetic variants associated with brugada syndrome. Circulation: Genomic and Precision Medicine 2020;13(4):e002797.

25. Tadros R, Tan HL, Investigators E-N, et al. Predicting cardiac electrical response to sodium-channel blockade and Brugada syndrome using polygenic risk scores. Eur Heart J 2019;40(37):3097–107.

26. Barc J, Tadros R, Glinge C, et al. Genome-wide association analyses identify new Brugada syndrome risk loci and highlight a new mechanism of sodium channel regulation in disease susceptibility. Nat Genet 2022;54(3):232–9.

27. Wilde AAM, Semsarian C, Márquez MF, et al. European heart rhythm association (EHRA)/Heart rhythm society (HRS)/Asia pacific heart rhythm society (APHRS)/Latin American heart rhythm society (LAHRS) expert consensus statement on the state of genetic testing for cardiac diseases. Heart Rhythm 2022;19(7):e1–60.

28. Wilde AA, Postema PG, Di Diego JM, et al. The pathophysiological mechanism underlying Brugada syndrome: depolarization versus repolarization. J Mol Cell Cardiol 2010;49(4):543–53.

29. Yan G-X, Antzelevitch C. Cellular basis for the brugada syndrome and other mechanisms of arrhythmogenesis associated with ST-segment elevation. Circulation 1999;100(15):1660–6.

30. Meregalli PG, Wilde AAM, Tan HL. Pathophysiological mechanisms of Brugada syndrome: depolarization disorder, repolarization disorder, or more? Cardiovasc Res 2005;67(3):367–78.

31. Hoogendijk MG, Opthof T, Postema PG, et al. The brugada ECG pattern. Circulation: Arrhythmia and Electrophysiology 2010;3(3):283–90.

32. Nademanee K, Raju H, de Noronha SV, et al. Fibrosis, connexin-43, and conduction abnormalities

in the brugada syndrome. J Am Coll Cardiol 2015; 66(18):1976–86.

33. Iacoviello M, Forleo C, Puzzovivo A, et al. Altered two-dimensional strain measures of the right ventricle in patients with Brugada syndrome and arrhythmogenic right ventricular dysplasia/cardiomyopathy. Eur J Echocardiogr 2011;12(10): 773–81.

34. Bastiaenen R, Cox AT, Castelletti S, et al. Late gadolinium enhancement in Brugada syndrome: a marker for subtle underlying cardiomyopathy? Heart Rhythm 2017/04/01/2017;14(4):583–9.

35. Ohkubo K, Watanabe I, Okumura Y, et al. Right ventricular histological substrate and conduction delay in patients with brugada syndrome. Int Heart J 2010;51(1):17–23.

36. Boukens BJ, Potse M, Coronel R. Fibrosis and conduction abnormalities as basis for overlap of brugada syndrome and early repolarization syndrome. Int J Mol Sci 2021;22(4):1570.

37. Behr ER, Ben-Haim Y, Ackerman MJ, et al. Brugada syndrome and reduced right ventricular outflow tract conduction reserve: a final common pathway? Eur Heart J 2021;42(11):1073–81.

38. Priori SG, Wilde AA, Horie M, et al. HRS/EHRA/APHRS Expert consensus statement on the diagnosis and management of patients with inherited primary arrhythmia syndromes: Document endorsed by HRS, EHRA, and APHRS in May 2013 and by ACCF, AHA, PACES, and AEPC in June 2013.. Heart Rhythm 2013;10(12):1932–63.

39. Brugada R, Brugada J, Antzelevitch C, et al. Sodium channel blockers identify risk for sudden death in patients with ST-segment elevation and right bundle branch block but structurally normal hearts. Circulation 2000;101(5):510–5.

40. Govindan M, Batchvarov VN, Raju H, et al. Utility of high and standard right precordial leads during ajmaline testing for the diagnosis of Brugada syndrome. Heart 2010;96(23):1904–8.

41. Viskin S, Rosso R, Friedensohn L, et al. Everybody has Brugada syndrome until proven otherwise? Heart Rhythm 2015;12(7):1595–8.

42. Tadros R, Nannenberg EA, Lieve KV, et al. Yield and pitfalls of ajmaline testing in the evaluation of unexplained cardiac arrest and sudden unexplained death: single-center experience with 482 families. JACC (J Am Coll Cardiol): Clinical Electrophysiology 2017;3(12):1400–8.

43. Viskin S, Rosso R. Read my lips: a positive ajmaline test does not always mean you have brugada syndrome. JACC (J Am Coll Cardiol): Clinical Electrophysiology 2017;3(12):1409–11.

44. Hasdemir C, Payzin S, Kocabas U, et al. High prevalence of concealed Brugada syndrome in patients with atrioventricular nodal reentrant tachycardia. Heart Rhythm 2015;12(7):1584–94.

45. Hasdemir C, Juang JJ, Kose S, et al. Coexistence of atrioventricular accessory pathways and drug-induced type 1 Brugada pattern. Pacing Clin Electrophysiol 2018;41(9):1078–92.

46. Probst V, Veltmann C, Eckardt L, et al. Long-term prognosis of patients diagnosed with brugada syndrome. Circulation 2010;121(5):635–43.

47. Havakuk O, Viskin S. A tale of 2 diseases: the history of long-QT syndrome and brugada syndrome. J Am Coll Cardiol 2016;67(1):100–8.

48. Kawada S, Morita H, Antzelevitch C, et al. Shanghai Score system for diagnosis of brugada syndrome: validation of the score system and system and reclassification of the patients. JACC (J Am Coll Cardiol): Clinical Electrophysiology 2018; 4(6):724–30.

49. Delise P. Risk stratification in Brugada syndrome: the challenge of the grey zone. Eur Heart J 2021;42(17): 1696–7.

50. Honarbakhsh S, Providencia R, Garcia-Hernandez J, et al. A primary prevention clinical risk score model for patients with brugada syndrome (BRUGADA-RISK). JACC Clin Electrophysiol 2021;7(2):210–22.

51. Sieira J, Ciconte G, Conte G, et al. Long-term prognosis of drug-induced Brugada syndrome. Heart Rhythm 2017;14(10):1427–33.

52. Sieira J, Conte G, Ciconte G, et al. A score model to predict risk of events in patients with Brugada Syndrome. Eur Heart J 2017;38(22):1756–63.

53. Probst V, Goronflot T, Anys S, et al. Robustness and relevance of predictive score in sudden cardiac death for patients with Brugada syndrome. Eur Heart J 2021;42(17):1687–95.

54. Postema PG, Wolpert C, Amin AS, et al. Drugs and brugada syndrome patients: review of the literature, recommendations, and an up-to-date website. Heart Rhythm 2009;6(9):1335–41. Available at: www.brugadadrugs.org.

55. Lambiase PD, Eckardt L, Theuns DA, et al. Evaluation of subcutaneous implantable cardioverter-defibrillator performance in patients with ion channelopathies from the EFFORTLESS cohort and comparison with a meta-analysis of transvenous ICD outcomes. Heart Rhythm O2 2020;1(5):326–35.

56. Nordkamp LRAO, Conte G, Rosenmöller BRAM, et al. Brugada syndrome and the subcutaneous implantable cardioverter-defibrillator. J Am Coll Cardiol 2016;68(6):665–6.

57. Dendramis G, Brugada P. Lights and shadows of subcutaneous implantable cardioverter-defibrillator in Brugada syndrome. Heart Rhythm 2022. https://doi.org/10.1016/j.hrthm.2022.09.016.

58. Hoogendijk MG, Potse M, Vinet A, et al. ST segment elevation by current-to-load mismatch: an experimental and computational study. Heart Rhythm 2011;8(1):111–8.

59. Belhassen B, Glick A, Viskin S. Efficacy of quinidine in high-risk patients with brugada syndrome. Circulation 2004;110(13):1731–7. https://doi.org/10.1161/01.CIR.0000143159.30585.90.

60. Anguera I, García-Alberola A, Dallaglio P, et al. Shock reduction with long-term quinidine in patients with brugada syndrome and malignant ventricular arrhythmia episodes. J Am Coll Cardiol 2016; 67(13):1653–4.

61. Belhassen B, Rahkovich M, Michowitz Y, et al. Management of brugada syndrome. Circulation: Arrhythmia and Electrophysiology 2015;8(6): 1393–402.

62. Andorin A, Gourraud J-B, Mansourati J, et al. The QUIDAM study: hydroquinidine therapy for the management of Brugada syndrome patients at high arrhythmic risk. Heart Rhythm 2017;14(8):1147–54.

63. Mazzanti A, Tenuta E, Marino M, et al. Efficacy and limitations of quinidine in patients with brugada syndrome. Circulation: Arrhythmia and Electrophysiology 2019;12(5):e007143.

64. Viskin S, Antzelevitch C, Márquez MF, et al. Quinidine: a valuable medication joins the list of 'endangered species'. EP Europace 2007;9(12):1105–6.

65. Viskin S, Wilde AAM, Guevara-Valdivia ME, et al. Quinidine, a life-saving medication for brugada syndrome, is inaccessible in many countries. J Am Coll Cardiol 2013;61(23):2383–7.

66. Priori SG, Blomström-Lundqvist C, Mazzanti A, et al. 2015 ESC guidelines for the management of patients with ventricular arrhythmias and the prevention of sudden cardiac death: the task force for the management of patients with ventricular arrhythmias and the prevention of sudden cardiac death of the European society of cardiology (ESC)endorsed by: association for European paediatric and congenital cardiology (AEPC). Eur Heart J 2015;36(41): 2793–867.

67. Belhassen B, Rahkovich M, Michowitz Y, et al. Management of brugada syndrome: thirty-three-year experience using electrophysiologically guided therapy with class 1A antiarrhythmic drugs. Circ Arrhythm Electrophysiol 2015;8(6):1393–402.

68. Haïssaguerre M, Extramiana F, Hocini M, et al. Mapping and ablation of ventricular fibrillation associated with long-QT and brugada syndromes. Circulation 2003;108(8):925–8.

69. Nademanee K, Veerakul G, Chandanamattha P, et al. Prevention of ventricular fibrillation episodes in Brugada syndrome by catheter ablation over the anterior right ventricular outflow tract epicardium. Circulation 2011;123(12):1270–9.

70. Pappone C, Brugada J, Vicedomini G, et al. Electrical substrate elimination in 135 consecutive patients with brugada syndrome. Circulation: Arrhythmia and Electrophysiology 2017;10(5):e005053.

71. Viskin S. Radiofrequency ablation of asymptomatic brugada syndrome. Circulation 2018;137(18): 1883–4.

72. Tung R, Michowitz Y, Yu R, et al. Epicardial ablation of ventricular tachycardia: an institutional experience of safety and efficacy. Heart Rhythm 2013; 10(4):490–8.

73. Nademanee K. Ablation in Brugada Syndrome for the Prevention of VF (BRAVE). Updated April 22, 2022. Available at: https://clinicaltrials.gov/ct2/show/NCT02704416. Accessed December 5, 2022.

Personalized Care in Long QT Syndrome
Better Management, More Sports, and Fewer Devices

Ciorsti J. MacIntyre, MD[a],*, Michael J. Ackerman, MD, PhD[a,b,c]

KEYWORDS

- Long QT syndrome • Genetics • QT interval

KEY POINTS

- Appropriate diagnosis, risk stratification and initiation of an appropriate phenotype-tailored and genotype-guided treatment strategy are of paramount importance in the care of patients with Long QT Syndrome.
- Most patients with long QT syndrome do not need and should not receive an ICD.
- In addition to beta blocker therapy, adjunctive therapies such as mexiletine, left cardiac sympathetic denervation surgery, or atrial pacing should be considered in appropriately selected patients.

INTRODUCTION

Long QT Syndrome (LQTS) is an inherited cardiac channelopathy affecting approximately 1 in 2000 people.[1] LQTS is characterized by predominantly autosomal dominant inheritance. The hallmark electrocardiographic (ECG) feature is prolongation of the heart rate corrected QT interval (QTc); however, approximately 20% to 25% of patients with genotype-confirmed LQTS have QTc values within the normal range.[2,3] Clinical expressivity is similarly variable with some patients having concealed, asymptomatic disease with minimal to no LQTS expressivity, whereas others may have a malignant course with arrhythmia-mediated syncope/seizures, sudden cardiac arrest (SCA), or sudden cardiac death (SCD) secondary to torsades de pointes (TdP) and subsequent ventricular fibrillation. Appropriate diagnosis, risk stratification, and initiation of an appropriate phenotype-tailored and genotype-guided treatment strategy are therefore of paramount importance.

THE GENETICS

Type 1, type 2, and type 3 LQTS are the 3 most common subtypes accounting for approximately 80% to 90% of all cases of LQTS.

Type 1 Long QT Syndrome

Type 1 long QT syndrome (LQT1) is the most common subtype accounting for 30% to 40% of LQTS.[4] It is caused by loss-of-function mutations in the *KCNQ1* gene. The classic ECG appearance includes a delayed T-wave upstroke, which creates a broad-based T wave. *KCNQ1* encodes the alpha-subunit of the potassium channel Kv7.1, which is responsible for generating I_{Ks}. I_{Ks}, along with I_{Kr}, underlie phase 3 of repolarization in ventricular myocytes. Within LQT1, there is now intragenic risk stratification, as mutations localizing to the transmembrane spanning domains are associated with higher clinical risk of LQT1-triggered cardiac events than those mutations localizing to the

[a] Department of Cardiovascular Medicine, Division of Heart Rhythm Services, Windland Smith Rice Genetic Heart Rhythm Clinic, Mayo Clinic, Rochester, MN, USA; [b] Department of Pediatric and Adolescent Medicine, Division of Pediatric Cardiology, Mayo Clinic, Rochester, MN, USA; [c] Department of Molecular Pharmacology & Experimental Therapeutics, Windland Smith Rice Sudden Death Genomics Laboratory, Mayo Clinic, Rochester, MN, USA
* Corresponding author.
E-mail address: macintyre.ciorsti@mayo.edu

Card Electrophysiol Clin 15 (2023) 285–291
https://doi.org/10.1016/j.ccep.2023.04.007

C-terminus. In addition, those mutations that damage Kv7.1 the most (dominant-negative ones) are associated with greater clinical risk than those mutations that produce so-called channel haploinsufficiency.[5] Under normal circumstances, I_{Ks} increases with sympathetic activation, which in turn shortens repolarization duration. In LQT1, I_{Ks} is impaired, and as such, the QT fails to adapt to increasing heart rates.[6,7] This translates to a predilection for malignant arrhythmias particularly in higher adrenergic states. This underlies the association between LQTS-attributable events and exercise or emotional stress in the patient with LQT1, particularly when previously undiagnosed and therefore untreated.[8]

Type 2 Long QT Syndrome

Type 2 long QT syndrome (LQT2) is the second most common subtype accounting for approximately 25% to 35% of LQTS.[4] LQT2 is caused by loss-of-function mutations in the KCNH2 gene. The classic ECG appearance includes lower-amplitude T waves in the limb leads and characteristically notched or bifid T waves, particularly in the precordial leads V4 to V6.[9] KCNH2 encodes the pore-forming alpha-subunit of the cardiac voltage-gated potassium channel Kv11.1, which is responsible for conducting I_{Kr}, the rapidly activating delayed rectifier potassium current that contributes to phase 3 repolarization.[10,11] Mutations located in the pore loop region of Kv11.1 exhibit a significantly higher risk of arrhythmia.[12] In view of the fact that the I_{Ks} current is preserved in LQT2, patients with LQT2 are less likely to have events during exercise compared with LQT1. Most events in LQT2 occur during periods of emotional stress or in response to auditory stimuli (often during arousal from sleep). Women with LQT2 are more likely to have events during the postpartum period than LQT1 women.[8,13,14]

Type 3 Long QT Syndrome

Type 3 long QT syndrome (LQT3) is the third most common subtype accounting for approximately 5% to 10% of LQTS. LQT3 is caused by so-called gain-of-function mutations in the SCN5A gene. The classic ECG appearance includes a prolonged ST segment with a late onset of the T wave. SCN5A encodes the alpha-subunit of the cardiac Na^+ channel Nav 1.5, which is responsible for generating the inward sodium current (INa) that results in phase 0 depolarization of the cardiac action potential. In LQT3, Nav 1.5 fails to inactivate, thereby contributing a persistent depolarizing Na^+ current, which, in turn, prolongs repolarization and

action potential duration.[15] Ventricular arrhythmias are more likely to occur at rest or during sleep.

RISK PREDICTION

Risk stratification is an integral component of LQTS management. Multiple factors must be considered during the risk-stratification process.

Degree of QT Prolongation

Longer QTc intervals carry increased arrhythmic risk.[2,3] The risk of cardiac events increases with progressive QT prolongation, and the risk is greatest above a QTc of 500 milliseconds.[2] Although genotype-positive individuals with normal range QTc values have a 10-fold higher event rate than their unaffected family members, their absolute risk of an LQTS-triggered cardiac event is very low.[3]

Sex

Independent of the QTc value on their resting, baseline ECG, boys with LQT1 are at increased risk of a first cardiac event during childhood, whereas women are at increased risk from puberty onward.[16] The QTc shortens by approximately 20 milliseconds in men after puberty. This is not observed in women. This likely reflects the inhibitory effect of estrogen on I_{Kr} current corresponding to the elevated event rates seen in LQT2 women after puberty, postpartum, and perimenopause.[17]

Genotype

LQT1 is associated with relatively shorter QTc values, a lower cumulative cardiac event rate, and lower incidence of SCA and SCD compared with LQT2 and LQT3.[2]

Age

Symptomatic infants typically manifest severe QT prolongation and have a significantly higher cumulative event rate later in life.[18] Cardiac events do continue to occur even in those above 40 years of age.[19]

Syncope

Recurrent arrhythmic syncope, particularly if recent (within the past 2 years), is associated with an increased risk of breakthrough cardiac events on therapy, including cardiac arrest.[16]

MANAGEMENT
Preventative Measures

Avoidance of QT prolonging medications
Nearly all medications that prolong the QTc block Kv11.1 channels, impairing I_{Kr} current and prolonging

action potential duration.[20] Although beta blockers provide excellent protection against arrhythmia, avoidance of QT prolonging medications remains of paramount importance. Among patients with LQTS treated with beta blockers, the 2 main causes of breakthrough cardiac events are beta blocker noncompliance and the use of a QT prolonging medication.[21] Indeed, the surest way to convert a low-risk patient with LQTS with a previously incompletely penetrant phenotype into a high-risk patient is with prescription of a QT prolonging medication. It is important to educate the patient with LQTS about resources, such as www.crediblemeds.org/ as a safety net to ensure that QT prolonging medications are not inadvertently prescribed. Importantly, a patient with LQTS should only be prescribed a medication on the QT drugs-to-avoid list with the explicit awareness and approval of his/her LQTS specialist.

Fever prevention strategies
Under normal circumstances, fever increases I_{Kr} current, thereby shortening repolarization. Patients with LQT2 are unable to increase I_{Kr}, which leads to an increase in QTc duration and, in turn, an increased risk for ventricular arrhythmias.[22] Fever-induced T-wave alternans has also been described in a patient with LQT1.[6] As such, it is prudent to advise fever prevention strategies at times of illness.

Avoidance/correction of electrolyte abnormalities
Extracellular potassium concentration can alter the QT duration in patients with and without LQTS. Hypokalemia can also potentiate QT prolongation in the context of fever. As such, it is important to advise attention to electrolyte status particularly at times where electrolytes may be disturbed, such as in the context of vomiting or diarrheal illness. There is conflicting evidence regarding the role of potassium supplementation in LQTS; however, there are some data to suggest that potassium supplementation corrects abnormal repolarization and improves the ECG in LQTS. There is likely a role for maintaining potassium levels at the upper limit of normal in certain high-risk patients with LQT2 through either supplementation of potassium or administration of spironolactone.[23–25]

Medications

Beta blockers
International guidelines advise universal beta-blocker therapy as either a class I recommendation for patients with prior symptoms or QTc values ≥470 milliseconds or as a class II recommendation for asymptomatic patients with QTc values less than 470 milliseconds.[26] Beta blockers remain the cornerstone of LQTS management and significantly reduce the likelihood of life-threatening cardiac events compared with untreated patients.[27]

Beta blockers work best in LQT1 in which abnormal I_{Ks} channel function makes patients more sensitive to catecholamines. Beta blockers reduce the rate of life-threatening cardiac events by 97% in patients with LQTS followed for more than 10 years. Beta-blocker nonadherence is a significant concern, as this represents the single most common root cause of "breakthrough" cardiac events.[21] Beta blockers are also first-line therapy in LQT2; however, there is a higher incidence of cardiac events (lethal and nonlethal) compared with LQT1. As such, in highly selected high-risk patients, intensification beyond beta-blocker monotherapy should be considered.[28] Previously, there was a misconception that beta blockers were harmful in patients with LQT3 on the basis of exacerbation of bradycardia and proarrhythmia. Ultimately, it was ascertained that beta blockers do indeed reduce cardiac events in LQT3 and are not associated with a signal for harm.[29]

Although beta blockers are fundamental to LQTS management, it should be noted that not all beta blockers are created equal. Nadolol and propranolol represent the preferred beta blockers for LQTS management. Although propranolol has more QTc shortening effect than nadolol and metoprolol, both nadolol and propranolol are equally effective in symptomatic patients with LQTS in reducing the likelihood of breakthrough cardiac events. In contrast, metoprolol is associated with a higher breakthrough cardiac event rate and should be avoided.[30] In general, nadolol is the beta blocker of choice for LQT1 and LQT2, whereas propranolol (because of its concomitant late sodium current blocking properties) is often preferred in LQT3.

Mexiletine
Although most patients are treated with a beta blocker in general and nadolol or propranolol in particular, genotype-specific pharmacologic treatments have emerged. Mexiletine first emerged as an effective treatment in combination with beta blockers in SCN5A-mediated LQT3 based on the observation that mexiletine significantly shortened the QTc among patients with LQT3.[31–33] This shortening of the QTc translated to the observation that there was also a major reduction in life-threatening arrhythmic events among patients with LQT3, making mexiletine an effective therapeutic strategy in high-risk patients.[34] In addition, mexiletine also reduces the QTc in a subset of

patients with potassium channel–mediated LQT2, suggesting that pharmacologic targeting of the physiologic late sodium current may provide added therapeutic efficacy to beta-blocker therapy alone in patients with LQT2 as well.[35]

Intentional nontherapy

There is growing recognition of patients who may be genotype positive but who have mild to no LQTS expressivity. As awareness for cascade family screening grows and as genetic testing becomes more widely available, there is a growing cohort of patients with concealed and asymptomatic disease coming to medical attention. Intentional nontherapy represents the least-aggressive treatment strategy in LQTS management. In this strategy, only the preventative measures of QT drug avoidance, fever prevention strategies, and correction of electrolyte disturbance are advised; however, after a thorough risk assessment, a decision is made between the patient and the genetic cardiologist not to pursue beta-blocker therapy, left cardiac sympathetic denervation (LCSD), or device implantation. This has been described as "intentional nontherapy." This strategy can be considered in very-low-risk patients after thorough assessment. The typical profile of this very-low-risk patient population includes asymptomatic, postpubertal men with normal resting QTc.[36]

Procedures

Left cardiac sympathetic denervation surgery

Videoscopic LCSD surgery is a minimally invasive therapy that effectively reduces the risk of ventricular arrhythmias in patients with LQTS, especially LQT1. There is a class I recommendation for LCSD as treatment intensification in patients with LQTS and breakthrough cardiac events on effective LQTS-directed pharmacotherapy or in patients in whom beta-blocker therapy is poorly tolerated as a means for possible dose reduction.[37–39] In highly selected patients intolerant of beta-blocker therapy, there may also be a role for LCSD as stand-alone therapy, although not yet endorsed by guidelines.[40] Patient selection is of critical importance if LCSD monotherapy is considered.[41]

Intentional permanent atrial pacing

In high-risk patients with LQTS, pacing effectively attenuates the QTc, prevents pause-dependent triggering of TdP, and decreases the breakthrough cardiac event rate. This effect was most marked in patients with recalcitrant LQT2 in which the reduction in average QTc and breakthrough event rate was greatest.[42] Typically, the lower rate limit for atrial pacing needs to be 80 to 90 beats per minute

to provide meaningful therapeutic efficacy. Algorithms that aim to minimize ventricular pacing by allowing pauses should be turned off to prevent pause-dependent triggering of TdP.

Implantable cardioverter defibrillators

Although there is general consensus about the implantation of an implantable cardioverter-defibrillator (ICD) following a resuscitated SCA in the patient with LQTS as secondary prevention,[37] there remains controversy about the indications for ICD implantation as primary prevention of SCD.

Although ICDs represent an important component of LQTS management in high-risk, highly selected patients, ICD therapy is not without risk. ICD implantation is associated with complications, including infection, lead fracture, lead dislodgment, device malfunction, and inappropriate shocks. There is also a potential psychological impact, including increased anxiety, depression, and even posttraumatic stress disorder. As such, avoiding both overdiagnosis of LQTS and overtreatment of LQTS is of utmost importance.

ICD implantation carries a significant risk of inappropriate shocks and device-related complications, particularly in young patients with LQTS. The ICD is also not generally an appropriate substitute for an appropriately tailored treatment program. Overall, among the leading LQTS destination centers throughout the world, approximately 10% to 20% of their patients are treated with a strategy that includes an ICD. In other words, most patients with LQTS do not need and should not receive an ICD.

Lifestyle Factors

To bench or not to bench?

Genotype-specific triggers have been well described in LQTS. For example, exercise in general and swimming in particular are known triggers in LQT1, again particularly in the previously undiagnosed and therefore untreated patient. There is no question that the sudden death of a young person, especially an athlete, is both shocking and devastating. The association between LQTS, sudden death, and exercise has previously led some of the major cardiology societies to recommend disqualification from essentially all competitive sports. In 2012, Mayo Clinic introduced the concept of return to play and shared decision making for athletes with LQTS after demonstrating for the first time that after correct diagnosis, risk stratification, and tailoring of therapy, LQTS-triggered events are very low, and lethality remains zero for more than 500 athletes with LQTS over the past 20 years.[43–46] Disqualification is not a benign intervention. For the athlete for whom sport participation is as "necessary as oxygen," disqualification can have a profoundly devastating impact. It is well established that regular aerobic activity is essential for health maintenance, obesity prevention, and overall cardiovascular health.[47] In addition to impacts on physical health, there are significant potential impacts to psychological health and well-being. Compared with their nonathlete peers, adolescent athletes score higher in mental, emotional, and social functioning.[48] Combining the favorable effects of exercise on mental and physical well-being with the low event rate in well-treated patients, complete disqualification from all aerobic activity should be discouraged. Instead, a patient-focused approach should be embraced inclusive of careful risk stratification and institution of appropriate LQTS-directed treatment strategies as part of a shared decision-making process that respects patient autonomy.

SUMMARY

The thoughtful management of patients with complex genetic heart disease, such as LQTS, requires a thorough understanding of the underlying disease substrate, the nuanced application of both phenotype and genotype in the personalized tailoring of their LQTS-directed treatment program. Comprehensive patient care also requires thoughtful consideration of the individual patient. Our mission is to not just formulate an appropriate LQTS-directed treatment strategy with evidence-based therapies but to give equal consideration to patient priorities and values so as to ensure that excellent quality care also leads to an excellent quality of life.

CLINICS CARE POINTS

- The care of patients with LQTS requires the nuanced application of both phenotype and genotype to tailor an appropriate treatment program.

REFERENCES

1. Schwartz PJ, Stramba-Badiale M, Crotti L, et al. Prevalence of the congenital long-QT syndrome. Circulation 2009;120:1761–7.
2. Priori SG, Schwartz PJ, Napolitano C, et al. Risk stratification in the long-QT syndrome. N Engl J Med 2003;348:1866–74.
3. Goldenberg I, Horr S, Moss AJ, et al. Risk for life-threatening cardiac events in patients with genotype-confirmed long-QT syndrome and normal range corrected QT intervals. J Am Coll Cardiol 2011;57:51–9.
4. Schwartz PJ, Crotti L, Insolia R. Long QT syndrome: from genetics to management. Circ Arrhythm Electrophysiol 2012;5:868–77.
5. Barshshet A, Goldenberg I, O-Uchi J, et al. Mutations in cytoplasmic loops of the KCNQ1 channel and the risk of life-threatening events: implications for mutation-specific response to beta-blocker therapy in type 1 long-QT syndrome. Circulation 2012;125:1988–96.
6. Moss AJ, Shimizu W, Wilde AA, et al. Clinical aspects of type-1 long-QT syndrome by location, coding type, and biophysical function of mutations involving the KCNQ1 gene. Circulation 2007;115(19):2481–9.
7. Etheridge SP, Asaki SY, Niu Mary CI. A personalized approach to long QT syndrome. Current Opinions in Cardiology 2019;34(1):46–2489.
8. Schwartz PJ, Priori SG, Spazzolini C, et al. Genotype-phenotype correlation in the long-QT syndrome: gene-specific triggers for life-threatening arrhythmias. Circulation 2001;103:89–95.
9. Moss AJ, Zareba W, Benhorin J, et al. ECG T-wave patterns in genetically distinct forms of the hereditary long QT syndrome. Circulation 1995;92:2929–34.
10. Trudeau MC, Warmke JW, Ganetzky B, et al. A human inward rectifier in the voltage-gated potassium channel family. Science 1995;269:92–5.
11. Sanguinetti MC, Jiang C, Curran ME, et al. A mechanistic link between an inherited and an acquired cardiac arrhythmia: HERG encodes the IKr potassium channel. Cell 1995;81:299–307.
12. Moss AJ, Zareba W, Kaufman ES, et al. Increased risk of arrhythmic events in long-QT syndrome with mutations in the pore region of the human ether-a-go-go-related gene potassium channel. Circulation 2022;105:794–9.
13. Wilde AA, Jongbloed RJ, Doevendans PA, et al. Auditory stimuli as a trigger for arrhythmic events differentiate HERG-related (LQTS2) patients from KvLQT1-related patients (LQTS1). J Am Coll Cardiol 1999;33:327–32.
14. Khositseth A, Tester DJ, Will ML, et al. Identification of a common genetic substrate underlying postpartum cardiac events in congenital long QT syndrome. Heart Rhythm 2004;1:60–4.
15. Amin AS, Pinto YM, Wilde AA. Long QT syndrome: beyond the causal mutation. J Physiol 2013;591:4125–39.
16. Goldenberg I, Moss AJ, Peterson DR, et al. Risk factors for aborted cardiac arrest and sudden cardiac death in children with the congenital long-QT syndrome. Circulation 2008;117:2184–91.

17. Abrams DJ, MacRae CA. Long QT syndrome. Circulation 2014;129:1524–9.
18. Spazzolini C, Mullally J, Moss AJ, et al. Clinical implications for patients with long QT syndrome who experience a cardiac event during infancy. J Am Coll Cardiol 2009;54:832–7.
19. Goldenberg I, Moss AJ, Bradley J, et al. Long-QT syndrome after age 40. Circulation 2009;117(17):2192–201.
20. Kannankeril P, Roden DM, Darbar D. Drug-induced long QT syndrome. Pharmacol Rev 2010;62:760–81.
21. Vincent GM, Schwartz PJ, Denjoy I, et al. High efficacy of beta-blockers in long-QT syndrome type 1: contribution of noncompliance and QT-prolonging drugs to the occurrence of beta-blocker treatment "failures. Circulation 2009;119:215–21.
22. Amin AS, Klemens CA, Verker AO, et al. Fever-triggered ventricular arrhythmias in Brugada syndrome and type 2 long-QT syndrome. Neth Heart J 2010;18:165–9.
23. Compton SJ, Lux RL, Ramsey MR, et al. Genetically defined therapy of inherited long-QT syndrome. Correction of abnormal repolarization by potassium. Circulation 1996;94:1018–22.
24. Etheridge SP, Compton SJ, Tristani-Firouzi M, et al. A new oral therapy for long QT syndrome: long-term oral potassium improves repolarization in patients with HERG mutations. J Am Coll Cardiolo 2003;42:1777–82.
25. Marstrand P, Almatlouh K, Kanters JK, et al. Effect of moderate potassium-elevating treatment in long QT syndrome: the TriQarr Potassium Study. Open Heart 2021;8(2):e001670.
26. Priori SG, Wilde AA, Horie M, et al. HRS/EHRA/APHRS expert consensus statement on the diagnosis and management of patients with inherited primary arrhythmia syndromes: document endorsed by HRS, EHRA, and APHRS in May 2013 and by ACCF, AHA, PACES and AEPC in June 2013. Heart Rhythm 2013;10:1932–63.
27. Moss AJ, Schwartz PJ, Crampton RS, et al. The long QT syndrome: a prospective international study. Circulation 1985;71:17–21.
28. Priori SG, Napolitano C, Schwartz PJ, et al. Association of long QT syndrome loci and cardiac events among patients treated with beta-blockers. JAMA 2004;292:1341–4.
29. Wilde AA, Moss AJ, Kaufman Es, et al. Clinical aspects of type 3 long-QT syndrome: an international multicenter study. Circulation 2016;134:872–82.
30. Chockalingam P, Crotti L, Girardengo G, et al. Not all beta-blockers are equal in the management of long QT syndrome types 1 and 2: higher recurrence of events under metoprolol. J Am Coll Cardiol 2012;60(20):2092–9.
31. Schwartz PJ, Priori SG, Locati EH, et al. Long QT syndrome patients with mutations of the SCN5A and HERG genes have differential responses to Na+ channel blockade and to increases in heart rate. Implications for gene-specific therapy. Circulation 1995;92:3381–6.
32. Priori SG, Napolitano C, Cantù F, et al. Differential response to Na+ channel blockade, beta-adrenergic stimulation, and rapid pacing in a cellular model mimicking the SCN5A and HERG defects present in the long-QT syndrome. Circ Res 1996;78:1009–15.
33. Blaufox AD, Tristani-Firouzi M, Seslar S, et al. Congenital long QT 3 in the pediatric population. Am J Cardiol 2012;109:1459–65.
34. Mazzanti A, Maragna R, Faragli A, et al. Gene-specific therapy with mexiletine reduces arrhythmic events in patients with long QT syndrome type 3. J Am Coll Cardiol 2016;67:1053–8.
35. Bos JM, Crotti L, Rohatgi RK, et al. Mexiletine shortens the QT interval in patients with potassium channel mediated type 2 long qt syndrome. Circulation: Arrhythmia and Electrophysiology 2019;12:e007280.
36. MacIntyre CJ, Rohatgi RK, Sugrue AM, et al. Intentional nontherapy in long QT syndrome. Heart Rhythm 2020;17:1147–50.
37. Al-Khatib SM, Stevenson WG, Ackerman MJ, et al. 2017 AHA/ACC/HRS guideline for management of patients with ventricular arrhythmias and the prevention of sudden cardiac death: a report of the American College of Cardiology/American Heart Association Task Force on clinical Practice guidelines and the Heart Rhythm Society. Circulation 2018;138:e272–391.
38. Schwartz PJ, Priori SG, Cerrone M, et al. Left cardiac sympathetic denervation in the management of high-risk patients affected by the long-QT syndrome. Circulation 2004;109:1826–33.
39. Collura CA, Johnson JN, Moir C, et al. Left cardiac sympathetic denervation for the treatment of long QT syndrome and catecholaminergic polymorphic ventricular tachycardia using video-assisted thoracic surgery. Heart Rhythm 2009;6:752–9.
40. Schwartz PJ, Ackerman MJ. Cardiac sympathetic denervation in the prevention of genetically mediated life-threatening ventricular arrhythmias. Eur Heart J 2022;43(22):2096–102 [Erratum in: Eur Heart J. 2022 Jul 08;: PMID: 35301528; PMCID: PMC9459868].
41. Niaz T, Bos JM, Sorensen KB, et al. Left cardiac sympathetic denervation monotherapy in patients with congenital long qt syndrome. Circulation: Arrhythmia and Electrophysiology 2020;13(12):e0008830.
42. Kowlgi G, Giudicessi JR, Barake W, et al. Efficacy of intentional permanent atrial pacing in the long-term management of congenital long QT syndrome. J Cardiovasc Electrophysiol 2021;32(3):782–9.
43. Johnson JN, Ackerman MJ. Competitive sports participation in athletes with congenital long QT syndrome. JAMA 2012;308(8):764–5.

44. Johnson JN, Ackerman MJ. Return to play? Athletes with congenital long QT syndrome. Br J Sports Med 2013;47(1):28–33.

45. Turkowski KL, Bos JM, Ackerman NC, et al. Return-to-Play for athletes with genetic heart diseases. Circulation 2018;137(10):1086–8.

46. Tolbert KE, Bos MJ, Garmany R, et al. Return-to-Play for athletes with long QT syndrome or genetic heart diseases Predisposing to sudden death. J Am Coll Cardiol 2021;78(6):594–605.

47. Kim BY, Choi DH, Jung CH, et al. Obesity and physical activity. J Obes Metab Syndr 2017;26:15–22.

48. Snyder AR, Martinez JC, Bay RC, et al. Health-related quality of life differs between adolescent athletes and adolescent nonathletes. J Sport Rehabil 2010;19:237–48.

Catecholaminergic Polymorphic Ventricular Tachycardia
A Review of Therapeutic Strategies

Auke T. Bergeman, MD[a,b], Arthur A.M. Wilde, MD, PhD[a,b],
Christian van der Werf, MD, PhD[a,b],*

KEYWORDS

- Catecholaminergic polymorphic ventricular tachycardia • Sudden cardiac death
- Therapeutic management • β-blockers • Flecainide • *RYR2*-specific compounds

KEY POINTS

- Therapeutic management choices in catecholaminergic polymorphic ventricular tachycardia (CPVT) have expanded in recent years and should be individualized.
- Nonselective β-blockers remain the foundation of treatment in CPVT, with flecainide and left cardiac sympathetic denervation (LCSD) being effective additions.
- The role of the ICD in CPVT is controversial, and new evidence suggesting a lack of mortality benefit should prompt clinicians to critically review the ICD indication.
- *RYR2*-specific compounds are a promising new modality for CPVT but clinical efficacy still needs to be assessed.

INTRODUCTION

Catecholaminergic polymorphic ventricular tachycardia (CPVT) is a rare malignant inherited arrhythmia syndrome, characterized by bidirectional or polymorphic ventricular arrhythmia induced by exercise or emotion in individuals with structurally normal hearts and a normal resting electrocardiogram (ECG).[1] These arrhythmias are often asymptomatic but may cause syncope or sudden cardiac arrest (SCA). The true prevalence of CPVT remains unknown but is estimated to be 1:10.000.[2] Following isolated case reports,[3,4] it was first described as a clinical syndrome in 1995.[5] At present, 7 genes (*RYR2*, *CASQ2*, *TRDN*, *TECRL*, *CALM1-3*) have been associated with CPVT, all of which encode proteins that are directly or indirectly involved in intracellular calcium homeostasis in cardiomyocytes.[6] The pathophysiological mechanism of CPVT involves inappropriate β-adrenergic receptor-mediated diastolic calcium release from the sarcoplasmic reticulum into the cytosol because of "leaky" cardiac ryanodine receptor (RyR2) channels, leading to delayed afterdepolarizations and triggered activity.[7] Despite tremendous advances in our understanding of the disease during the past decades, numerous uncertainties regarding therapeutic management persist and new questions continue to emerge. Additionally, there is a need to develop new therapies because some patients remain symptomatic despite all available options and existing therapies are associated with significant side effects. In this review, we summarize the current state of knowledge on therapeutic management in CPVT, outline

[a] Department of Cardiology, Heart Centre, Amsterdam UMC Location Academic Medical Centre, University of Amsterdam, Meibergdreef 9, Amsterdam, the Netherlands; [b] Amsterdam Cardiovascular Sciences, Heart Failure and Arrhythmias, Amsterdam, the Netherlands
* Corresponding author. Department of Cardiology, Heart Centre, Amsterdam UMC Location Academic Medical Centre, University of Amsterdam, Meibergdreef 9, Amsterdam, the Netherlands.
E-mail address: c.vanderwerf@amsterdamumc.nl

Card Electrophysiol Clin 15 (2023) 293–305
https://doi.org/10.1016/j.ccep.2023.04.002
1877-9182/23/© 2023 Elsevier Inc. All rights reserved.

our approach to treatment, and discuss new developments in chronic treatment options as well as future areas of research.

GENERAL TREATMENT CONSIDERATIONS

There is general agreement that symptomatic and phenotype-positive patients should receive intensive pharmacological treatment. Current guidelines recommend that treatment with β-blockers should also be considered in patients without clinical manifestations including a normal exercise stress test, such as genetically positive relatives identified through cascade screening.[8] In specific patients regarded as very-low risk, that is, asymptomatic patients who were identified through cascade screening and who have no or very limited ventricular ectopy, we and others use a strategy of active monitoring using repeated exercise stress tests without medication, in particular in very young children and middle age adults. However, there are limited data available about the predictors of arrhythmic events in CPVT, which makes identifying truly low-risk patients challenging. In genotype-positive, phenotype-negative relatives, sudden cardiac death is very rare.[9]

We primarily evaluate therapeutic efficacy using consecutive exercise stress tests. If this is not possible, for example in very young children, Holter monitoring may be used. There are limited data on the acceptable level of residual ventricular arrhythmia on exercise stress test. In one study, the presence of couplets or more severe ventricular arrhythmia was associated with arrhythmic events.[10] As a general rule, we consider frequent isolated or bigeminal premature ventricular contractions (PVCs) or more complex ventricular ectopy a reason to intensify treatment. Naturally, the occurrence of arrhythmic events is also a reason for uptitration. It is important to acknowledge that ventricular arrhythmia complexity may not be completely reproducible on exercise stress test even when repeated on the exact same treatment regimen.[11] Despite this limitation, the exercise stress test is the most suitable test for monitoring treatment adequacy in CPVT.[12] Burst exercise testing may more readily unveil a CPVT phenotype as compared with the Bruce protocol.[13] We typically schedule follow-up every 3 to 6 months for high-risk patients, and on an annual basis for all other patients.

LIFESTYLE MODIFICATIONS

Although the avoidance of epinephrine and related compounds is noncontroversial in CPVT, even in the setting of a SCA,[14] there is substantial uncertainty surrounding lifestyle modifications. The European Society of Cardiology (ESC) guidelines endorse a blanket recommendation to limit or avoid exercise, competitive sports, and stressful environments in all patients with CPVT, for both probands and asymptomatic genotype-positive relatives.[8] Although similarly strict overall, guidelines by the American Heart Association and American College of Cardiology also state that participation in (competitive) sports may be considered for asymptomatic, phenotype-negative patients under certain preconditions.[15] These recommendations are based on expert opinion, and the extent of benefit conferred has not been studied extensively. The degree to which exercise should be limited is not specified but we think it may be reasonable to limit the maximum permitted heart rate to the value at which ventricular arrhythmia starts to occur during exercise stress testing, as we do in our center.

The benefits of exercise on physical and mental health have been documented abundantly,[16] and some experts have questioned whether strict limitations are necessary in all patients with CPVT.[17,18] One small observational study found that among well-treated patients, the likelihood of arrhythmic events was equal in athletes and nonathletes.[18] Although the paucity of data on risk stratification in CPVT makes it difficult to identify low-risk patients in whom a more lenient approach might be justified, some risk factors have been identified.[19] Patients with concomitant neurodevelopmental disorders seem to be a high-risk subgroup with a malignant phenotype.[20] We think an approach involving discussion of risks, consideration of all aspects of a patient's presentation, and shared decision-making should be used to make individualized recommendations. In high-risk patients, we strongly advise patients who are not perceived as low-risk to only engage in swimming or other forms of exercise in the presence of others. Most importantly, more research is needed on the risk of exercise and outcomes associated with exercise restriction in CPVT.

PHARMACOLOGICAL THERAPY

Fig. 1 illustrates the cellular mechanisms of the discussed treatment strategies.

β-Blockers

The first reports of β-blocker efficacy emerged soon after recognition of the disease entity and the role of sympathetic activation in arrhythmogenesis.[8,19] Indeed, life-long use of β-blockers without intrinsic sympathomimetic activity in the highest tolerated dose is the undisputed

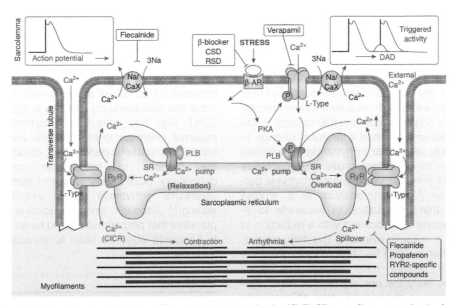

Fig. 1. The cellular mechanism of action of treatment strategies in CPVT. CSD, cardiac sympathetic denervation; DAD, delayed afterdepolarization; RSD, renal sympathetic denervation. (*Adapted from* Priori SG, Chen SR. Inherited dysfunction of sarcoplasmic reticulum Ca2+ handling and arrhythmogenesis. Circ Res. 2011;108(7):871-883; with permission.)

foundation of therapeutic management in those with a clinical diagnosis of CPVT,[8,19,21] and their use should be considered in genotype positive, phenotype negative patients.[8]

A number of studies attempted to evaluate which β-blocker type is most effective. The largest study by Peltenburg and colleagues,[22] being the result of a collaboration between the Pediatric & Congenital Electrophysiology Society (PACES) and the International CPVT Registry, studied a symptomatic pediatric CPVT population of 329 patients carrying *RYR2* variants. We found that β1-selective β-blockers were associated with a significantly higher risk of arrhythmic events than nonselective β-blockers (hazard ratio [HR] 2.04, $P = .002$). This difference was mostly driven by the efficacy of nadolol. Specifically, when comparing individual nonselective β-blockers, the risk of arrhythmic events was higher in patients treated with atenolol, bisoprolol, and metoprolol than in those treated with nadolol but this was not found for propranolol. Mazzanti and colleagues[23] studied the outcomes of a cohort of 216 *RYR2* variant-carrying patients with CPVT using β-blockers and found that the risk of arrhythmic events was higher in those taking β1-selective β-blockers as compared with nadolol (HR 5.8, $P = .001$). Here, there was no significant difference between propranolol and nadolol. A smaller prospective study used consecutive exercise stress tests before and after the initiation of β-blocker treatment and found that arrhythmia

severity was significantly lower during treatment with nadolol as compared with β1-selective β-blockers.[24] In conclusion, there is compelling evidence that nadolol is superior to its β1-selective counterparts, although the mechanism explaining this difference has not entirely been resolved. We and others think that in countries where nadolol is unavailable, such as in the Netherlands, another nonselective β-blocker (ie, propranolol) should be the preferred option.

Strict adherence to β-blockers is of crucial importance and should be emphasized to patients, as a substantial proportion of arrhythmic events occur due to nonadherence.[19,22,25] However, side-effects challenge medication adherence and limit the ability to reach an optimal dose. Additionally, profound bradycardia can limit β-blocker therapy, which may be compounded by the relative sinus bradycardia often seen in patients with a severe phenotype.[26]

Flecainide

Another well-established therapeutic option is flecainide, a class Ic antiarrhythmic drug that has been used for other indications for decades, and has seen its role expand to CPVT since 2009, when it was discovered that it potentially inhibits ryanodine-receptor mediated sarcoplasmic reticulum calcium release.[27] Since then, multiple clinical studies have demonstrated flecainide to be clinically effective. In an international collaborative study, we retrospectively studied the safety and efficacy of flecainide in a cohort of 33 CPVT patients from 8 academic centers and found that flecainide reduced the complexity of ventricular arrhythmia on exercise stress test in 76% of patients.[28] In the sole randomized controlled trial (RCT), which was initially designed with ventricular tachycardia (VT) or appropriate ICD therapy as the primary endpoint and had a protocol change to evaluate only ventricular arrhythmias on exercise testing due to enrollment challenges, flecainide reduced the severity of ventricular arrhythmia during exercise.[13] A meta-analysis of 8 studies confirmed that the addition of flecainide to β-blocker therapy is associated with a reduction of the risk of arrhythmic events.[29] The main mechanism of action in CPVT had been a topic of debate but recent studies have shown that RyR2 blockade is likely the primary mechanism.[30] Flecainide's sodium channel blocking efficacy may also play a role as is evident by the fact that flecainide also seems to be effective in genotype-negative CPVT.[31]

Flecainide is now the first-line additional therapeutic option on top of β-blockers, and should be added in the event of breakthrough arrhythmic events on β-blocker, or when significant ventricular arrhythmia persists on exercise testing.[8] In our view, however, initiation of both flecainide and a β-blocker simultaneously should be considered in patients presenting with SCA or a particularly severe phenotype. The recommended dosage of flecainide is 2 to 3 mg/kg/d. Although usually well tolerated, clinicians should be mindful of QRS complex prolongation during exercise and the associated potential proarrhythmia. At older age, patients should be informed about complaints compatible with ischemic heart disease as flecainide is contraindicated in this setting. The use of flecainide as monotherapy has been described in a small group of patients with moderately positive results[25,32] but is, in our experience, less effective than combination therapy with a β-blocker. Larger studies are necessary to corroborate the efficacy of flecainide in the absence of β-blockers.

Propafenone

Similar to flecainide, propafenone is a class Ic sodium channel blocking agent that also has minor β-adrenoceptor and calcium antagonist properties.[33] Unlike flecainide, propafenone is seldomly used in CPVT and has not been the focus of research efforts. Animal CPVT models have been used to establish that propafenone inhibits calcium waves caused by increased *RYR2*

activity.[34,35] Case reports noted one patient with recurring syncope in whom propafenone was started before CPVT was described as a disease entity. The patient, who was subsequently appreciated to have CPVT, continued this treatment for decades and remained asymptomatic.[36] Propafenone was also markedly effective in a patient with CPVT who had refractory arrhythmia despite maximal pharmacological therapy and bilateral cardiac sympathetic denervation, greatly reducing the number of implantable cardioverter-defibrillator (ICD) discharges and eliminating all ventricular arrhythmia during exercise stress testing.[34] Although limited evidence, it seems plausible that propafenone could be an alternative to flecainide when the latter is unavailable or not tolerated.

Verapamil

There is limited literature about the efficacy of non-dihydropyridine calcium channel blockers in patients with CPVT. The initial small studies were cautiously optimistic, showing that adding verapamil to β-blockers attenuated the severity and onset of ventricular arrhythmia on exercise stress testing in patients that remain symptomatic on β-blocker monotherapy.[37–39] However, longer term results showed that 3 out of 6 patients treated with the combination of verapamil and β-blocker experienced arrhythmic events during a mean follow-up of 37 months.[40] These studies are insufficient to come to any conclusions, and research into the efficacy of verapamil seems to have been largely abandoned. As a result, verapamil is scarcely used for CPVT in clinical practice,[19] and we do not prescribe it at our center. Considering the efficacy of other therapeutic options, it would arguably be unethical to perform a prospective trial on verapamil, and a larger retrospective study is infeasible owing to its minimal usage.

Ivabradine

Ivabradine inhibits the cardiac pacemaker or "funny" current (I_f), responsible for the automaticity observed in the sinoatrial node, thereby slowing the heart rate.[41] It is currently used for treatment of angina, heart failure with reduced ejection fraction, and inappropriate sinus tachycardia.[42] There have been some studies devoted to ivabradine in CPVT, some of which could be viewed as contradictory. Case reports describe clinically successful use of ivabradine in a patient with CPVT and ventricular arrhythmia refractory to the combination of nadolol, flecainide, and LCSD,[43] and in patients in whom nadolol and flecainide were not tolerated.[44] Bueno-Levy and colleagues studied the effects of ivabradine in human-induced pluripotent stem cell-derived cardiomyocytes and a transgenic mouse model, both carrying the homozygous CASQ2 p.D307H mutation.[45] They found that the administration of ivabradine reduced neither delayed afterdepolarizations in isolated cardiomyocytes nor delayed ventricular arrhythmias in their mouse model, leading the authors to conclude that ivabradine should not be used as treatment of CPVT. One may speculate that an explanation for this apparent discrepancy could be the difference in studied genotype, as the available case reports describe patients with *RYR2*-mediated CPVT. Nevertheless, it would be premature to come to conclusions from these data, and at present, the use of ivabradine in CPVT is not recommended.

Novel RYR2-Specific Compounds

Certain drugs exhibit ryanodine receptor-specific mechanisms of action, which, although most of these are currently preclinical, make them interesting as potential future therapeutic options in CPVT. At present, trials to evaluate the clinical effects of some of these compounds in CPVT are ongoing.

Dantrolene is one example of such a medication that is already available in clinical practice for other indications. Dantrolene is a hydantoin derivative that is used as a muscle relaxant to treat malignant hyperthermia, a disease related to mutations in skeletal muscle ryanodine receptors (*RYR1*) resulting in abnormal calcium release due to leaky *RYR1* channels.[46] It was later discovered that dantrolene can bind to *RYR2* as well but it seems to bind only in certain diseased conditions.[47] In vitro and mouse model studies have demonstrated that dantrolene attenuates abnormal calcium handling in *RYR2*-mutated cardiomyocytes.[48–50] Consequently, there is a basis to be cautiously optimistic but studies in human patients are warranted before dantrolene should be applied. However, hepatotoxicity is a major limitation to its chronic use, which, in contrast to malignant hyperthermia, would be required in CPVT, although it may have a role in the management of electrical storm. A dantrolene derivative that is more RyR2-selective might potentially be safer.[46]

Derivatives of tetracaine, another sodium channel blocker and RyR2 blocker, are a recently developed category of medications targeting leaky RyR2 channels. Of this group, EL9 and EL20 have shown encouraging results in the context of CPVT. EL9 was demonstrated to reduce spontaneous calcium sparks in cardiomyocytes isolated from RyR2-mutated mice without affecting heart rate, conduction velocity, or ventricular contractility.[51] Selective inhibition of RyR2 only when calmodulin is absent was shown to be the mechanism of EL20 in mice with CPVT1,[52] and normalization of calcium handling was observed in human-induced pluripotent stem cell-derived cardiomyocytes.[53]

Benzothiazepine derivatives are a group of compounds mostly in preclinical phase of development for CPVT. Using multiple animal models, it was found that K201 restored the calcium leak from RyR2 channels. This effect may be dependent on mutation location in RyR2 domains. S107, a derivative of K201, was similarly effective in mice models.[54] It remains to be determined whether any of these investigational compounds will prove useful and safe in human patients.

NONPHARMACOLOGICAL THERAPY
Cardiac Sympathetic Denervation

Left cardiac sympathetic denervation (LCSD) is a highly effective surgical treatment option in CPVT.[55–57] The procedure comprises thoracoscopic dissection of the stellate ganglion and a number of upper thoracic ganglia (usually T2 through T4).[58] Its fascinating, now more than a century-old history has been documented in detail elsewhere.[59] In 2008, Wilde and colleagues[55] reported highly successful use of LCSD in 3 patients with CPVT who remained symptomatic despite pharmacological therapy but became fully asymptomatic for years subsequently. In a larger series of 13 patients, all but 1 remained event-free after LCSD during median follow-up of 0.8 years.[56] The largest (multicenter) series on LCSD in CPVT, including 63 patients, was described in 2015 by De Ferrari and colleagues.[57] It was found that 79% had no arrhythmic events during the median post-LCSD follow-up of 37 months. The antiarrhythmic mechanism of LCSD entails limiting the release of norepinephrine in the ventricular myocardium during sympathetic neural activation, and increasing the ventricular fibrillation threshold.[60] Complications, including ptosis, Horner syndrome, harlequin flushing, pneumothorax, and neuropathic pain, are uncommon and often transient.[55,61] A distinct advantage of this procedure over pharmacological therapy is that its effects are permanent and not dependent on patient adherence.

Although there can be little doubt about the efficacy of LCSD, its place within the contemporary arsenal of therapeutic modalities in CPVT is subject of discussion. Accumulating reports of its efficacy have pushed LCSD ever further from being a "last resort option," as it once was. It is now uncontroversial that consideration of LCSD should come before an ICD.[57,61] Some experts have advocated instituting "triple therapy" (ie, nadolol, flecainide, and LCSD) in patients with a sentinel SCA before diagnosis.[61] However, it is our opinion that LCSD should follow after evidence of treatment failure on β-blocker and flecainide because many patients are well protected by this combination, unless an arrhythmic event occurs in the setting of nonadherence or the risk of nonadherence is considered to be significant.

Right-sided or bilateral cardiac sympathetic denervation is much more unconventional. Schwartz and Ackerman recently reported that only a fraction of their patients with an LCSD performed had undergone right cardiac sympathetic denervation (RCSD) as well,[61] which matches our experience. One reason for this is the effectiveness of LCSD, rendering an additional right-sided procedure unnecessary. Removal of the compensation of right-sided cardiac innervation after LCSD, causing a reduction in heart rate control and ventricular contractility, is a specific downside of bilateral cardiac sympathetic denervation.[60] For these reasons, we only consider RCSD after demonstration of insufficient protection by LCSD.

Renal Sympathetic Denervation

Primarily used for the management of hypertension, renal sympathetic denervation (RSD) is a percutaneous procedure in which renal artery nerves undergo catheter ablation, decreasing sympathetic nerve activity.[62] Given the involvement of the autonomic nervous system in the pathophysiological mechanism, there are theoretical grounds to conceptualize a possible beneficial role in CPVT. There have been a number of trials demonstrating a positive effect of RSD in ventricular arrhythmias caused by ischemic and nonischemic cardiomyopathies[63] but in CPVT, the experience is limited to a small number of case reports.[64,65] We have performed RSD in one of our patients, with moderate effect. Further research is needed to elucidate its risk and benefit in CPVT.

Implantable Cardioverter-Defibrillators

The ICD is considered to be the ultimate protection against sudden cardiac death in inherited cardiac arrhythmia syndromes but its role in patients with CPVT is controversial and studies have shown contrasting results. Recently, Mazzanti and colleagues performed a large cohort study of 216 patients with RYR2-mediated CPVT treated with β-blockers, of whom 79 received an ICD. They found that patients with an ICD had more life-threatening arrhythmic events but such events were more often lethal in those without an ICD

than in those with an ICD (4 of 10 vs 0 of 18, $P = .01$).[23] The authors concluded that the ICD is associated with mortality benefit. This article, however, contains some important limitations. First, the authors did not provide any information on the indications to insert an ICD and on the proportion of patients with appropriate ICD shocks who were adequately treated with nadolol. In addition, it is unclear why patients were not treated with flecainide and/or LCSD. Second, their endpoint of "life-threatening arrhythmic event" was a composite of sudden cardiac death, SCA, and hemodynamically nontolerated ventricular tachycardia. Bidirectional ventricular tachycardia is usually the only type of hemodynamically tolerable ventricular tachycardia that may occur in patients with CPVT, so presumably these events were not included in the study endpoint. However, the authors state that the "ICD successfully terminated the life-threatening arrhythmic event in 18 of 21 cases (86%). Overall, all 15 episodes of ventricular tachycardia were successfully interrupted, while only 3 of 6 episodes (50%) of hemodynamically unstable, polymorphic fast ventricular tachycardia were terminated." Therefore, it remains unclear if the 15 aforementioned ventricular tachycardia episodes concerned hemodynamically nontolerated bidirectional ventricular tachycardia or were in fact ventricular tachycardia episodes that did not meet their definition of the study endpoint.

In a global collaboration (the International CPVT Registry), we studied 136 patients with CPVT who presented with a sentinel SCA and found that the ICD was not associated with an improved survival.[66] Over the median follow-up of 4.8 years, 3 of the 79 patients with an ICD died suddenly, whereas none had died in the no-ICD group ($P = .1$). It should be noted that the no-ICD group received more nadolol/propranolol than the patients with an ICD, which may have been a confounding factor. Importantly, a significant proportion of patients with and without an ICD who experienced a nonfatal arrhythmic event during follow-up were not optimally treated. Thus, the arrhythmic event rates in patients presenting with SCA and treated with nadolol or propranolol, flecainide and/or LCSD remains unknown.

This conflicting evidence illustrates that the question of whether to implant an ICD in patients with CPVT is far from straightforward. Within the context of CPVT, ICD therapy has a number of specific drawbacks (**Fig. 2**). The first consideration is that the pain and fear caused by ICD shocks, whether appropriate or inappropriate, can provoke or exacerbate arrhythmia because of catecholamine surge, which may be lethal.[67,68] Second, inappropriate ICD shocks occur more often in CPVT than in other

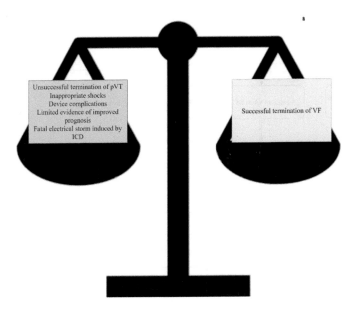

Unsuccessful termination of pVT
Inappropriate shocks
Device complications
Limited evidence of improved prognosis
Fatal electrical storm induced by ICD

Successful termination of VF

Fig. 2. Advantages and disadvantages of ICDs in patients with CPVT. ICD, implantable cardioverter-defibrillator; pVT, polymorphic ventricular tachycardia; VF, ventricular fibrillation.

inherited heart diseases due to frequent atrial tachyarrhythmias and nonsustained VT episodes.[69,70] In addition, shocks delivered for polymorphic VT and bidirectional VT are usually unsuccessful, although conversion success for ventricular fibrillation is extremely high.[70,71] Finally, patients with CPVT are often young at the time of ICD implantation and therefore more prone to complications during their lifetime. The rate of complications, not including inappropriate shocks, is substantial, at 17% to 32%.[66,67,71] Aggravating these concerns is the observation that many ICD recipients receive suboptimal medical treatment.[71]

These considerations have caused a shift in the once liberal attitude to ICD implantation in CPVT. Still, both the American Heart Association/American College of Cardiology/Heart Rhythm Society guidelines and the recently updated ESC guidelines conclude that it is premature to demote ICD implantation and maintain a class I indication for patients with aborted SCA.[8,72] However, we strongly believe an ICD should be considered as a last resort for the rare patient in whom the combination of nadolol/propranolol, flecainide, and LCSD has proved inadequate. The 2021 PACES expert consensus statement is the first published guideline to suggest that a treatment strategy without an ICD is possible in some patients with a history of aborted SCA.[73] If implanted, the ICD should be programmed with the longest possible time to detection to minimize the chance of delivering shocks for episodes of polymorphic VT that have a very high probability of self-terminating. Importantly, data evaluating outcomes in CPVT patients with optimally programmed ICDs are not available. Software improvements to distinguish polymorphic VT from VF could lead to a better safety profile but may be technically challenging. In addition to this restrictive implantation policy, we occasionally explant ICDs in patients with no clear indication, after ample discussion with the patient and colleagues.

Ablation

Catheter ablation for ventricular arrhythmia in CPVT is difficult, given the multifocal origin of trigger PVCs and the mechanism of triggered activity, which is likely the reason why it is rarely attempted. The cellular foci of trigger PVCs remain uncertain but may be ventricular cardiomyocytes located near Purkinje cells.[74] There is only a single study of 5 patients who had undergone ablation, and although the incidence of arrhythmic events was lower after ablation, all but 1 patient experienced one or more recurrences.[75]

OUR RECOMMENDED CHRONIC TREATMENT ALGORITHM

Determining the risk category of an individual patient is the first step in our treatment algorithm (**Fig. 3**). Those who are asymptomatic and display no significant ventricular ectopy, usually family members identified through cascade screening, constitute the low-risk category. In general, we recommend prophylactic treatment with nadolol (1–2 mg/kg/d), or propranolol (2–3 mg/kg/d) if nadolol is unavailable, in these patients. However, as discussed previously, certain patient characteristics, such as a very young or older age, a lower

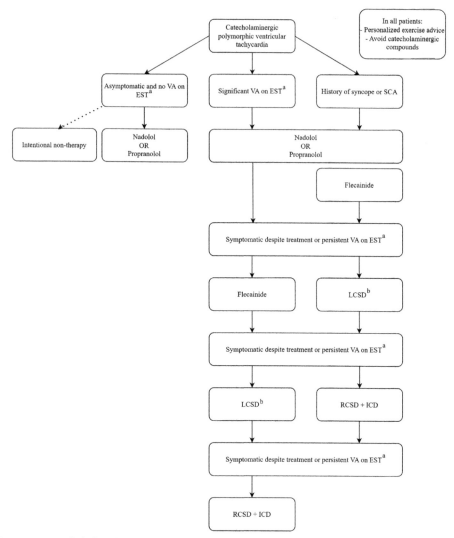

Fig. 3. Our recommended chronic treatment algorithm. EST, exercise stress test; ICD, implantable cardioverter-defibrillator; LCSD, left cardiac sympathetic denervation; RCSD, right cardiac sympathetic denervation; VA, ventricular arrhythmia. [a]Frequent isolated PVCs or worse. [b]LCSD may be considered earlier in the algorithm if the risk of nonadherence is significant.

level of physical activity and the patient's choice, may justify an approach of intentional nontherapy with regular monitoring.

We divide all other patients into 2 categories for the purpose of therapy: those with a history of SCA or syncope and those without such a history but who nonetheless exhibit (asymptomatic) ventricular arrhythmias. Our treatment algorithm follows a similar pattern in both, the difference being that in the first group, we immediately start flecainide (2–3 mg/kg/d) along with nadolol or propranolol, rather than starting with β-blocker monotherapy. If the patient has persistent ventricular arrhythmia on exercise despite adequate doses of nadolol or propranolol and flecainide, LCSD is the next

step. In the rare case of continued therapy refractoriness, RCSD and an ICD should be considered. The settings of the ICD should be optimized to minimize the chance of inappropriate shocks, with long detection delays. Advice regarding exercise restrictions should be individualized and guided by exercise test parameters. All other therapeutic options have insufficient evidence to recommend them in clinical practice.

ACUTE MANAGEMENT OF VENTRICULAR ARRHYTHMIAS

Treatment of electrical storm in patients with CPVT can be challenging, and there is little guidance

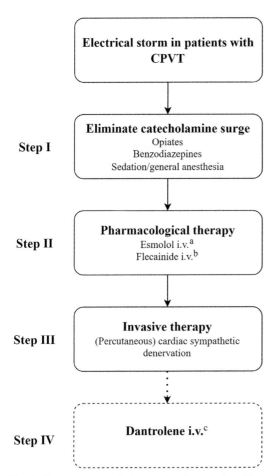

Fig. 4. Our recommended acute treatment algorithm. CPVT, catecholaminergic polymorphic ventricular tachycardia. [a]Recommended esmolol dosage: 500 μg/kg loading dose during 1 min, followed by 50 μg/kg/min continuous infusion uptitrated in steps of 50 μg/kg/min every 4 min until the desired effect is achieved, to a maximum of 200 μg/kg/min. [b]Recommended flecainide dosage: 2 mg/kg bolus during 30 min, followed by continuous infusion of 0.1–0.2 mg/kg/h. [c]Recommended dantrolene dosage: 2.5 mg/kg bolus, repeated as required until the maximal cumulative dose of 10 mg/kg has been reached.

available on this subject in the guidelines and literature; however, it is fortunately extremely rare. Administration of intravenous β-blockers should be a priority. From its rapid onset of effects and short half-life, esmolol may be the most suitable choice in emergency situations, although we are not aware of any published data in CPVT. Esmolol may be combined with intravenous flecainide. Benzodiazepines could be useful to reduce stress and opiates are helpful to reduce pain in patients with repeated ICD shocks. Administration of general anesthesia is highly effective in drug-refractory electrical storms in our experience and allows time to optimally titrate therapy. If ventricular arrhythmia persists despite these interventions, percutaneous stellate ganglion block, which is essentially a temporary CSD, should be considered.[76] Finally, dantrolene may be considered as a last-resort option but there is much uncertainty surrounding its effectiveness (**Fig. 4**).

MANAGEMENT OF ATRIAL ARRHYTHMIAS

Atrial arrhythmias are common in patients with CPVT[5,77] and should not be disregarded because they may cause bothersome symptoms and most importantly, inappropriate ICD shocks.[78] The prognostic significance of the occurrence of atrial arrhythmia in CPVT is unknown. In the absence of CPVT-specific studies, it is reasonable to manage supraventricular arrhythmias as one would in non-CPVT patients, the details of which are outside the scope of this review. Mainstays of CPVT drug therapy such as β-blockers and especially flecainide are well known to attenuate atrial arrhythmia as well. One case report of successful ablation for supraventricular arrhythmia in CPVT is available.[79] Studies evaluating the prognostic value and treatment options of atrial arrhythmias in CPVT are needed.

DRUG-INDUCED CATECHOLAMINERGIC POLYMORPHIC VENTRICULAR TACHYCARDIA

It is widely recognized that certain drugs can cause an acquired phenotype in susceptible individuals and can aggravate the existing phenotype in certain inherited arrhythmia syndromes. Clear examples of this phenomenon are long QT syndrome, and Brugada syndrome.[80] The finding that the tricyclic antidepressant amitriptyline was associated with an increased risk of sudden cardiac death prompted Chopra and colleagues to investigate the mechanism of its proarrhythmic effects in isolated cardiomyocytes. They found that amitriptyline causes calcium leak by activating RyR2 channels, mimicking the arrhythmogenic mechanism of CPVT.[81] Whether this form of what one might call "drug-induced CPVT" is associated with clinical manifestations is unknown, and other drugs with this mechanism have not been reported.

TRIAL DESIGN ISSUES

There is a lack of robust evidence for most interventions in CPVT, reflected by a level of evidence C, or expert opinion, for all recommendations in the recent ESC guidelines because of numerous challenges in study design. With the notable exception of the flecainide RCT by Kannankeril and colleagues,[12] no other prospective randomized trials have been performed. The overarching obstacle in CPVT is the difficulty of recruiting a sufficient number of patients. The rarity of the disease certainly contributes but the main issue is that patients and clinicians are, often for good reason, reluctant to temporarily withhold or discontinue interventions that are considered effective based on available retrospective observational data. Nevertheless, we think it is worth pursuing a higher quality of evidence.

In order to achieve a higher level of evidence, innovative trial designs and international collaboration are needed. Although it is largely unknown to which degree the level of residual ventricular arrhythmia on exercise stress test predicts future arrhythmic events, we think this outcome to be the most suitable for future trials, given that evaluating hard endpoints (ie, arrhythmic events) is infeasible. A crossover, or aggregated N-of-1 design using multiple crossovers in multiple individual patients, can significantly reduce sample size and is suitable due to the chronic nature of CPVT.[82]

SUMMARY

Despite the remarkable growth of knowledge in CPVT during the past decades, many unanswered questions remain, and the number of options and the complexity of management decisions have increased. Care for patients with CPVT should be individualized, and choices must be made scrupulously, balancing freedom from ventricular arrhythmia and maximizing quality of life.

CLINICS CARE POINTS

- Therapeutic efficacy of various therapies in patients with CPVT should be evaluated primarily by means of consecutive exercise stress tests
- Nonselective β-blockers (nadolol and propranolol) are the preferred first-line therapy in patients with CPVT
- Management of electrical storm in patients with CPVT should simultaneously include eliminating catecholamine surge and instituting CPVT-specific therapies

CONFLICT OF INTEREST

None declared.

FUNDING

This study was supported by the ZonMW Priority Medicines for Rare Diseases and Orphan Drugs (grant 113304045 to Dr C. Van der Werf), eRare (E-rare 3–Joint Call 2015 to Dr A.A.M. Wilde), and the Netherlands CardioVascular Research Initiative: the Dutch Heart Foundation, Dutch Federation of University Medical Centres, Netherlands, the Netherlands Organisation for Health Research and Development and the Royal Netherlands Academy of Sciences (PREDICT2 to Dr A.A.M. Wilde).

REFERENCES

1. Baltogiannis GG, Lysitsas DN, di Giovanni G, et al. CPVT: arrhythmogenesis, therapeutic management, and future perspectives. A brief review of the literature. Front Cardiovasc Med 2019;6:92.
2. Leenhardt A, Denjoy I, Guicheney P. Catecholaminergic polymorphic ventricular tachycardia. Circ Arrhythm Electrophysiol 2012;5(5):1044–52.
3. Reid DS, Tynan M, Braidwood L, et al. Bidirectional tachycardia in a child. A study using His bundle electrography. Br Heart J 1975;37(3):339–44.
4. Coumel P, Fidelle J, Lucet V, et al. Catecholamine-induced severe ventriculae arrhythmias with Adams Stockes syndrome in children: report of four cases. Br Heart J 1978;40:28–37.
5. Leenhardt A, Lucet V, Denjoy I, et al. Catecholaminergic polymorphic ventricular tachycardia in children. A 7-year follow-up of 21 patients. Circulation 1995;91(5):1512–9.
6. Walsh R, Adler A, Amin AS, et al. Evaluation of gene validity for CPVT and short QT syndrome in sudden arrhythmic death. Eur Heart J 2022;43(15):1500–10.
7. Wleklinski MJ, Kannankeril PJ, Knollmann BC. Molecular and tissue mechanisms of catecholaminergic polymorphic ventricular tachycardia. J Physiol 2020;598(14):2817–34.
8. Zeppenfeld K, Tfelt-Hansen J, de Riva M, et al. 2022 ESC Guidelines for the management of patients with ventricular arrhythmias and the prevention of sudden cardiac death. Eur Heart J 2022;43(40):3997–4126.
9. van der Werf C, Nederend I, Hofman N, et al. Familial evaluation in catecholaminergic polymorphic ventricular tachycardia: disease penetrance and expression in cardiac ryanodine receptor mutation-carrying relatives. Circ Arrhythm Electrophysiol 2012;5(4):748–56.
10. Hayashi M, Denjoy I, Extramiana F, et al. Incidence and risk factors of arrhythmic events in catecholaminergic polymorphic ventricular tachycardia. Circulation 2009;119(18):2426–34.
11. Peltenburg PJ, Kallas D, Bos JM, et al. An International Multicenter Cohort Study on β-Blockers for

the Treatment of Symptomatic Children With Cate-cholaminergic Polymorphic Ventricular Tachycardia. Circulation 2022;145(5):333–44.

12. Kannankeril PJ, Moore JP, Cerrone M, et al. Efficacy of flecainide in the treatment of catecholaminergic polymorphic ventricular tachycardia: a randomized clinical trial. JAMA Cardiol 2017;2(7):759–66.

13. Roston TM, Kallas D, Davies B, et al. Burst exercise testing can unmask arrhythmias in patients with incompletely penetrant catecholaminergic polymor-phic ventricular tachycardia. JACC Clin Electrophy-siol 2021;7(4):437–41.

14. Bellamy D, Nuthall G, Dalziel S, et al. Catecholamin-ergic polymorphic ventricular tachycardia: the car-diac arrest where epinephrine is contraindicated. Pediatr Crit Care Med 2019;20(3):262–8.

15. Ackerman MJ, Zipes DP, Kovacs RJ, et al. Eligibility and disqualification recommendations for competi-tive athletes with cardiovascular abnormalities: task force 10: the cardiac channelopathies: a scientific statement from the American Heart Association and American College of Cardiology. J Am Coll Car-diol 2015;66(21):2424–8.

16. Etheridge SP, Saarel EV, Martinez MW. Exercise participation and shared decision-making in pa-tients with inherited channelopathies and cardiomy-opathies. Heart Rhythm 2018;15(6):915–20.

17. Pflaumer A, Wilde AAM, Charafeddine F, et al. 50 years of catecholaminergic polymorphic ventricu-lar tachycardia (CPVT) - time to explore the dark side of the moon. Heart Lung Circ 2020;29(4): 520–8.

18. Ostby SA, Bos JM, Owen HJ, et al. Competitive sports participation in patients with catecholamin-ergic polymorphic ventricular tachycardia: a single center's early experience. JACC Clin Electrophysiol 2016;2(3):253–62.

19. Kallas D, Roston TM, Franciosi S, et al. Evaluation of age at symptom onset, proband status, and sex as predictors of disease severity in pediatric catechol-aminergic polymorphic ventricular tachycardia. Heart Rhythm 2021;18(11):1825–32.

20. Lieve KVV, Verhagen JMA, Wei J, et al. Linking the heart and the brain: neurodevelopmental disorders in patients with catecholaminergic polymorphic ven-tricular tachycardia. Heart Rhythm 2019;16(2): 220–8.

21. van der Werf C, Zwinderman AH, Wilde AA. Thera-peutic approach for patients with catecholaminergic polymorphic ventricular tachycardia: state of the art and future developments. Europace 2012;14(2): 175–83.

22. Peltenburg PJ, Kallas D, Bos JM, et al. An interna-tional multicenter cohort study on β-blockers for the treatment of symptomatic children with catechol-aminergic polymorphic ventricular tachycardia. Cir-culation 2022;145(5):333–44.

23. Mazzanti A, Kukavica D, Trancuccio A, et al. Outcomes of patients with catecholaminergic poly-morphic ventricular tachycardia treated with β-blockers. JAMA Cardiol 2022;7(5):504–12.

24. Leren IS, Saberniak J, Majid E, et al. Nadolol de-creases the incidence and severity of ventricular ar-rhythmias during exercise stress testing compared with β1-selective β-blockers in patients with cate-cholaminergic polymorphic ventricular tachycardia. Heart Rhythm 2016;13(2):433–40.

25. Roston TM, Vinocur JM, Maginot KR, et al. Catechol-aminergic polymorphic ventricular tachycardia in children: analysis of therapeutic strategies and out-comes from an international multicenter registry. Circ Arrhythm Electrophysiol 2015;8(3):633–42.

26. Postma AV, Denjoy I, Kamblock J, et al. Catechol-aminergic polymorphic ventricular tachycardia: RYR2 mutations, bradycardia, and follow up of the patients. J Med Genet 2005;42(11):863–70.

27. Watanabe H, Chopra N, Laver D, et al. Flecainide prevents catecholaminergic polymorphic ventricular tachycardia in mice and humans. Nat Med 2009; 15(4):380–3.

28. van der Werf C, Kannankeril PJ, Sacher F, et al. Fle-cainide therapy reduces exercise-induced ventricu-lar arrhythmias in patients with catecholaminergic polymorphic ventricular tachycardia. J Am Coll Car-diol 2011;57(22):2244–54.

29. Wang G, Zhao N, Zhong S, et al. Safety and efficacy of flecainide for patients with catecholaminergic polymorphic ventricular tachycardia: a systematic review and meta-analysis. Medicine (Baltim) 2019; 98(34):e16961.

30. Kryshtal DO, Blackwell DJ, Egly CL, et al. RYR2 channel inhibition is the principal mechanism of fle-cainide action in CPVT. Circ Res 2021;128(3): 321–31.

31. Watanabe H, van der Werf C, Roses-Noguer F, et al. Effects of flecainide on exercise-induced ventricular arrhythmias and recurrences in genotype-negative patients with catecholaminergic polymorphic ven-tricular tachycardia. Heart Rhythm 2013;10(4): 542–7.

32. Padfield GJ, AlAhmari L, Lieve KV, et al. Flecainide monotherapy is an option for selected patients with catecholaminergic polymorphic ventricular tachy-cardia intolerant of β-blockade. Heart Rhythm 2016;13(2):609–13.

33. Bryson HM, Palmer KJ, Langtry HD, et al. A reappraisal of its pharmacology, pharmacoki-netics and therapeutic use in cardiac arrhythmias. Drugs 1993;45(1):85–130.

34. Hwang HS, Hasdemir C, Laver D, et al. Inhibition of cardiac Ca2+ release channels (RyR2) determines efficacy of class I antiarrhythmic drugs in catechol-aminergic polymorphic ventricular tachycardia. Circ Arrhythm Electrophysiol 2011;4(2):128–35.

35. Savio-Galimberti E, Knollmann BC. Channel activity of cardiac ryanodine receptors (RyR2) determines potency and efficacy of flecainide and R-propafenone against arrhythmogenic calcium waves in ventricular cardiomyocytes. PLoS One 2015;10(6): e0131179.

36. Marx A, Lange B, Nalenz C, et al. A 35-year effective treatment of catecholaminergic polymorphic ventricular tachycardia with propafenone. HeartRhythm Case Rep 2018;5(2):74–7.

37. Valdivia HH, Valdivia C, Ma J, et al. Direct binding of verapamil to the ryanodine receptor channel of sarcoplasmic reticulum. Biophys J 1990;58(2): 471–81.

38. Swan H, Laitinen P, Kontula K, et al. Calcium channel antagonism reduces exercise-induced ventricular arrhythmias in catecholaminergic polymorphic ventricular tachycardia patients with RyR2 mutations. J Cardiovasc Electrophysiol 2005;16(2):162–6.

39. Rosso R, Kalman JM, Rogowski O, et al. Calcium channel blockers and beta-blockers versus beta-blockers alone for preventing exercise-induced arrhythmias in catecholaminergic polymorphic ventricular tachycardia. Heart Rhythm 2007;4(9):1149–54.

40. Rosso R, Kalman J, Rogowsky O, et al. Long-term effectiveness of beta blocker and calcium blocker combination therapy in patients with CPVT. Heart Rhythm 2010;7:S423.

41. Baruscotti M, Bucchi A, Difrancesco D. Physiology and pharmacology of the cardiac pacemaker ("funny") current. Pharmacol Ther 2005;107(1): 59–79.

42. Koruth JS, Lala A, Pinney S, et al. The clinical use of ivabradine. J Am Coll Cardiol 2017;70(14):1777–84.

43. Kohli U, Aziz Z, Beaser AD, et al. Ventricular arrhythmia suppression with ivabradine in a patient with catecholaminergic polymorphic ventricular tachycardia refractory to nadolol, flecainide, and sympathectomy. Pacing Clin Electrophysiol 2020; 43(5):527–33.

44. Vaksmann G, Klug D. Efficacy of ivabradine to control ventricular arrhythmias in catecholaminergic polymorphic ventricular tachycardia. Pacing Clin Electrophysiol 2018;41(10):1378–80.

45. Bueno-Levy H, Weisbrod D, Yadin D, et al. The hyperpolarization-activated cyclic-nucleotide-gated channel blocker ivabradine does not prevent arrhythmias in catecholaminergic polymorphic ventricular tachycardia. Front Pharmacol 2020;10:1566.

46. Szentandrássy N, Magyar ZÉ, Hevesi J, et al. Therapeutic approaches of ryanodine receptor-associated heart diseases. Int J Mol Sci 2022; 23(8):4435.

47. Paul-Pletzer K, Yamamoto T, Ikemoto N, et al. Probing a putative dantrolene-binding site on the cardiac ryanodine receptor. Biochem J 2005;387(Pt 3): 905–9.

48. Jung CB, Moretti A, Mederos y Schnitzler M, et al. Dantrolene rescues arrhythmogenic RYR2 defect in a patient-specific stem cell model of catecholaminergic polymorphic ventricular tachycardia. EMBO Mol Med 2012;4(3):180–91.

49. Kobayashi S, Yano M, Uchinoumi H, et al. Dantrolene, a therapeutic agent for malignant hyperthermia, inhibits catecholaminergic polymorphic ventricular tachycardia in a RyR2(R2474S/+) knock-in mouse model. Circ J 2010;74(12):2579–84.

50. Penttinen K, Swan H, Vanninen S, et al. Antiarrhythmic effects of dantrolene in patients with catecholaminergic polymorphic ventricular tachycardia and replication of the responses using iPSC models. PLoS One 2015;10(5):e0125366.

51. Li N, Wang Q, Sibrian-Vazquez M, et al. Treatment of catecholaminergic polymorphic ventricular tachycardia in mice using novel RyR2-modifying drugs. Int J Cardiol 2017;227:668–73.

52. Klipp RC, Li N, Wang Q, et al. EL20, a potent antiarrhythmic compound, selectively inhibits calmodulin-deficient ryanodine receptor type 2. Heart Rhythm 2018;15(4):578–86.

53. Word TA, Quick AP, Miyake CY, et al. Efficacy of RyR2 inhibitor EL20 in induced pluripotent stem cell-derived cardiomyocytes from a patient with catecholaminergic polymorphic ventricular tachycardia. J Cell Mol Med 2021;25(13):6115–24.

54. Connell P, Word TA, Wehrens XHT. Targeting pathological leak of ryanodine receptors: preclinical progress and the potential impact on treatments for cardiac arrhythmias and heart failure. Expert Opin Ther Targets 2020;24(1):25–36.

55. Wilde AA, Bhuiyan ZA, Crotti L, et al. Left cardiac sympathetic denervation for catecholaminergic polymorphic ventricular tachycardia. N Engl J Med 2008;358(19):2024–9.

56. Coleman MA, Bos JM, Johnson JN, et al. Videoscopic left cardiac sympathetic denervation for patients with recurrent ventricular fibrillation/malignant ventricular arrhythmia syndromes besides congenital long-QT syndrome. Circ Arrhythm Electrophysiol 2012;5(4):782–8.

57. De Ferrari GM, Dusi V, Spazzolini C, et al. Clinical management of catecholaminergic polymorphic ventricular tachycardia: the role of left cardiac sympathetic denervation. Circulation 2015;131(25): 2185–93.

58. Collura CA, Johnson JN, Moir C, et al. Left cardiac sympathetic denervation for the treatment of long QT syndrome and catecholaminergic polymorphic ventricular tachycardia using video-assisted thoracic surgery. Heart Rhythm 2009;6(6):752–9.

59. Schwartz PJ, De Ferrari GM, Pugliese L. Cardiac sympathetic denervation 100years later: jonnesco would have never believed it. Int J Cardiol 2017; 237:25–8.

60. Dusi V, De Ferrari GM, Pugliese L, et al. Cardiac sympathetic denervation in channelopathies. Front Cardiovasc Med 2019;6:27.

61. Schwartz PJ, Ackerman MJ. Cardiac sympathetic denervation in the prevention of genetically mediated life-threatening ventricular arrhythmias. Eur Heart J 2022;43(22):2096–102.

62. Akinseye OA, Ralston WF, Johnson KC, et al. Renal sympathetic denervation: a comprehensive review. Curr Probl Cardiol 2021;46(3):100598.

63. Garg J, Shah S, Shah K, et al. Renal sympathetic denervation for the treatment of recurrent ventricular arrhythmias-ELECTRAM investigators. Pacing Clin Electrophysiol 2021;44(5):865–74.

64. Aksu T, Güler TE, Özcan KS, et al. Renal sympathetic denervation assisted treatment of electrical storm due to polymorphic ventricular tachycardia in a patient with cathecolaminergic polymorphic ventricular tachycardia. Turk Kardiyol Dernegi Arsivi 2017;45(5):441–9.

65. Aksu T, Guler E. Percutaneous renal sympathetic denervation in catecholaminergic polymorphic ventricular tachycardia. J Arrhythm 2017;33(3):245.

66. van der Werf C, Lieve KV, Bos JM, et al. Implantable cardioverter-defibrillators in previously undiagnosed patients with catecholaminergic polymorphic ventricular tachycardia resuscitated from sudden cardiac arrest. Eur Heart J 2019;40(35):2953–61.

67. Pizzale S, Gollob MH, Gow R, et al. Sudden death in a young man with catecholaminergic polymorphic ventricular tachycardia and paroxysmal atrial fibrillation. J Cardiovasc Electrophysiol 2008;19(12): 1319–21.

68. Palanca V, Quesada A, Trigo A, et al. Arrhythmic storm induced by AICD discharge in a patient with catecholaminergic polymorphic ventricular tachycardia. Rev Esp Cardiol 2006;59:1079–80.

69. Miyake CY, Webster G, Czosek RJ, et al. Efficacy of implantable cardioverter defibrillators in young patients with catecholaminergic polymorphic ventricular tachycardia: success depends on substrate. Circ Arrhythm Electrophysiol 2013;6(3):579–87.

70. Roses-Noguer F, Jarman JW, Clague JR, et al. Outcomes of defibrillator therapy in catecholaminergic polymorphic ventricular tachycardia. Heart Rhythm 2014;11(1):58–66.

71. Roston TM, Jones K, Hawkins NM, et al. Implantable cardioverter-defibrillator use in catecholaminergic polymorphic ventricular tachycardia: a systematic review. Heart Rhythm 2018;15(12):1791–9.

72. Al-Khatib SM, Stevenson WG, Ackerman MJ, et al. 2017 AHA/ACC/HRS guideline for management of patients with ventricular arrhythmias and the prevention of sudden cardiac death: executive summary: a report of the American College of Cardiology/American Heart Association Task Force on Clinical Practice Guidelines and the Heart Rhythm Society. J Am Coll Cardiol 2018;72(14):1677–749.

73. Shah MJ, Silka MJ, Silva JNA, et al. 2021 PACES expert consensus statement on the indications and management of cardiovascular implantable electronic devices in pediatric patients. Cardiol Young 2021;31(11):1738–69.

74. Blackwell DJ, Faggioni M, Wleklinski MJ, et al. The Purkinje-myocardial junction is the anatomic origin of ventricular arrhythmia in CPVT. JCI Insight 2022; 7(3):e151893.

75. Kaneshiro T, Nogami A, Kato Y, et al. Effects of catheter ablation targeting the trigger beats in inherited catecholaminergic polymorphic ventricular tachycardia. JACC Clin Electrophysiol 2017;3(9):1062–3.

76. Tian Y, Wittwer ED, Kapa S, et al. Effective use of percutaneous stellate ganglion blockade in patients with electrical storm. Circ Arrhythm Electrophysiol 2019;12(9):e007118.

77. Sumitomo N, Sakurada H, Taniguchi K, et al. Association of atrial arrhythmia and sinus node dysfunction in patients with catecholaminergic polymorphic ventricular tachycardia. Circ J 2007;71(10):1606–9.

78. Sy RW, Gollob MH, Klein GJ, et al. Arrhythmia characterization and long-term outcomes in catecholaminergic polymorphic ventricular tachycardia. Heart Rhythm 2011;8(6):864–71.

79. Kawada S, Morita H, Watanabe A, et al. Radiofrequency catheter ablation for drug-refractory atrial tachyarrhythmias in a patient with catecholaminergic polymorphic ventricular tachycardia: a case report. J Cardiol Cases 2018;19(1):36–9.

80. Krahn AD, Behr ER, Hamilton R, et al. Brugada syndrome. JACC Clin Electrophysiol 2022;8(3): 386–405.

81. Chopra N, Laver D, Davies SS, et al. Amitriptyline activates cardiac ryanodine channels and causes spontaneous sarcoplasmic reticulum calcium release. Mol Pharmacol 2009;75(1):183–95.

82. Guyatt G, Sackett D, Adachi J, et al. A clinician's guide for conducting randomized trials in individual patients. CMAJ (Can Med Assoc J) 1988;139(6): 497–503.

Investigation of Unexplained Cardiac Arrest: Phenotyping and Genetic Testing

Abdulelah H. Alsaeed, MBBS[a], Wael Alqarawi, MD, MSc[a,b,*]

KEYWORDS

- Unexplained cardiac arrest • Idiopathic ventricular fibrillation • Diagnosis • Investigation
- Approach • Review article

KEY POINTS

- Unexplained cardiac arrest (UCA) is a working diagnosis that should be replaced by a final diagnosis once evaluation is completed.
- Cardiac magnetic resonance imaging, exercise treadmill test, and sodium-channel blocker challenge are high-yield tests that should be performed in all patients with UCA.
- The care of patients with UCA should be delivered in specialized clinics utilizing a multidisciplinary team with access to important services such as clinical psychology and clinical genetic testing.

INTRODUCTION

Unexplained cardiac arrest (UCA) is defined as cardiac arrest of presumed cardiac etiology with no cause identified on initial evaluation [coronary assessment, echocardiogram, and 12-lead electrocardiogram (ECG)]. It is important to note that UCA is a working diagnosis that should be replaced by a final diagnosis once evaluation is completed. If no cause is identified despite complete evaluation, the diagnosis of [idiopathic ventricular fibrillation (IVF)] should then be made. In essence, IVF is UCA with no cause identified despite complete evaluation.

Epidemiology

Out-of-hospital cardiac arrest (OHCA) is a leading cause of mortality and morbidity worldwide.[1] It is commonly caused by coronary artery disease and cardiomyopathies; however, about 1 out of 10 OHCA cases are initially unexplained.[2] Waldmann and colleagues[2] reported that 12.3% of OHCA in the Paris Sudden Death Expertise Center (Paris-SDEC) registry remained unexplained after ECG, echo, and coronary angiography (ie, UCA).

Adult patients with UCA are typically in their 30s and 40s with a slight male predominance.[3] In real world settings, only a minority of patients with UCA receive complete evaluation.[2] Indeed, Waldmann and colleagues[2] showed that 84% of patients with UCA in the Paris-SDEC registry did not receive complete evaluation that included provocative testings.

Importance of Investigating Unexplained Cardiac Arrest

Identifying the specific cause of UCA is a crucial step in management of these patients for several reasons. First, it guides choosing the correct therapy to prevent and treat recurrent arrhythmias. For example, the empiric use of beta-blockers to treat recurrent implantable cardioverter-defibrillator (ICD) shocks due to ventricular arrhythmias in an UCA patient will not be effective if the diagnosis of Brugada syndrome (BrS) is made, whereas quinidine would be quite effective had the diagnosis

[a] Department of Cardiac Sciences, College of Medicine, King Saud University, Riyadh, Saudi Arabia;
[b] University of Ottawa Heart Institute, University of Ottawa, Ottawa, Canada
* Corresponding author. Department of Cardiac Sciences, College of Medicine, King Saud University, Riyadh, Saudi Arabia.
E-mail address: Walqarawi@ksu.edu.sa

Card Electrophysiol Clin 15 (2023) 307–318
https://doi.org/10.1016/j.ccep.2023.04.003
1877-9182/23/© 2023 Elsevier Inc. All rights reserved.

been made. Similarly, the use of flecainide as an added therapy to beta-blockers may be entertained if the diagnosis of catecholaminergic polymorphic ventricular tachycardia (CPVT) or long QT syndrome (LQTS) type 3 is made.[4] Second, it informs the assessment of family members. Given that many of the causes of UCA are potentially inherited, identifying the cause can guide family screening and therapeutic interventions to reduce the risk of cardiac arrest. Lastly, it helps discover new conditions that carry a risk of cardiac arrest in the general population. Indeed, BrS and calcium release deficiency syndrome (CRDS), for example, were only discovered as a result of evaluation of patients with UCA.[5,6] Additionally, the observation that mitral valve prolapse (MVP) was overrepresented in patients with UCA led to the better characterization of arrhythmic MVP (AMVP), which is now recognized as an important potential cause of cardiac arrest and sudden cardiac death (SCD) in the community.[7,8]

The Yield of Unexplained Cardiac Arrest Evaluation

Multiple studies examined the yield of comprehensive evaluation in identifying the cause of UCA.[3] We have recently performed a systematic review of these studies and meta-analyzed the proportion of patients who were eventually found to have a cause of their UCA after evaluation.[3] Most of these studies were multicenter registries that included all age groups and were done in referral centers. Several points were learnt from this review:

1. The overall diagnostic yield was high [43% (95% CI 39% to 48%)].
2. Most of the yield was obtained by performing 3 tests: cardiac magnetic resonance imaging (CMR), exercise treadmill test (ETT), and sodium-channel blocker challenge (SCB).
3. Some tests performed during the evaluation resulted in high rates of abnormal results; however, the clinical significance of these results was unclear. These tests include systematic genetic testing, electrophysiology study (EPS), and coronary spasm provocation (CSP).
4. The use of pre-specified criteria for diagnosis was associated with reduced yield. This raised a concern about inaccurate diagnoses which is not surprising given the lack of standardized definitions for most conditions associated with UCA.

DIAGNOSTIC TESTS

Table 1 summarizes the 3 most important diagnostic tests that are associated with a high yield in identifying the cause of UCA.

Exercise Treadmill Test

The main goal of ETT in this population is to look for concealed LQTS and CPVT. **Fig. 1** depicts a simple algorithm that incorporates resting and 4-min recovery QTc, which was found to have a high degree of accuracy in detecting concealed LQTS.[9] This algorithm was validated in families with LQTS and its use was associated with unmasking LQTS in a large proportion of patients with UCA.[9,10] Using a cut off value of $\geq$480 ms at 4-min recovery was more specific and is incorporated in the updated LQTS risk score.[11] CPVT is suspected when ETT reveals exercise-induced ventricular tachycardia or premature ventricular beats in the right clinical context.

Fig. 2 shows an example of a patient with concealed LQTS, which was revealed by a positive ETT.

Sodium-Channel Blocker Challenge

The goal of SCB is to provoke a type 1 Brugada pattern in those with normal baseline ECG or nondiagnostic Brugada patterns (type 2 and 3). High precordial lead placement should be performed at baseline and during SCB to increase the sensitivity of detecting a type 1 Brugada pattern.[12] Multiple sodium-channel blockers have been used, with the most common ones being procainamide, flecainide, and ajmaline. These agents have varying degrees of sodium-channel blockade potency which, at least in part, explains their relative likelihood of provoking a type 1 Brugada pattern.[13] Although the choice of agent is typically limited by the availability, it is important to note the different response to these agents to better interpret the literature. Cheung and colleagues[13] compared rates of positive response to procainamide versus ajmaline in a large cohort of patients with a family history of cardiac arrest, SCD, or BrS. They found a significant difference in the rates of positive response where Ajmaline was 6 times more likely to induce a type 1 Brugada pattern than procainamide (26% vs 4%, $P < .001$). Moreover, in a multivariate analysis, the use of ajmaline was an independent predictor of a positive response after adjustment for baseline ECG, gender, and ethnicity.[13]

In this context, sensitivity and specificity are important considerations for SCB provocation. The rates of false positive results of SCB using ajmaline and flecainide have been reported to be 4% to 16%.[14–18] As such, careful interpretation of a positive SCB, especially with the use of more potent SCB such as ajmaline, and incorporating other findings from the complete evaluation is crucial before diagnosing BrS based solely on SCB results. It is believed that procainamide is

Table 1
High-yield tests for unexplained cardiac arrest

Test	Main Conditions	Protocols	Positive Results	Notes
ETT	LQTS CPVT	Bruce or modified Bruce protocol. In recovery, ECGs are performed at 1-min intervals during a 6-min recovery phase.	LQTS: QTc ≥ 445 ms at 4 min. See **Fig. 1**. CPVT: Exercise-induced ventricular arrhythmias including bigeminy, couplets, polymorphic VT and bidirectional VT.	• A cut-off of ≥ 480 ms at 4-min recovery is more specific and has been incorporated in the Schwartz score. • Other findings from ETT can be helpful in diagnosing other conditions such as ARVC with inducing right ventricular tachycardia during exercise and BrS by revealing type 1 Brugada pattern. • Epinephrine challenge can be used in the context of suspected CPVT if the patient cannot exercise. • Resting PVCs even if it gets worse with exercise are not typical of CPVT and could be seen in arrhythmogenic cardiomyopathies.

SCB	BrS	15 mg/kg procainamide infusion for 20 min (to a maximum of 1 g)
		Or
		1 mg/kg ajmaline infused at 5–10 min (maximum 100 mg)
		Or
		Flecainide 2 mg/kg over 10 min) (maximum 150 mg).
			Type 1 Brugada pattern (coved ST segment elevation displaying J wave amplitude of ≥2 mm, followed by a negative T-wave, with little or no isoelectric separation in one of the right precordial leads.	• High precordial leads (second and third intercostal space) should be recorded to increase sensitivity.
				• Test should be terminated if:
				  ○ Positive (type 1 pattern)
				  ○ QRS prolongation (≥130%)
				  ○ Premature ventricular complexes or ventricular arrhythmias.

CMR	Cardiomyopathies • ARVC • ALVC/myocarditis • HCM • LVNC	NA	NA	• It is preferable to have cardiac imaging specialist(s) with special interest/training dedicated to reading scans to minimize inaccurate diagnoses.

Abbreviations: ALVC, arrhythmogenic left ventricular cardiomyopathy; ARVC, arrhythmogenic right ventricular cardiomyopathy; BrS, Brugada syndrome; CMR, cardiac magnetic resonance imaging; CPVT, catecholaminergic polymorphic ventricular tachycardia; ETT, exercise treadmill test; HCM, hypertrophic cardiomyopathy; LQTS, long QT syndrome; LVNC, left ventricular non-compaction; PVC, premature ventricular contraction; SCB, sodium-channel blocker challenge; VT, ventricular tachycardia.

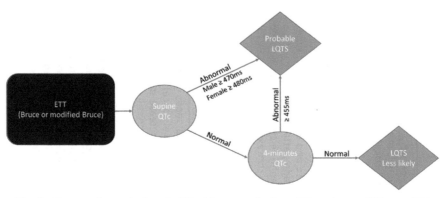

Fig. 1. Algorithm for the use of exercise treadmill test to screen for long QT syndrome. ETT, exercise treadmill test; LQTS, long QT syndrome.

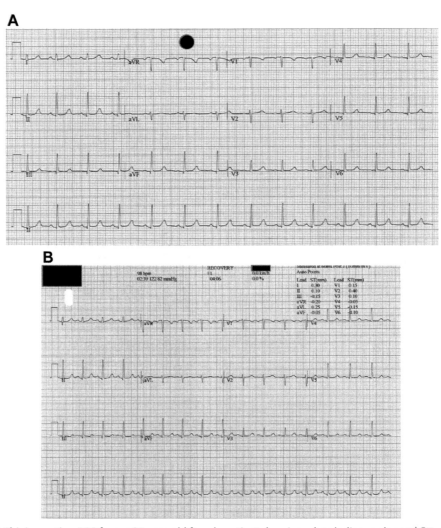

Fig. 2. (*A*) This is a resting ECG from a 31-year-old female patient showing a borderline prolonged QTc at rest. The QT is 400 ms (QTc = 465 ms). (*B*) Same patient at 4-min recovery. QT is 360 ms (QTc = 483 ms). Values ≥ 445 ms at 4-min recovery is suggestive of LQTS. Note that at rest (*A*), the QT is normal, which highlights the important role of exercise in diagnosing concealed LQTS (confirmed with a pathogenic variant in KCNQ1 gene in this case).

less sensitive but more specific than ajmaline and flecainide, although no systematic study has examined test characteristics of these 3 agents, notwithstanding also the difficulty in interpreting SCB given the lack of a gold standard test for BrS.

Fig. 3 shows an example of a patient with UCA who had a normal baseline ECG, type 2 Brugada pattern on a high-lead ECG, and a positive procainamide challenge test.

Cardiac Magnetic Resonance Imaging

The main goal of CMR is to detect concealed structural changes that can be missed on echocardiograms, such as early changes in arrhythmogenic right ventricular cardiomyopathy (ARVC) and myocarditis. It is known, for example, that patients with definite ARVC can have a normal echocardiogram, especially at early stages.[19] In one study, only 50% of patients with definite ARVC with a positive CMR fulfilled a minor or major Task Force Criteria (TFC) for ARVC by echocardiogram.[19] In addition, late gadolinium enhancement (LGE) is a major advantage of CMR that could reveal the diagnosis of healed myocarditis or early signs of cardiomyopathies before overt systolic dysfunction.[20] However, interobserver variability in interpreting CMR features is well-documented and caution needs to be taken when relying solely on CMR, especially when read by an inexperience observer

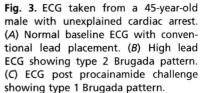

Fig. 3. ECG taken from a 45-year-old male with unexplained cardiac arrest. (A) Normal baseline ECG with conventional lead placement. (B) High lead ECG showing type 2 Brugada pattern. (C) ECG post procainamide challenge showing type 1 Brugada pattern.

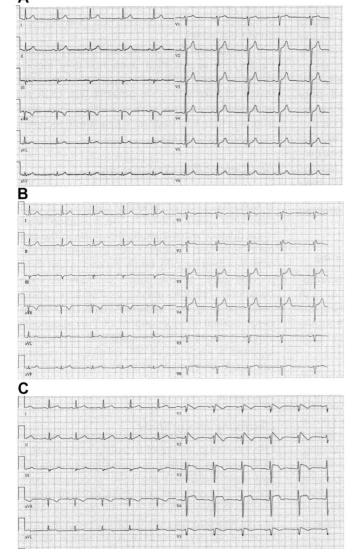

and in the presence of borderline changes.[21,22] Tandri and colleagues[23] assessed the interobserver variability of CMR features of ARVC. Despite having a standardized protocol, only including cases with good imaging quality and having 2 experienced readers, the interobserver kappa score for fat infiltration was found to be 0.74. The other important challenge with CMR is the overcautious reporting of findings that can be seen in healthy subjects, which can lead to inaccurate diagnoses.[24] It is preferable to have certain CMR readers involved in UCA cases to build experience and avoid inaccurate diagnoses.

Epinephrine Challenge Test

The goal of epinephrine challenge test is to diagnose concealed LQTS and CPVT. Two major protocols have been used: Shimizu protocol (bolus and brief infusion) and Mayo protocol (gradually escalating doses).[25,26] However, difficulty measuring QT during epinephrine infusion, especially with abnormal T-wave morphologies, renders intra- and interobserver agreement poor and increases the potential for false-positive results.[27,28] Additionally, the potential for QT prolongation in response to epinephrine challenge among patients without LQTS has brought its clinical utility as a diagnostic tool for LQTS assessment into question.[28] As such, it should likely only be used as an alternative to ETT in patients who cannot exercise in patients with a suspected diagnosis of CPVT.[27,28]

Ambulatory Electrocardiogram Monitoring

Although the yield of ambulatory electrocardiogram monitoring in identifying the cause of UCA is low, it can aid other tests in establishing the cause of UCA.[3] In our view, the findings from the ambulatory electrocardiogram monitoring in UCA can be categorized into 2 groups:

- "Diagnostic" findings: these are findings that are diagnostic for certain conditions. For example, documenting polymorphic ventricular tachycardia (PMVT) initiated by a premature ventricular contraction (PVC) with a coupling interval of less than 350 ms is diagnostic for short coupled ventricular fibrillation (SCVF) in the absence of confounding causes.[29] Another example is documentation of transient ischemic changes and PMVT during angina due to coronary spasm in patients with no obstructive CAD.
- "Suggestive" findings: these are findings that might be suggestive of certain conditions and can guide further evaluation. Examples

of this category include torsade de pointes (suggestive of LQTS), frequent PVCs (arrhythmogenic cardiomyopathies), and exercise-induced VT or PVCs (CPVT).

The utility of Holter monitor to diagnose LQTS is unclear. Some studies suggested minimal diagnostic value, whereas others reported certain QT intervals obtained from Holter monitor to discriminate between LQTS and healthy controls.[30–32] Similarly, Holter monitor has been shown to increase detection of intermittent type 1 Brugada pattern as compared to repeated 12-lead ECGs.[33,34] However, no studies examined the value of Holter in detecting LQTS or BrS with negative provocative tests (ie, ETT and SCB). If Holter is used to diagnose LQTS or BrS, it needs to be performed by experienced readers who specialize in inherited arrhythmias to avoid inaccurate diagnoses.

It is important to note that ambulatory electrocardiogram examination does not only include Holter monitors, but in fact should include a careful review of telemetry while patients with UCA are admitted and a careful review of intracardiac electrograms from ICD tracings in cases with recurrent ventricular arrhythmias.

First-Degree Relative Screening

Family screening to initiate preventative measures is essential once an inherited condition is diagnosed in a patient with UCA. The evaluation needs to be guided by the specific diagnosis in the proband. However, in patients with UCA with no diagnosis reached (ie, IVF), family screening can rarely provide clues to the cause of UCA or, more commonly, provides reassurance to family members. The prognosis of family members who undergo screening independent of their diagnostic status is excellent.[35] Steinberg and colleagues[35] reported a follow-up of 186 relatives of patients with UCA where none of them experienced cardiac arrest or SCD after a median follow-up of 24 months.

Electrophysiology Study

EPS has the potential of revealing rare causes of UCA such as bundle branch reentrant ventricular tachycardia (BBRVT) and latent accessory pathways.[36,37] Long-short ventricular extra-stimuli are needed to screen for BBRVT. Although supraventricular tachycardias (SVT) have been suspected to be the primary cause of UCA in few case reports, complete evaluation should be performed to ensure the absence of other causes. The ongoing study titled, "The Role of Electrophysiology Testing in Survivors of Unexplained Cardiac Arrest" (ClinicalTrials.gov identifier: NCT03079414) will provide more insight into the role and proper interpretation of EPS in patients with UCA.

Coronary Spasm Provocation

Coronary spasm can be provoked by administering vasoconstrictor agents during coronary angiography (most common agents: ergonovine and acetylcholine). Different definitions of a positive response have been proposed, but all include a specified reduction in luminal diameter accompanying symptoms and/or ischemic ECG changes.[3] In our recent meta-analysis, the pooled proportion of patients with UCA with a positive CSP from 4 studies that performed CSP as part of the evaluation of UCA was found to be 23% (95% CI 8% to 43%).[3] However, this does not necessarily mean that coronary spasm was the cause of their UCA given the reported overlap with other conditions such as early repolarization syndrome (ERS) and BrS.[38,39] For example, Komatsu and colleagues[39] reported that 50% (8/16) patients with UCA who had type 1 Brugada pattern tested positive with CSP. As such, careful and expert interpretation of CSP that takes into account other findings needs to be exercised.

Genetics

Genetic testing for patients with UCA is essential when a specific diagnosis is suspected based on phenotypic features. This can help confirm the diagnosis, inform prognosis, and guide family screening.[40] However, the role of genetic testing to reveal the cause of UCA in patients without a clear phenotype is questionable. Just recently, Grondin and colleagues[41] reported the yield of systematic whole-exome sequencing in patients with UCA. They found that 6% of patients with definite IVF (ie, no clear explanation for UCA despite complete phenotypic evaluation) had a pathogenic/likely pathogenic (P/LP) variant in previously reported cardiovascular disease genes.[41] Most of these patients were diagnosed with "unclassified arrhythmogenic cardiomyopathy" based on their genetic findings and the absence of structural changes on echo and CMR.[41] This is consistent with previous smaller studies reporting a high proportion of P/LP variants in cardiomyopathy genes in patients with UCA, suggesting an important role of "concealed cardiomyopathy" in patients with IVF.[3] However, this came at a cost of a frequent finding of variants of unknown significance (VUS) which was identified in 40% of patients. In addition, 8% of P/LP variants were judged to be incidental findings, highlighting the paramount importance of a multidisciplinary team approach for proper interpretation and management of these findings.[3] Another important finding from this study was the substantial increase in the rate of VUS with larger genetic panels with no significant change in the rate of P/LP variants.[3] Indeed, the rate of VUS dropped down to 20% without a difference in the rate of P/LP when only 45 genes were included in their secondary analysis [these 45 genes were classified by the Clinical Genome Resource (ClinGen) cardiovascular panel as having ≥ moderate evidence in any of the curated arrhythmia syndromes and/or cardiomyopathies].[3]

CAUSES OF UNEXPLAINED CARDIAC ARREST

Fig. 4 depicts conditions associated with UCA. LQTS, BrS, CPVT, and cardiomyopathies are the most common conditions revealed after evaluation.[3] Certain conditions are only recently described and require the exclusion of other causes and/or do not have an established definition that renders making the diagnosis difficult. These include AMVP, ERS, SCVF, CRDS, and IVF which will be described below.

Early Repolarization Syndrome

ERS is diagnosed in patients with unexplained cardiac arrest who have J-point elevation of ≥ 1 mm in ≥ 2 contiguous inferior and/or lateral leads.[4] J-point is where QRS ends, and ST segment starts. Importantly, in the cardiac arrest survivors with preserved ejection fraction registry (CASPER), a third of patients with UCA and early repolarization were found to have an alternative diagnosis.[42] As such, ERS should only be considered in patients with UCA who underwent complete evaluation with no diagnosis reached.[43,44]

Patients with ERS are usually males in their 30s to 50s who present with cardiac arrest during sleep or minimal activity. Most of these patients have intermittent J-point elevation, underlining the importance of examining multiple ECGs. The risk of recurrent arrhythmias in ERS is higher than IVF with a reported risk of recurrence of 40% within a mean follow-up of 5 years.[44] Higher amplitude of J-point elevation has been linked to a higher risk of recurrence and quinidine has been shown to be effective in eliminating arrhythmias.[44]

Short-Coupled Ventricular Fibrillation

SCVF is diagnosed by documenting VF or polymorphic VT initiated by a PVC with a coupling interval of less than 350 ms in the absence of electrical or myocardial disease.[29] Similar to ERS, a complete evaluation needs to be performed before

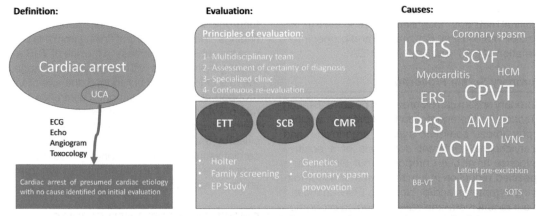

Fig. 4. Overview of unexplained cardiac arrest including definition, evaluation, and potential etiologies. ACMP, arrhythmogenic cardiomyopathy; AMVP, arrhythmic mitral valve prolapse; BBRVT, bundle branch reentrant ventricular tachycardia; BrS, Brugada syndrome; CMR, cardiac magnetic resonance imaging; CPVT, catecholaminergic polymorphic ventricular tachycardia; ECG, electrocardiogram; EP study, electrophysiology study; ERS, early repolarization syndrome; ETT, exercise treadmill test; HCM, hypertrophic cardiomyopathy; IVF, idiopathic ventricular fibrillation; LQTS, long QT syndrome; LVNC, left ventricular noncompaction cardiomyopathy; SCB, sodium-channel blocker challenge; SCVF, short-coupled ventricular fibrillation; SQTS, short QT syndrome; UCA, unexplained cardiac arrest.

entertaining the diagnosis of SCVF. This is particularly important in SCVF because other conditions are well described to cause short-coupled PVCs such as ESR, BrS, and myocarditis.[44–46] By virtue of its definition, documenting the initiation of the arrest rhythm is necessary to establish the diagnosis and, as such, most of the diagnoses are made during follow-up by examining the initiation of recurrent ventricular arrhythmias on intracardiac tracings. However, the diagnosis can be made at the time of arrest in patients with VF storms or those having runs of nonsustained polymorphic VT, which can be made by carefully examining telemetry strips in patients with UCA during their initial admission. Quinidine has been shown to be effective in those with recurrent ventricular arrhythmias.[29]

Arrhythmic Mitral Valve Prolapse

AMVP refers to the subset of patients with MVP who are at risk for developing malignant ventricular arrhythmias such as cardiac arrest or arrhythmic death in large part independent of LV dysfunction.[47] In patients with UCA, AMVP should be diagnosed in those with MVP and no cause identified despite complete evaluation. Typically, these patients have bileaflet prolapse, mitral annular disjunction, and/or frequent and complex PVCs.[7,48] Similar to ERS, due to the prevalence of MVP in the general population of (1%–3%), it is expected to be found in patients with UCA and might not be the primary cause of arrest.[49] Indeed, In CASPER, 17% of patients with UCA and MVP

were found to have an alternative diagnosis for their arrest, highlighting the point that complete evaluation of patients with UCA and MVP should be performed before diagnosing AMVP.[50]

Calcium Release Deficiency Syndrome

CRDS is a newly reported form of inherited heart disease that manifests secondary to *RyR2* loss of function.[6] In contrast to CPVT, which arises secondary to *RyR2* gain of function, patients with CRDS most often have normal treadmill tests with no evidence of ventricular ectopy on exertion. Standard clinical testing is most often normal in patients with CRDS.[51–53] Because of the absence of a clinical test for CRDS, diagnosis can only be confirmed following *in vitro* confirmation that the *RyR2* rare variant results in a loss of function. At present, our limited insight into the condition renders management of probands and asymptomatic family members carrying these variants particularly challenging.

Idiopathic Ventricular Fibrillation

IVF is diagnosed when complete evaluation does not reveal any cause of UCA. However, there is no clear guidance as to what constitutes a complete evaluation. In order to standardize the terminology used, we proposed using the probability of missing an alternative diagnosis to grade the certainty of IVF diagnosis into definite, probable, or possible IVF.[3] The probability of missing an alternative diagnosis is determined by the number of high-yield tests that are not performed (**Fig. 5**).

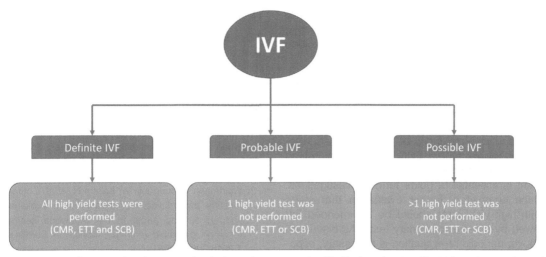

Fig. 5. Proposed criteria for the strength of idiopathic ventricular fibrillation diagnosis based on the number of high-yield tests were performed. CMR, cardiac magnetic resonance imaging; ETT, exercise treadmill test; IVF, idiopathic ventricular fibrillation; SCB, sodium-channel blocker challenge.

This is important because conditions such as ERS, AMVP, and SCVF should only be diagnosed after a complete evaluation (ie, definite IVF). It is likely that more conditions within the IVF cohort will be discovered in the future and, as such, having a uniform IVF definition will help guide the evaluation of these patients.

APPROACH TO PATIENTS WITH UNEXPLAINED CARDIAC ARREST

The approach to patients with UCA should be guided by the following principles:

1. Patients should be managed by a multidisciplinary team that includes, at least, an electrophysiologist, medical geneticist, and a genetic counselor.[54] These specialized clinics should have links to important services such as clinical psychology and molecular genetics.

2. Conditions diagnosed during evaluation should be assessed for the certainty of diagnosis. Established criteria for the strength of diagnosis should be utilized (eg, TFC for ARVC/Schwartz score for LQTS) and pre-specified criteria based on best available evidence should be developed and updated for conditions without established criteria.[55] This is to help avoid inaccurate diagnoses and assess the likelihood of alternative diagnoses when 2 or more conditions are suspected.

3. Patients should undergo periodic examination with re-evaluation of their diagnosis. This is important for 2 reasons. First, diagnoses can emerge during follow-up due to new findings in probands or their family members. Indeed, in CASPER, 7% of patients with UCA were found to have a cause during follow-up despite a negative initial evaluation.[10] Second, new evidence continues to describe new conditions

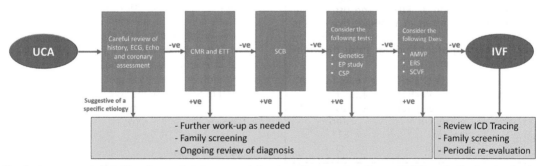

Fig. 6. A proposed algorithm for evaluating unexplained cardiac arrest patients. AMVP, arrhythmic mitral valve prolapse; CMR, cardiac magnetic resonance imaging; CSP, coronary spasm provocation; ECG, electrocardiogram; EP study, electrophysiology study; ERS, early repolarization syndrome; ETT, exercise treadmill test; ICD, implantable cardioverter-defibrillator; IVF, idiopathic ventricular fibrillation; SCB, sodium-channel blocker challenge; SCVF, short-coupled ventricular fibrillation; UCA, unexplained cardiac arrest.

that are distinct from IVF which affects family screening, managing recurrent arrhythmia, and prognosis. Examples of that include CRDS, AMVP, and SCVF.[8,29]

Fig. 6 shows our proposed algorithm for evaluating patients with UCA. It should start by a careful review of clinical information including clinical characteristics, pre-arrest symptoms, family history, and circumstances of cardiac arrest. Also, critical review of the ECG (including high-lead ECG), echocardiogram, and the coronary assessment is essential to guide further investigations. Once completed, further evaluation that starts with high-yield tests should be commenced followed by other discretionary tests. As discussed above, periodic re-evaluation is necessary, especially in those diagnosed with IVF.

CLINICS CARE POINTS

- Pearl: The evaluation process of unexplained cardiac arrest (UCA) should start with careful review of clinical information, electrocardiogram (ECG), echocardiogram, and the coronary assessment. Afterwards, further evaluation using the following high-yield diagnostic tests can be helpful: cardiac magnetic resonance imaging (CMR), exercise treadmill test (ETT), and sodium-channel blocker (SCB) challenge.

- Pearl: CMR can detect concealed structural changes that can be missed on echocardiograms. These include arrhythmogenic right ventricular cardiomyopathy (ARVC), hypertrophic cardiomyopathy (HCM), left ventricular non-compaction (LVNC), and myocarditis.

- Pearl: SCB challenge can induce a type 1 Brugada pattern in patients with normal baseline ECG or nondiagnostic Brugada patterns (type 2 and 3). Pitfall: The use of SCB challenge can result in false-positive results and should be interpreted with caution by incorporating other findings from the complete evaluation.

- Pitfall: Resting ECG alone may miss long QT syndrome and catecholaminergic polymorphic ventricular tachycardia, as these conditions may have concealed or intermittent ECG abnormalities. Therefore, an ETT should be considered in the evaluation of UCA.

DISCLOSURE

The authors have nothing to disclose.

FUNDING

This research received no specific grant from any funding agency in the public, commercial, or not-for-profit sectors.

REFERENCES

1. Berdowski J, Berg RA, Tijssen JGP, et al. Global incidences of out-of-hospital cardiac arrest and survival rates: systematic review of 67 prospective studies. Resuscitation 2010;81(11):1479–87.
2. Waldmann V, Bougouin W, Karam N, et al. Characteristics and clinical assessment of unexplained sudden cardiac arrest in the real-world setting: focus on idiopathic ventricular fibrillation. Eur Heart J 2018;39(21):1981–7.
3. Alqarawi W, Dewidar O, Tadros R, et al. Defining idiopathic ventricular fibrillation: a systematic review of diagnostic testing yield in apparently unexplained cardiac arrest. Heart Rhythm 2021;18(7):1178–85.
4. Priori SG, Wilde AA, Horie M, et al. HRS/EHRA/APHRS expert consensus statement on the diagnosis and management of patients with inherited primary arrhythmia syndromes: document endorsed by HRS, EHRA, and APHRS in May 2013 and by ACCF, AHA, PACES, and AEPC in June 2013. Heart Rhythm 2013;10(12):1932–63.
5. Brugada P, Brugada J. Right bundle branch block, persistent ST segment elevation and sudden cardiac death: a distinct clinical and electrocardiographic syndrome. A multicenter report. J Am Coll Cardiol 1992;20(6):1391–6.
6. Sun B, Yao J, Ni M, et al. Cardiac ryanodine receptor calcium release deficiency syndrome. Sci Transl Med 2021;13(579). https://doi.org/10.1126/scitranslmed.aba7287.
7. Sriram CS, Syed FF, Ferguson ME, et al. Malignant bileaflet mitral valve prolapse syndrome in patients with otherwise idiopathic out-of-hospital cardiac arrest. J Am Coll Cardiol 2013;62(3):222–30.
8. Sabbag A, Essayagh B, Barrera JDR, et al. EHRA expert consensus statement on arrhythmic mitral valve prolapse and mitral annular disjunction complex in collaboration with the ESC Council on valvular heart disease and the European Association of Cardiovascular Imaging endorsed cby the Heart Rhythm Society, by the Asia Pacific Heart Rhythm Society, and by the Latin American Heart Rhythm Society. Europace 2022. https://doi.org/10.1093/europace/euac125.
9. Sy RW, van der Werf C, Chattha IS, et al. Derivation and validation of a simple exercise-based algorithm for prediction of genetic testing in relatives of LQTS probands. Circulation 2011;124(20):2187–94.
10. Herman ARM, Cheung C, Gerull B, et al. Outcome of apparently unexplained cardiac arrest: results from

investigation and follow-up of the prospective cardiac arrest survivors with preserved ejection fraction registry. Circ Arrhythm Electrophysiol 2016;9(1). https://doi.org/10.1161/CIRCEP.115.003619.

11. Schwartz PJ, Crotti L. QTc behavior during exercise and genetic testing for the long-qt syndrome. Circulation 2011;124(20):2181–4.

12. Govindan M, Batchvarov VN, Raju H, et al. Utility of high and standard right precordial leads during ajmaline testing for the diagnosis of Brugada syndrome. Heart 2010;96(23):1904–8.

13. Cheung CC, Mellor G, Deyell MW, et al. Comparison of ajmaline and Procainamide provocation tests in the diagnosis of brugada syndrome. JACC Clin Electrophysiol 2019;5(4):504–12.

14. Peters S, Trümmel M, Denecke S, et al. Results of ajmaline testing in patients with arrhythmogenic right ventricular dysplasia-cardiomyopathy. Int J Cardiol 2004;95(2–3):207–10.

15. Peters S. Arrhythmogenic right ventricular dysplasia-cardiomyopathy and provocable coved-type ST-segment elevation in right precordial leads: clues from long-term follow-up. Europace 2008;10(7):816–20.

16. Meregalli PG, Ruijter JM, Hofman N, et al. Diagnostic value of flecainide testing in unmasking SCN5A-related Brugada syndrome. J Cardiovasc Electrophysiol 2006;17(8):857–64.

17. Hong K, Brugada J, Oliva A, et al. Value of electrocardiographic parameters and ajmaline test in the diagnosis of Brugada syndrome caused by SCN5A mutations. Circulation 2004;110(19):3023–7.

18. Tadros R, Nannenberg EA, Lieve Kv, et al. Yield and pitfalls of ajmaline testing in the evaluation of unexplained cardiac arrest and sudden unexplained death: single-center experience with 482 families. JACC Clin Electrophysiol 2017;3(12):1400–8.

19. Borgquist R, Haugaa KH, Gilljam T, et al. The diagnostic performance of imaging methods in ARVC using the 2010 task force criteria. Eur Heart J Cardiovasc Imaging 2014;15(11):1219–25.

20. Holmström M, Kivistö S, Heliö T, et al. Late gadolinium enhanced cardiovascular magnetic resonance of lamin A/C gene mutation related dilated cardiomyopathy. J Cardiovasc Magn Reson 2011;13(1). https://doi.org/10.1186/1532-429X-13-30.

21. Domenech-Ximenos B, Sanz-De La Garza M, Prat-González S, et al. Prevalence and pattern of cardiovascular magnetic resonance late gadolinium enhancement in highly trained endurance athletes. J Cardiovasc Magn Reson 2020;22(1). https://doi.org/10.1186/s12968-020-00660-w.

22. Lücke C, Karthe D, Matthias G, et al. Frequency and variability of late gadolinium "mid-wall" enhancement(MLE) depending on observer experience, image quality and underlying disease. J Cardiovasc Magn Reson 2011;13(S1):P286.

23. Tandri H, Castillo E, Ferrari VA, et al. Magnetic resonance imaging of arrhythmogenic right ventricular dysplasia. Sensitivity, specificity, and observer variability of fat detection versus functional analysis of the right ventricle. J Am Coll Cardiol 2006;48(11):2277–84.

24. Sievers B, Addo M, Franken U, et al. Right ventricular wall motion abnormalities found in healthy subjects by cardiovascular magnetic resonance imaging and characterized with a new segmental model. J Cardiovasc Magn Reson 2004;6(3):601–8.

25. Shimizu W, Noda T, Takaki H, et al. Diagnostic value of epinephrine test for genotyping LQT1, LQT2, and LQT3 forms of congenital long QT syndrome. Heart Rhythm 2004;1(3):276–83.

26. Ackerman MJ, Khositseth A, Tester DJ, et al. Epinephrine-induced QT interval prolongation: a gene-specific paradoxical response in congenital long QT syndrome. Mayo Clin Proc 2002;77(5):413–21.

27. Churet M, Luttoo K, Hocini M, et al. Diagnostic reproducibility of epinephrine drug challenge interpretation in suspected long QT syndrome. J Cardiovasc Electrophysiol 2019;30(6):896–901.

28. Krahn AD, Healey JS, Chauhan VS, et al. Epinephrine infusion in the evaluation of unexplained cardiac arrest and familial sudden death: from the Cardiac Arrest Survivors with Preserved Ejection Fraction Registry. Circ Arrhythm Electrophysiol 2012;5(5):933–40.

29. Steinberg C, Davies B, Mellor G, et al. Short-coupled ventricular fibrillation represents a distinct phenotype among latent causes of unexplained cardiac arrest: a report from the CASPER registry. Eur Heart J 2021;42(29):2827–38.

30. Mauriello DA, Johnson JN, Ackerman MJ. Holter monitoring in the evaluation of congenital long QT syndrome. Pacing Clin Electrophysiol 2011;34(9):1100–4.

31. Neyroud N, Maison-Blanche P, Denjoy I, et al. Diagnostic performance of QT interval variables from 24-h electrocardiography in the long QT syndrome. Eur Heart J 1998;19(1):158–65.

32. Tamr Agha MK, Fakhri G, Ahmed M, et al. QTc interval on 24-hour holter monitor: to trust or not to trust? Ann Noninvasive Electrocardiol 2022;27(1). https://doi.org/10.1111/anec.12899.

33. Shimeno K, Takagi M, Maeda K, et al. Usefulness of multichannel holter ECG recording in the third intercostal space for detecting type 1 brugada ECG: comparison with repeated 12-lead ECGs. J Cardiovasc Electrophysiol 2009;20(9):1026–31.

34. Gray B, Kirby A, Kabunga P, et al. Twelve-lead ambulatory electrocardiographic monitoring in Brugada syndrome: potential diagnostic and prognostic implications. Heart Rhythm 2017;14(6):866–74.

35. Steinberg C, Padfield GJ, Champagne J, et al. Cardiac abnormalities in first-degree relatives of unexplained cardiac arrest victims. Circ Arrhythm Electrophysiol 2016;9(9). https://doi.org/10.1161/CIRCEP.115.004274.

36. Foo FS, Stiles MK, Heaven D. Unmasking latent pre-excitation of a right-sided accessory pathway with intravenous adenosine after unexplained sudden cardiac arrest. J Arrhythm 2020;36(5):939–41.

37. Roberts JD, Gollob MH, Young C, et al. Bundle branch Re-entrant ventricular tachycardia: novel genetic mechanisms in a life-threatening arrhythmia. JACC Clin Electrophysiol 2017;3(3):276–88.

38. Kamakura T, Wada M, Ishibashi K, et al. Significance of coronary artery spasm diagnosis in patients with early repolarization syndrome. J Am Heart Assoc 2018;7(4). https://doi.org/10.1161/JAHA.117.007942.

39. Komatsu M, Takahashi J, Fukuda K, et al. Usefulness of testing for coronary artery spasm and programmed ventricular stimulation in survivors of out-of-hospital cardiac arrest. Circ Arrhythm Electrophysiol 2016;9(9). https://doi.org/10.1161/CIRCEP.115.003798.

40. Wilde AAM, Semsarian C, Márquez MF, et al. European heart rhythm association (EHRA)/Heart rhythm society (HRS)/Asia pacific heart rhythm society (APHRS)/Latin American heart rhythm society (LAHRS) expert consensus statement on the state of genetic testing for cardiac diseases. Europace 2022;24(8):1307–67.

41. Grondin S, Davies B, Cadrin-Tourigny J, et al. Importance of genetic testing in unexplained cardiac arrest. Eur Heart J 2022;43(32):3071–81.

42. Derval N, Simpson CS, Birnie DH, et al. Prevalence and characteristics of early repolarization in the CASPER registry: cardiac arrest survivors with preserved ejection fraction registry. J Am Coll Cardiol 2011;58(7):722–8.

43. Malhi N, So PP, Cheung CC, et al. Early repolarization pattern inheritance in the cardiac arrest survivors with preserved ejection fraction registry (CASPER). JACC Clin Electrophysiol 2018;4(11):1473–9.

44. Haïssaguerre M, Derval N, Sacher F, et al. Sudden cardiac arrest associated with early repolarization. N Engl J Med 2008;358(19):2016–23.

45. Kakishita M, Kurita T, Matsuo K, et al. Mode of onset of ventricular fibrillation in patients with Brugada syndrome detected by implantable cardioverter defibrillator therapy. J Am Coll Cardiol 2000;36(5):1646–53.

46. Marume K, Ishibashi K, Noda T, et al. Short coupled Torsade de pointes with myocardial injury: a possible sequela of myocarditis. J Cardiol Cases 2019;19(2):62–5.

47. Essayagh B, Sabbag A, Antoine C, et al. Presentation and outcome of arrhythmic mitral valve prolapse. J Am Coll Cardiol 2020;76(6):637–49.

48. Hourdain J, Clavel MA, Deharo JC, et al. Common phenotype in patients with mitral valve prolapse who experienced sudden cardiac death. Circulation 2018;138(10):1067–9.

49. Freed LA, Levy D, Levine RA, et al. Prevalence and clinical outcome of mitral-valve prolapse. N Engl J Med 1999;341(1):1–7.

50. Alqarawi W, Cheung CC, Roberts JD, et al. Mitral valve prolapse among patients with an unexplained cardiac arrest. Heart Rhythm 2020;17(5 Supplement):S666.

51. Roston TM, Wei J, Guo W, et al. Clinical and functional characterization of ryanodine receptor 2 variants implicated in calcium-release deficiency syndrome. JAMA Cardiol 2022;7(1):84–92.

52. Li Y, Wei J, Guo W, et al. Human RyR2 (ryanodine receptor 2) loss-of-function mutations: clinical phenotypes and in vitro characterization. Circ Arrhythm Electrophysiol 2021;14(9):874–85.

53. Ormerod JOM, Ormondroyd E, Li Y, et al. Provocation testing and therapeutic response in a newly described channelopathy: RyR2 calcium release deficiency syndrome. Circ Genom Precis Med 2022;15(1):E003589.

54. Stiles MK, Wilde AAM, Abrams DJ, et al. 2020 APHRS/HRS expert consensus statement on the investigation of decedents with sudden unexplained death and patients with sudden cardiac arrest, and of their families. Heart Rhythm 2021;18(1):e1–50.

55. Davies B, Roberts JD, Tadros R, et al. The hearts in rhythm organization: a Canadian national cardiogenetics network. CJC Open 2020;2(6):652–62.

Calcium Release Deficiency Syndrome
A New Inherited Arrhythmia Syndrome

Dania Kallas, MS[a], Jason D. Roberts, MD, MAS[b], Shubhayan Sanatani, MD[a],
Thomas M. Roston, MD, PhD[c],*

KEYWORDS

- Ryanodine receptor • RyR2 • Calcium release deficiency syndrome • Inherited arrhythmia
- Sudden death • Idiopathic ventricular fibrillation
- Catecholaminergic polymorphic ventricular tachycardia

KEY POINTS

- Calcium release deficiency syndrome (CRDS) is characterized by cardiac ryanodine receptor (RyR2) loss-of-function and is distinct from catecholaminergic polymorphic ventricular tachycardia (CPVT).
- In contrast to CPVT, patients with CRDS appear to have no or minimal ventricular arrhythmias during exercise stress test.
- Early afterdepolarizations are the underlying triggering mechanism that leads to ventricular arrhythmias in CRDS.
- An electrophysiology study consisting of a long burst, long pause, and short-coupled extra-stimulus ("LBLPS") appears to induce polymorphic ventricular arrhythmias in CRDS, but not CPVT.

INTRODUCTION

Sudden cardiac arrest (SCA) in the young is a rare, devastating event. Following comprehensive evaluation, the etiology remains unexplained in up to half of survivors and is termed unexplained cardiac arrest (UCA).[1–3] Contemporary advancements in clinical testing and genetic sequencing have standardized our approach to the established primary arrhythmia syndromes that predispose to SCA. These include long QT syndrome, Brugada syndrome, short QT syndrome, early repolarization syndrome, catecholaminergic polymorphic ventricular tachycardia (CPVT), and now a newly recognized condition known as calcium release deficiency syndrome (CRDS). Up until recently, most cases of CRDS were classified as idiopathic ventricular fibrillation (IVF) or labelled as atypical CPVT due to several apparent similarities between the conditions, including a common gene and predisposition to sudden arrhythmic death. However, CRDS is caused by loss-of-function (LOF) variants in the cardiac ryanodine receptor (RyR2) and contrasts from CPVT which occurs secondary to RyR2 gain-of-function (GOF) variants. Their distinct pathophysiologies align with observed differences in their respective clinical phenotypes. RyR2-associated CPVT manifests with bidirectional and polymorphic ventricular arrhythmias during exercise, but such adrenergic-induced ventricular ectopy is generally absent in CRDS. Instead, a specific pattern of induced or spontaneous ectopy

[a] Department of Pediatrics, Division of Cardiology, BC Children's Hospital, Heart Center, 4480 Oak Street, Vancouver, British Columbia V6H 3V4, Canada; [b] Population Health Research Institute, McMaster University and Hamilton Health Sciences, C3-111, 237 Barton Street East, Hamilton, Ontario L8L 2X2, Canada; [c] Division of Cardiology and Centre for Cardiovascular Innovation, The University of British Columbia, 1081 Burrard Street, 4th Floor – Burrard Building, Vancouver, British Columbia V6Z 1Y6, Canada
* Corresponding author
E-mail address: rostontm@alumni.ubc.ca
Twitter: @Daniakallas2 (D.K.)

Card Electrophysiol Clin 15 (2023) 319–329
https://doi.org/10.1016/j.ccep.2023.05.003
1877-9182/23/© 2023 Elsevier Inc. All rights reserved.

appears to be needed to trigger CRDS-related arrhythmias. As such, substantial evidence now exists to define CRDS as a unique inherited arrhythmia syndrome caused by pathogenic LOF variants in RyR2.[4,5] In this review, we summarize the existing molecular, clinical, and therapeutic data on CRDS, and compare it to CPVT.

MOLECULAR MECHANISM: CRDS VERSUS CPVT

RyR2 is a large tetrameric ion channel located on the sarcoplasmic reticulum (SR) which controls the release of Ca^{2+} from the SR lumen to the cytosol. Excitation–contraction coupling (ECC) in cardiac myocytes is regulated by changes in intracellular Ca^{2+}. In normal ECC, depolarization of the sarcolemma and T-tubules trigger the release of Ca^{2+} from L-type Ca^{2+} channels. An increase in cytosolic Ca^{2+} triggers the spontaneous release of Ca^{2+} from the SR in a process called calcium-induced calcium release (CICR), which in turn leads to the downstream contraction of cardiomyocytes. In CPVT, GOF RyR2 variants lead to diastolic leakage of Ca^{2+} from the SR into the cytoplasm and promote delayed afterdepolarizations (DADs) as a result of a leaky RyR2 channel.[6] It is hypothesized that RyR2 variants enhance the channel's sensitivity to the luminal Ca^{2+} concentration reducing the threshold for spontaneous SR Ca^{2+} through a store overload-induced Ca^{2+} release (SOICR) mediated mechanism.[6]

In contrast, patients with LOF RyR2 variants leading to CRDS ultimately have depressed response to luminal Ca^{2+} and low open RyR2 probability state in the presence of agonists such as cytosolic Ca^{2+} and caffeine.[7] In 2007, Jiang and colleagues proposed that the ineffective autoregulation of SR Ca^{2+} release, as a result of diminished luminal Ca^{2+} sensitivity and reduced SR Ca^{2+} overload, increases the propensity for Ca^{2+} alternans and electromechanical alternans. This concept was further advanced by Zhao and colleagues who identified through a RyR2 p.A4860G$^{+/-}$ mouse model that early afterdepolarizations (EADs), as opposed to DADs, inhibited the Ca^{2+} dependent Ca^{2+} channel inactivation.[8,9] EADs occur when the action potential duration is increased. The proposed mechanism of EAD pathogenesis in the presence of a LOF *RYR2* variant is as follows (**Fig. 1**): (1) The depolarization of the sarcolemma opens L-type Ca^{2+} channels which induces the activation of RyR2 via cytosolic Ca^{2+}; (2) The lack of luminal Ca^{2+} sensitivity and low open probability state of RyR2, coupled with consecutive pulses of Ca^{2+} currents, increases SR Ca^{2+} load; (3) Once the luminal Ca^{2+} threshold

is reached, SR Ca^{2+} is unloaded into the cytosol; (4) The release of Ca^{2+} from the SR during systole occurs in a decreased, but prolonged manner, which inhibits CICR; (5) Simultaneously, the sodium–calcium exchanger (NCX) generates an inward current (during the plateau and descending phase of an action potential) which enhances the prolonged Ca^{2+} release from the SR inducing EADs; (6) These EADs increase the likelihood that re-entrant arrhythmias lead to ventricular arrhythmias and thus, the risk of SCA.[10]

The reduced response to Ca^{2+} sensitivity as a result of LOF RyR2 variants has been postulated to be a result of a defective gating mechanism of RyR2.[11] The stabilization of the channel in the closed and open states are controlled by the interactions near the channel pore (central domain) or surrounding region.[11] Mutations affecting the interaction between the U-motif (a key component for channel opening), S2-S3 linker domains, S1-S2 or S2-S3 interface of RyR2 can disrupt channel sensitivity and opening, which leads to the diminished or complete loss of function of RyR2.[11] In addition, LOF variants such as RyR2 p.D3291V, which decreases the S2808 phosphorylation levels of RyR2, may affect intra/inter domain interactions, important for channel gating, which in turn affects luminal Ca^{2+} sensitivity and/or conductance.[12] In the simplest of terms, the mechanism of CRDS appears to be the direct "opposite" to that of CPVT, despite the clinical entities appearing similar.

A recently devised electrophysiology test has become a promising diagnostic maneuver to identify CRDS based on in vitro and clinical studies, termed the long burst, long pause, short-coupled ventricular extra-stimulus (LBLPS) protocol.[4] In mutant mice experiments, this specifically consisted of a long burst of 20 beats at 60-ms cycle length, then a long-coupled ventricular extrastimulus of 122-ms, and a subsequent short-coupled ventricular extrastimulus, which was progressively reduced from 78-ms to 18-ms in 4-ms increments.[4] In RyR2 LOF mutant mice, this specific stimulation sequence was able to induce ventricular arrhythmias, but did not result in any arrhythmias in RyR2 GOF mutant mice or WT control mice. It is hypothesized that the aberrantly large Ca^{2+} flux during the long-pause beat after rapid tachycardia, either spontaneously occurring or pacing-induced in the lab, increases the likelihood for the short-coupled extra stimulus to trigger EADs and EAD-mediated re-entrant arrhythmia.[10] No other commonly used protocols could induce CRDS-related arrhythmias. These important findings were replicated in CRDS patient studies which showed a similar pattern of ectopy to the LBLPS protocol preceding spontaneous events.[4]

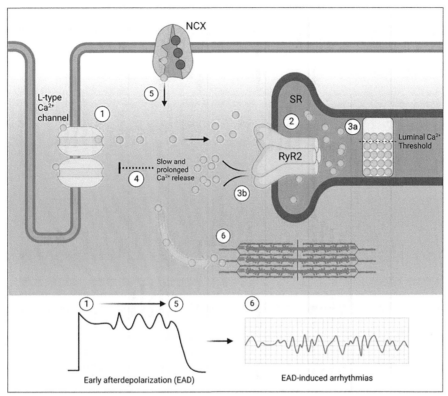

Fig. 1. *Mechanism of early afterdepolarization (EAD) as a result of a loss of function RyR2 mutation.* (1) Depolarization of L-type Ca^{2+} channels induces Ca^{2+}-induced Ca^{2+} release (CICR) from sarcoplasmic reticulum (SR); (2) Consecutive pulses of Ca^{2+} currents increases SR Ca^{2+} load; (3) Once the luminal Ca^{2+} threshold is reached, SR Ca^{2+} is unloaded into the cytosol in a prolonged manner (3b); (4) Ca^{2+} released from the SR inhibits CICR; (5) The Na^+/Ca^{2+} exchanger (NCX) generates an inward current prolonging the action potential and thus developing EADs; (6) EADs lead to ventricular arrhythmias.

PRESENTATIONS AND SYMPTOMS: CRDS VERSUS CPVT

Despite the novelty of CRDS, much has been learned from the individual cases described thus far. In the seminal study identifying RyR2 as the primary gene associated with CPVT, 4 of 30 (13%) patients carried a referring diagnosis of "catecholaminergic idiopathic ventricular fibrillation," a term used to describe cardiac arrest victims with a normal exercise stress test (EST).[13] One of these patients was a 7-year old girl with a family history of premature SUD in her mother and maternal uncle who harbored the RyR2 p.A4860G variant. She survived a catecholamine-stimulated cardiac arrest, and was then treated with a β-blocker and an implantable cardioverter defibrillator (ICD). Because her EST was entirely normal, she was classified as having an atypical form of CPVT. Further investigation of the RyR2 p.A4860G variant in cellular[7] and mice models[9] identified this to be the first known LOF variant in RyR2.[13] Several years later, a RyR2 p.S4938F

LOF variant [8] was reported in a patient who had short-coupled torsades de pointes.[8] These findings raised the possibility that these cases represented a condition that was phenotypically and genetically distinct from traditional CPVT.[5] Since then, many more cases of CRDS have emerged in the literature,[4,10,14,15] substantiating this early hypothesis.

The variants identified to date and associated phenotypes of LOF RyR2 variants are described in **Table 1**. A total of 33 patient-specific RyR2 variants with in vitro data confirmatory of LOF have been reported in 12 publications to date. The two largest studies of CRDS were published in 2021; the first led by Sun and colleagues[4] focused on evidence for disease-causation and arrhythmia inducibility via the LBLPS protocol in 6 families, and the second[14] was a multicenter international initiative that identified 19 individuals (6 probands and 13 family members) with RyR2 LOF variants. While disease penetrance remains uncertain, both studies reported multigenerational sudden cardiac arrest, death, and syncope in several

Table 1
Phenotype and genotype of cases with known loss of function RyR2 variants

RyR2 Variant Protein Change	RyR2 Hotspot	Age of Symptom-Onset	Sex	Symptoms	Circumstance Preceding Symptoms	Phenotype/ Working Diagnosis	Last Prescribed Therapy	ICD Appropriate Shock (for VT/VF)	Worst Arrhythmia on EST or ECG	Known Affected Individuals and Respective Phenotype	RyR2 Variant Carriers[a]	Reference
										(Family/Relatives)		
A4860G	4	7	F	Syncope	Exercise and Emotion	"Catecholaminergic IVF"	Nadolol and ICD	3	None	2 SCD	2 carriers: 1 asymptomatic and 1 obligate carrier	Jiang et al,[7] 2007
I4855M	4	10	F	SCA	Exertion	Pre-excitation, LVNC	Carvedilol and ICD	None	Bigeminy	3 SUD/SCD/QT prolongation/ LVNC with normal ejection fraction	2 carriers: 1 symptomatic and 1 obligate carrier	Roston et al,[16] 2017
S4938F	4	13	M	Syncope	Exertion	scTdP (230-ms), VF induced by PVCs	Verapamil and ICD	Yes (unknown number)	None	None	2 carriers: 1 asymptomatic and 1 obligate carrier	Fuji et al,[8] 2017 and Hirose et al,[18] 2022
A4142T	3	22	M	SCA	Rest	None	ICD	1	Isolated VEs and single ventricular couplet	4 SCD/SCA	17 carriers: 13 symptomatic	Ormrod et al,[15] 2022
Q3774L	NH	12	F	SCA	Emotion	None	Propranolol, Flecainide, ICD	1	None	None	3 asymptomatic carriers	Sun et al,[4] 2021
I3995V	3	52	F	Syncope	Watching TV	None	Metoprolol and ICD	No but PVT/VF recorded	None	4 SUD/SCD	7 carriers: 3 asymptomatic carriers	
D4112N	3	15	M	SCA	Exertion	VF	Nadolol and ICD	3	None	4 SCD/SCA	6 carriers: 2 asymptomatic carriers	
T4196I	3	17	F	Syncope, SCD (19 y)	Exertion	None	None	N/a	None	2 SCD	2 symptomatic carriers	
D4646A	4	39	F	SCA, Syncope	Emotion	IVF	Metoprolol and ICD	1	None	5 SCD	6 gene carriers: 2 asymptomatic	
Q4879H	4	11	M	SCA	Emotion	VF	ICD	None	None	None	None	
K4594R/ I2075T	4/NH	13	F	SCA	Unknown	None	ICD	None	None	7 SCA/SCD and seizures	7 mutation carriers	

Variant		Age	Sex	Symptoms	Trigger	ECG/Clinical	Treatment		Arrhythmia	Family history	Carriers	Reference
Homozygous, biallelic tandem duplication, RYR2's 5' UTR/ promoter region, and exons 1–4 of RYR2	N/a	15	F	Syncope, SCD	Exercise	None	Unknown	N/a	None	14 SCD and SCA <30 y	14 symptomatic carriers (some heterozygous and some homozygous)	Tester et al,[20,21] 2020
D3291V	NH	Family 1: 10 Family 2: 20 Family 3: 10	Family 1: F Family 2: F Family 3: F	Family 1: Syncope, SCD (14 y) Family 2: Syncope Family 3: SCD	Family 1: Emotion/ moderate hypokalemia Family 2: Not reported Family 3: Exercise	Family 1: Initially diagnosed with CPVT Family 2 and 3: None	Unknown	N/A	Family 1 and 3: Unknown Family 2: PVCs and ventricular bigeminy	Family 1: 8 SCDs <30 y of age, some were homozygous and others heterozygous for variant Family 2: 2 SCD Family 3: No family inquiry made	Family 1: 39 carriers Family 2: 6 carriers Family 3: unknown	Blancard et al,[12] 2021
K4594Q	4	10	F	Syncope	Exercise	LQTS (QTc: 485-ms)	Unknown	N/a	Unknown	Unknown	Unknown	Hirose et al,[18] 2022
S4168P	3	Before birth	M	Asymptomatic	N/a	Bradycardia and LQTS (QTc: 514-ms)	Mexiletine	N/a	Unknown	1 Syncope/epilepsy	1	
E4146D	3	0.2	F	SCA and Syncope	Emotion	VF, TdP, short coupled PVCs and LQTS (QTc: 506-ms)	Carvedilol and flecainide, ICD	1	Unknown	None	None	
G570D	NH	34	Not reported	SCA	Normal daily activity	None	ICD	2	PVCs during recovery	1 SCD	Unknown	Li et al,[10] 2021
R4147K	4	14	F	SCA, Syncope	Unknown	VF	Metoprolol and ICD	1	Unable to perform	Unknown	4 asymptomatic carriers	
A4203V	NH	25	F	Seizure	Unknown	IVF	ICD and flecainide	Unknown	Unknown	Unknown	Unknown	
Q3925E	3	Unknown	Unknown	SCD	Unknown	Unknown	Unknown Amiodarone and quinidine	Unknown	Unknown	Unknown	Unknown	
M4109R	3	31	F	SCA	Emotion	None		N/A	None	3 SCD/SCA/VF	6	
A4204V	NH	16	F	SCA, syncope	Exertion (running to school bus/stairs)	VF, acute myocarditis, prolonged QTc (490-ms)	Carvedilol and ICD	1	None	Unknown	Unknown	
E1127G	NH	25	F	SCA	Emotion/Rest	None	ICD	Unknown	None	1 SCD	1 asymptomatic carrier	Kobayshi et al,[11] 2022
A3442E	NH	16	F	Pre-syncope and syncope	Emotion	None	Nadolol and ICD	Unknown	Couplets and bidirectional triplets	Unknown	Unknown	
I3476T	NH	2	F	Syncope	Emotion	PVT/TdP, Prolonged QT (QT not reported)	Unspecified β-blocker	N/a	Polymorphic ventricular couplets and triplets	None	1 asymptomatic carrier	

(continued on next page)

Table 1
(continued)

RYR2 Variant Protein Change	RyR2 Hotspot	Age of Symptom-Onset	Sex	Symptoms	Circumstance Preceding Symptoms	Phenotype/ Working Diagnosis	Last Prescribed Therapy	ICD Appropriate Shock (for VT/VF)	Worst Arrhythmia on EST or ECG	Known Affected Individuals and Respective Phenotype	RYR2 Variant Carriers[a]	Reference
						Proband					Family/Relatives	
Q2275H	2	22 (IQR: 8-34)	F	SCA, Syncope	Normal daily activity	SVT	Metoprolol and ICD	Yes (unknown number)	None	Unknown	Unknown	Roston et al,[14] 2022
E4415del	NH		F	SUD	Unknown	None	None	N/a	Unable to perform	Unknown	2 asymptomatic carriers	
F4499C	4		F	Syncope	Emotion	Atrial fibrillation	Nadolol and ICD	Yes (unknown number)	Isolated PVCs	Unknown	1 symptomatic carrier	
V4606E	4		F	Syncope, Seizure	Normal daily activity	Atrial tachycardia, dilated cardiomyopathy	Metoprolol and flecainide	N/a	Isolated PVCs and 1 monomorphic couplet	Unknown	Unknown	
R4608Q	4		M	Palpitations, SUD	Emotion and Exertion	None	None	N/a	Unable to perform	Unknown	10 carriers: 8 asymptomatic	
R4608W	4		F	SCA	Exertion	None	Bisoprolol and ICD	None	None	Unknown	Unknown	
E4146K	3	14	M	SUD	Sleep	None	Unknown	N/a	Unknown	SCD	Unknown	Zhong et al,[19] 2021
G4935R	4	4	F	Loss of consciousness and SCD (8 y)	Exertion	Bradycardia in utero	Unknown	N/a	None	Seizures	Unknown	

Abbreviations: CPVT, catecholaminergic polymorphic ventricular tachycardia; F, female; ICD, implantable cardioverter defibrillator; IVF, idiopathic ventricular fibrillation; LVNC, left ventricular non-compaction; M, male; N/a, not applicable; NH, not in hotspot; SCA, sudden cardiac arrest; SCD, sudden cardiac death; SUD, sudden unexpected death; SVT, supraventricular tachycardia; scTdP, short-coupled torsades de pointes; VF, ventricular fibrillation; VT, ventricular tachycardia; EST, exercise stress test; ECG, electrocardiogram; PVC, premature ventricular complex; LQTS, long QT syndrome.

[a] Excluding the proband but inclusive of obligate carriers.

CRDS families (see **Table 1**). Like CPVT, 4 of 33 (12%) patients who had a confirmed LOF-RyR2 variant experienced atrial arrhythmias. However, breakthrough cardiac events was less frequent among CRDS cases than CPVT. Finally, these studies also reported that the majority of CRDS variants occurred in the C-terminus of RyR2, which may indicate the direct relationship between mutations affecting the pore region and LOF. It is however important to recognize that the C-terminus also comprises disease-associated "Hotspot 3" and "Hotspot 4" in CPVT, making variant localization likely an insensitive marker for differentiating CRDS from CPVT.

There are several other clinical findings in CRDS warranting discussion. Two RyR2 LOF variants, p.I4855M[16] and p.V4606E,[14] have been associated with non-compaction and dilated cardiomyopathy, respectively. In the case of RyR2 p.V4606E, the resulting impact of the variant in vitro is a total loss of channel function even at extremely high concentrations of caffiene activation. Whether the degree of LOF may affect myocardial development or function remains to be investigated further. Based on these two cases, it may be beneficial to follow patients with CRDS with serial echocardiography. Similarly, albeit likely through a different mechanism, RyR2 exon 3 deletion syndrome can also cause non-compaction cardiomyopathy, which is due to a GOF-RyR2 variant, not a LOF-RyR2 variant.[17] In other cases of CRDS, QTc prolongation (mean 499-ms) and/or bradycardia have also been reported in patients with RyR2 LOF variants, p.K4594Q, p.S4168P, p.E4146D, p.A4204V, p.I3476T, and p.G4935R.[10,11,18,19] It is speculated that the slow Ca^{2+} release from the SR prolongs phase 2 of the cardiac action potential thereby, supressing the inactivation of L-type Ca^{2+} channels, which may manifest as a prolongation of the QT interval.[20] Bradycardia is thought to be the result of an impaired "Ca^{2+} clock" which regulates pacemaker activity in sinoatrial nodal cells.[18] A familial report by Tester and colleagues also suggested that copy number variant testing may also help identify novel LOF RyR2 variants. These authors identified two seemingly unrelated Amish families with large homozygous tandem duplications of 344,085 base pairs involving 26,000 base pairs of intergenic sequence spanning *RYR2* 5'UTR/promoter region and exon 1 to 4.[21] There were penetrant family histories of exercise-associated SCDs during childhood and adolescence: 22 of 23 were symptomatic and 18 of 23 experienced SCD.[21] These individuals had intermittently prolonged QTc intervals (466-ms) or prominent U waves and normal ESTs, epinephrine

challenges, and ambulatory monitors.[21] Functional analysis revealed that the tandem duplication caused a 70% to 80% reduction in RyR2 mRNA transcript and RyR2 protein expression in induced pluripotent stem cells derived cardiomyocytes (iPSC-CM). This was reported to lead to diminished Ca^{2+} handling and a CICR apparatus that was insensitive to catecholamines and caffeine.[20] Importantly, this autosomal recessive inherited condition may differ from the wider descriptions of CRDS, which is caused by autosomal dominant RyR2-LOF variants.

DIAGNOSTIC CONSIDERATIONS IN CRDS

CRDS should be considered as a possible diagnosis whenever a potentially damaging RyR2 variant, particularly in the C-terminus (amino acids 3778–4959), is identified in a patient with a life-threatening arrhythmia. However, standard clinical testing is usually normal in CRDS, meaning that it has an electrocardiographic phenotype distinct from that of classic CPVT, particularly with respect to an EST (**Fig. 2**). **Table 1** summarizes EST findings associated with the RyR2 LOF variants implicated in CRDS, as well as the triggers that precede CRDS events. Exertion and emotion were the most common circumstances preceding symptom onset in patients, but were not universally observed. There were 7 cases where rest and/or normal daily activity (watching TV, sleep) preceded the onset of a life-threatening arrhythmic event. Thus, the circumstances preceding events are alone not useful in predicting RyR2 mechanism. Nevertheless, in some cases, patients with CRDS do manifest isolated ventricular ectopy during exercise. However, these extrasystoles do not resemble the crescendo pattern of bidirectional or polymorphic ventricular tachycardia (PVT) with increasing workload that is considered to be diagnostic of CPVT. Rather, non-sustained ventricular arrhythmias during EST may be monomorphic in nature and occur mainly during recovery from exercise in CRDS. These ventricular arrhythmias seen after an adrenergic-triggered event, especially when an RyR2 variant is found, can easily be mistaken for CPVT.[14] In patients without a classic CPVT phenotype during EST, it may be worthwhile to order a burst protocol[22] EST to rule out latent CPVT, before considering CRDS. Accordingly, clinicians may be particularly vulnerable to misdiagnosing CRDS as CPVT when the variant is ascertained through the molecular autopsy in a victim of exertional SCA, or when an EST is not performed.

The most promising diagnostic test for CRDS at present is the LBLPS. The LBLPS protocol, first

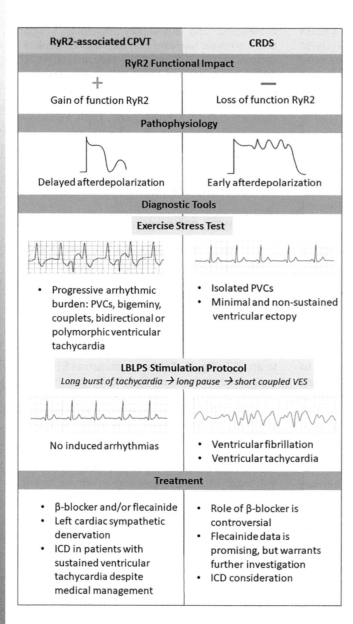

Fig. 2. Comparison of functional studies, pathophysiology, diagnostic tools, arrhythmias, and treatments between CRDS and CPVT.

proposed by Sun and colleagues in 2021,[4] was effective in inducing arrhythmias in mice with LOF variants, but not in WT or CPVT mice. In this study, the authors also demonstrated that LBLPS could induce polymorphic ventricular arrhythmias in two patients harboring different RyR2 LOF variants (p.I3995V$^{+/-}$ and p.T4196I$^{+/-}$). A later study by Ormerod and colleagues[15] applied the LBLPS protocol to 9 individuals who harbored the RyR2 p.A4142T LOF variant. This led to monomorphic ventricular tachycardia (VT) degenerating into VF or PVT/torsades de pointes in 7 of 9 the CRDS subjects tested. The ease of inducibility appeared to correlate with the severity of disease

expression, suggesting both a potential diagnostic and prognostic utility of the LBLPS protocol. There is also emerging evidence indicating that some spontaneous CRDS events appear to be induced by a pattern of ectopy reminiscent of the LBLPS. In the largest multicenter CRDS cohort study,[14] the LBLPS-like pattern preceding VF/PVT was captured on a device recording in a proband (RyR2 p.Q2275H) and a relative (RyR2 p.F4499C) affected by CRDS. The spontaneous capture of an LBLPS-like pattern was also seen in patients with CRDS who harbored the RyR2 p.R4147K variant.[10] Specifically, an ICD electrogram showed a period of sinus tachycardia, ventricular triplet, a long-pause and a short coupled premature ventricular complex (PVC) before the onset of VF.[10] In this study, another patient with the p.A4203V LOF variant had sinus tachycardia followed by a PVC and a subsequent sinus beat prior to the initiation of VF. Based on these observations, it is important to recognize that although atrial/sinus tachycardia may be the initial stimulus required for the development of spontaneous VT or VF in CRDS, the complex arrhythmic "set-up" for CRDS (ie, LBLPS) is very unlikely to be reproducible with repeated exercise provocation.

THERAPEUTIC OPTIONS

Effective therapies for CRDS have not yet been established, but owing to a frequent misdiagnosis of CPVT, the greatest clinical experience is with β-blockers and flecainide. In vitro studies have helped to guide candidate medications for clinical use, including quinidine, β-blockers, and flecainide. In mutated (RyR2 LOF duplication variant) iPSC-CMs, nadolol, and propranolol successfully reduced erratic beating frequency.[20] Additionally, treatment with flecainide alone significantly reduced arrhythmic activity, although the response was not complete.[20] Reducing excessive Na^+ and Ca^{2+} currents may also be an effective strategy.[4,9] An amiloride derivative, CB-DMB used to block the NCX currents, was remarkably able to decrease EADs by decreasing the action potential duration in RyR2 p.A4860G$^{+/-}$ iPSC-CMs. In RyR2 p.D4646A$^{+/-}$ CRDS mice, quinidine sulfate and flecainide reduced the duration and incidence of LBLPS-induced polymorphic ventricular arrhythmias, which may be secondary to their inhibitory action on both outward and inward Na^+, Ca^{2+} and K^+ currents.[4] Although these pre-clinical findings are insightful, appropriately designed clinical studies will be necessary to determine the best therapies for CRDS. Notably, it would be convenient if β-blockers and/or flecainide were demonstrated to be effective, since so many patients with CRDS are likely misdiagnosed and treated as CPVT.

Demonstrating the benefit of candidate CRDS therapies has been hindered by the small population of patients with CRDS identified to date and the relatively low number of life-time events recorded in most cases. In the recent multicentre CRDS study, 16 of 18 patients diagnosed while alive received β-blockers (94%). Three of the 16 (19%) who were adherent had life-threatening breakthrough arrhythmia over 8 years (IQR 6–20); however, there was no comparison group because almost all patients were on treatment. Bisoprolol dominated as the β-blocker of choice because the largest family affected resided in an area where access to nadolol has been historically challenging.[14] Flecainide was only used in a single patient. ICDs were implanted in 4 patients (3 probands and 1 relative), 3 of whom had a successful shock for VF.[14] In one large CRDS kindred described recently by Ormerod and colleagues, intravenous flecainide monotherapy (50–100 mg) decreased the inducibility of ventricular arrhythmias, specifically the frequency and duration of non-sustained VT among 8 of 9 patients with CRDS. In some individuals (4 of 9), adding intravenous metoprolol on top of flecainide resulted increased inducibility of arrhythmias.[15] However, it is important to consider that the potential for β-blockers to suppress the burst of sinus/atrial tachycardia that sets up the spontaneous LBLPS-like pattern cannot be studied in a protocol that relies on pacing to simulate adrenergic stimulation. Therefore, the role of β-blockers, particularly their safety in concert with flecainide, warrants further clinical investigation in humans. Similarly, human data on quinidine are lacking, but should be pursued based on in vitro data suggesting a potential benefit in CRDS iPSCs. Finally, the lack of known effective medical therapy for CRDS may prompt the use of primary prevention ICDs in this population. No reasonable quality of evidence exists to support or refute this practice, and it remains a challenging area to navigate with patients, particularly asymptomatic relatives who carry a known CRDS susceptibility variant.

AREAS OF FUTURE RESEARCH

CRDS has become a newly established inherited arrhythmia syndrome over the past several years, but much still needs to be learned about its penetrance, expressivity, inducibility, and suppressibility. From a translational perspective, it is not known whether the degree of LOF correlates to disease severity, or why certain individuals and families appear to be more severely affected by recurrent events and rarely seen cardiomyopathies. Studies using human-derived iPSCs are limited, and may be better to characterize individual and family phenotypes. The LBLPS is a promising diagnostic tool, however, it is invasive, and the need to induce VF for a positive test is potentially dangerous. The degree of LBLPS inducibility appears to correlate with risk in one family,[15] but this experience may not extend to other variants and patients. Additionally, it is unclear how sensitive or specific the LBLPS is for CRDS in humans, despite promising animal data suggesting it distinguished CRDS from CPVT and normal controls. Further human studies are needed to establish its test characteristics. Flecainide is supported by encouraging data in the treatment of CRDS because of its ability to suppress LBLPS-induced arrhythmias in stem cells, mice, and humans, but its impact as a chronic therapy needs to be adjudicated in larger and ideally prospective studies. As is the case for CPVT, novel small molecule therapies may have promise, and should be designed to increase RyR2 function and/or repair the channel's sensitivity to Ca^{2+} in order to normalize SOICR activity. However, excessive RyR2 opening needs to be avoided to prevent drug-induced CPVT. Studying the gating mechanisms and phosphorylation sites of RyR2 may also identify novel therapeutic targets. Lastly, the incidence of CRDS is wholly unknown, particularly since the majority of CRDS cases appear to have been misdiagnosed with CPVT in the past or labeled as IVF or unexplained cardiac arrest.[1] Thus, patients with existing atypical CPVT diagnoses should have their phenotypes re-examined considering the emerging data. Additionally, individuals without a diagnosis (ie, IVF) now need to be re-evaluated for potential CRDS by performing genetic testing and conducting a functional assessment of identified RyR2 variants. Finally, the identification of CRDS more firmly establishes the potentially important role of molecular autopsy post-sudden unexplained death, since CRDS would otherwise be an entirely elusive diagnosis in the proband. Prospective studies on the diagnostic yield of molecular autopsies may help establish the true incidence of CRDS in SUD cohorts, with a special effort to characterize novel RyR2 variants in vitro to determine the likelihood of LOF. It is to be expected that the clinical and genetic spectrum of CRDS may evolve as more cases are diagnosed and reported, similar to any new disease entity that is first established.

SUMMARY

CRDS should be regarded as a novel form of inherited arrhythmia defined by ventricular arrhythmias secondary to damaging LOF RyR2 variants, which prolong Ca^{2+} release from the SR, leading to EADs and VF or PVT. Patients with CRDS have a phenotype distinct from CPVT devoid of progressive bidirectional or PVT during high workloads. LBLPS stimulation protocol can induce VT/VF in affected individuals, but data on its sensitivity and specificity, and correlation with arrhythmic risk are not established yet. Data on therapies are notably lacking, but there are promising advances in this area, with flecainide emerging as potentially the best option.

CLINICS CARE POINTS

- Genetic testing alone is not sufficient to diagnose CRDS, nor does it inform optimal treatment.
- The possibility of CRDS as the underlying disease entity should be carefully considered in patients with IVF who have a normal EST or an EST that is not indicative of CPVT.
- SUD can be caused by CRDS, but the diagnosis may only be suspected if molecular autopsy is pursued, leading to the detection of an RyR2 variant.
- In vitro characterization and confirmation of *RyR2* loss-of-function is necessary to conclude a CRDS diagnosis in the context of IVF and SUD.

DISCLOSURES

The authors have nothing to disclose.

REFERENCES

1. Antonio F, Konstantinos V, Takeshi K, et al. Long-term follow-up of idiopathic ventricular fibrillation in a pediatric population: clinical characteristics, management, and complications. J Am Heart Assoc 2019; 8(9). https://doi.org/10.1161/JAHA.118.011172.
2. Taylor C, Roston 2 TM, Sonia F, et al. Initially unexplained cardiac arrest in children and adolescents: a national experience from the Canadian Pediatric Heart Rhythm Network. Heart Rhythm 2020;17(6). https://doi.org/10.1016/j.hrthm.2020.01.030.
3. Herman AR, Cheung C, Gerull B, et al. Outcome of apparently unexplained cardiac arrest: results from investigation and follow-up of the prospective cardiac arrest survivors with preserved ejection fraction registry. Circ Arrhythm Electrophysiol 2016;9(1). https://doi.org/10.1161/CIRCEP.115.003619.
4. Sun B, Yao J, Ni M, et al. Cardiac ryanodine receptor calcium release deficiency syndrome. Sci Transl Med 2021;13:579.
5. Roston TM, Sanatani S, Chen SR. Suppression-of-function mutations in the cardiac ryanodine receptor: emerging evidence for a novel arrhythmia syndrome? Heart Rhythm 2017;14(1):108–9.
6. Priori SG, Chen SR. Inherited dysfunction of sarcoplasmic reticulum Ca2+ handling and arrhythmogenesis. Circ Res 2011 2011;108(7). https://doi.org/10.1161/CIRCRESAHA.110.226845.

7. Jiang D, Chen W, Wang R, et al. Loss of luminal Ca2+ activation in the cardiac ryanodine receptor is associated with ventricular fibrillation and sudden death. Proc Natl Acad Sci U S A 2007;104(46): 18309–14.

8. Yusuke F, Hideki I, Seiko O, et al. A type 2 ryanodine receptor variant associated with reduced Ca2+ release and short-coupled torsades de pointes ventricular arrhythmia. Heart Rhythm 2017;14(1). https://doi.org/10.1016/j.hrthm.2016.10.015.

9. Zhao YT, Valdivia CR, Gurrola GB, et al. Arrhythmogenesis in a catecholaminergic polymorphic ventricular tachycardia mutation that depresses ryanodine receptor function. Proc Natl Acad Sci U S A 2015; 112(13):E1669–77.

10. Li Y, Wei J, Guo W, et al. Human RyR2 (ryanodine receptor 2) loss-of-function mutations: clinical phenotypes and in vitro characterization. Circ Arrhythm Electrophysiol 2021. https://doi.org/10.1161/CIRCEP. 121.010013.

11. Kobayashi T, Tsutsumi A, Kurebayashi N, et al. Molecular basis for gating of cardiac ryanodine receptor explains the mechanisms for gain- and loss-of function mutations. OriginalPaper. Nat Commun 2022;13(1):1–15.

12. Malorie B, Touat-Hamici Z, Aguilar-Sanchez Y, et al. A type 2 ryanodine receptor variant in the helical domain 2 associated with an impairment of the adrenergic response. J Personalized Med 2021; 11(6). https://doi.org/10.3390/jpm11060579.

13. Priori SG, Napolitano C, Memmi M, et al. Clinical and molecular characterization of patients with catecholaminergic polymorphic ventricular tachycardia. Circulation 2002;106(1). https://doi.org/10.1161/01.cir. 0000020013.73106.d8.

14. Roston TM, Wei J, Guo W, et al. Clinical and functional characterization of ryanodine receptor 2 variants implicated in calcium-release deficiency syndrome. JAMA cardiology 2022;7(1). https://doi. org/10.1001/jamacardio.2021.4458.

15. Ormerod JOM, Ormondroyd E, Li Y, et al. Provocation testing and therapeutic response in a newly described channelopathy: RyR2 calcium release deficiency syndrome. Circ Genom Precis Med 2022;15(1). https://doi.org/10.1161/CIRCGEN.121. 003589.

16. Roston TM, Guo W, Krahn AD, et al. A novel RYR2 loss-of-function mutation (I4855M) is associated with left ventricular non-compaction and atypical catecholaminergic polymorphic ventricular tachycardia. J Electrocardiol 2017;50(2):227–33.

17. Campbell MJ, Czosek RJ, Hinton RB, et al. Exon 3 deletion of ryanodine receptor causes left ventricular noncompaction, worsening catecholaminergic polymorphic ventricular tachycardia, and sudden cardiac arrest. Am J Med Genet 2015;167A(9). https://doi.org/10.1002/ajmg.a.37140.

18. Hirose S, Murayama T, Tetsuo N, et al. Loss-of-function mutations in cardiac ryanodine receptor channel cause various types of arrhythmias including long QT syndrome. Europace 2022;24(3). https://doi. org/10.1093/europace/euab250.

19. Zhong X, Guo W, We J, et al. Identification of loss-of-function RyR2 mutations associated with idiopathic ventricular fibrillation and sudden death. Biosci Rep 2021;41(4). https://doi.org/10.1042/BSR20210209.

20. Tester DJ, Kim CSJ, Hamrick SK, et al. Molecular characterization of the calcium release channel deficiency syndrome. JCI insight 2020;5(15). https://doi. org/10.1172/jci.insight.135952.

21. Tester DJ, Bombei HM, Fitzgerald KK, et al. Identification of a novel homozygous multi-exon duplication in RYR2 among children with exertion-related unexplained sudden deaths in the amish community. JAMA Cardiol 2020;5(3):13–8.

22. Roston T, Kallas D, Davies B, et al. Burst exercise testing can unmask arrhythmias in patients with incompletely penetrant catecholaminergic polymorphic ventricular tachycardia. JACC Clinical electrophysiology 2021;7(4). https://doi.org/10.1016/j. jacep.2021.02.013.

Short-Coupled Ventricular Fibrillation

Christian Steinberg, MD

KEYWORDS

- Short-coupled ventricular fibrillation • Idiopathic ventricular fibrillation
- Premature ventricular contraction • Unexplained cardiac arrest

KEY POINTS

- Short-coupled ventricular arrhythmia (SCVF) represents a distinct phenotype accounting for at least 7-14% of IVF cases.
- Documentation of the VF onset is crucial to establish the diagnosis of SCVF.
- SCVF is characterized by a high risk of VF recurrence. Quinidine is highly effective and is the first-line antiarrhythmic medication.

INTRODUCTION AND DEFINITION

Idiopathic ventricular fibrillation (IVF) is a rare form of ventricular arrhythmia with unknown prevalence. Although it is estimated that IVF accounts for less than 10% of ventricular fibrillation (VF) episodes in the general population, it represents a major cause of unexplained cardiac arrest in otherwise healthy individuals.[1,2]

By definition, IVF is a diagnosis of exclusion describing documented VF or polymorphic ventricular tachycardia that remains unexplained after extensive cardiac evaluation. The large historic pool of IVF has significantly narrowed over time with the identification and characterization of multiple distinct primary electrical disorders, such as Brugada syndrome, short-QT syndrome, or early repolarization syndrome (**Fig. 1**).[3–7]

Short-coupled ventricular fibrillation (SCVF) describes a specific phenotype of IVF and has recently been identified as a distinct primary electrical disorder accounting for at least 7% to 14% of unexplained cardiac arrest (UCA).[8,9]

The particular phenotype of SCVF was first described by Leenhardt and colleagues[10] in 1994 in a small case series, who used the term "short-coupled torsades-de-pointes" for their observations. Considering the pathophysiologic and genetic differences and to avoid confusion with true long-QT syndrome or pause-/bradycardia-dependent torsades de pointes, the term SCVF has been proposed.[9]

The hallmark of SCVF is VF initiation by a trigger premature ventricular contraction (PVC) with a short-coupling interval (<350 milliseconds) in the absence of a spontaneous or inducible type 1 Brugada or early repolarization pattern, prolonged QTc intervals, or preceding pause (**Box 1**; **Fig. 2**).[9]

CLINICAL MANIFESTATIONS AND ELECTROPHYSIOLOGY OF SHORT-COUPLED VENTRICULAR FIBRILLATION

In contrast to many other primary electrical disorders, individuals with SCVF have a normal resting electrocardiogram (ECG).[9,10] Exercise treadmill testing in patients with SCVF shows normal QTc dynamics and absence of stress-induced ventricular arrhythmia.[9] The diagnosis of SCVF is challenging given the fact that documented VF onset is the sole diagnostic criteria at this point. As a consequence, up to 79% of patients with SCVF are diagnosed during follow-up at the time of VF recurrence, which occurs in up to 92% of cases. The median time to VF recurrence after the index cardiac event is about 30.6 months (8.6, 70.7;

Funding sources: Fonds de Recherche du Québec–Santé.
Conflict of interests: none.
Institut universitaire de cardiologie et pneumologie de Québec (IUCPQ-UL), Laval University, 2725 Chemin Ste-Foy, Quebec, QC, G1V 4G5, Canada
E-mail address: christian.steinberg@criucpq.ulaval.ca

Card Electrophysiol Clin 15 (2023) 331–341
https://doi.org/10.1016/j.ccep.2023.05.004

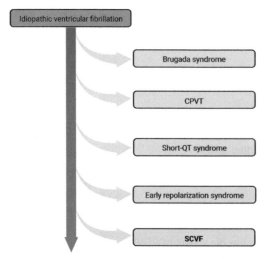

Fig. 1. Evolution of the diagnosis of IVF over time. CPVT, catecholaminergic polymorphic ventricular tachycardia.

range, 0.3–124 months), which is much more common compared with Brugada syndrome or early repolarization syndrome (ERS).[7,9] In addition, up to 21% to 32% of SCVF cases present with electrical storm at the time of the diagnosis, illustrating the malignant phenotype of this particular disorder.[8,9] SCVF typically occurs during nonadrenergic states (rest, sleep, or low-intensity activities) at normal heart rates, which is similar to Brugada syndrome or early repolarization syndrome.[11–13] The onset of SCVF is not bradycardia- or pause-dependent.[14] In contrast to classic torsades de pointes in the context of QT prolongation, SCVF is not associated with an electrical prodrome of T-wave alternans or giant T-U waves.[9]

As outlined above, VF initiation by trigger PVCs with a coupling interval of less than 350 milliseconds has been proposed as a diagnostic cutoff value for SCVF.[9] This was based on the observation of an average coupling interval at 274 ± 31 milliseconds (range, 234–350 milliseconds) in the SCVF cohort of the Cardiac Arrest in Cardiac Arrest Survivors With Preserved Ejection Fraction Registry (CASPER) and the fact that 92% of all patients with SCVF presented coupling intervals within a z score of −1 to 1.5.[9] Similar observations have been reported by other groups showing that the interval of the trigger PVC in SCVF is typically between 250 and 300 milliseconds, and within 40 to 60 milliseconds of the peak of the preceding T wave.[10,14–16] Interestingly, up to 18% of patients with SCVF may on occasion also present VF initiation with coupling intervals greater than 350 milliseconds.[8] The electrophysiologic explanations for this "dual mode" of VF

Box 1
Proposed diagnostic criteria of short-coupled ventricular arrhythmia[9]

Documentation of VF or polymorphic VT initiated by a PVC with a coupling interval of less than 350 milliseconds

AND

The presence of *all* of the following:

1. Absence of QTc prolongation according to current definitions.

2. Absence of pause-dependent torsades de pointes (preceding R-R interval before the trigger PVC greater than 1500 milliseconds in individuals without pacemaker/ICD or greater than 1300 milliseconds in individuals with pacemaker/ICD) following a stable baseline rhythm.[a]

3. Absence of type 1 Brugada pattern (spontaneous or inducible), early repolarization pattern, or short-QT at the index cardiac arrest or during follow-up.

4. Absence of catecholaminergic polymorphic ventricular tachycardia according to current definitions.

5. Absence of structural heart disease (no active ischemia or coronary artery disease with >50% stenosis, no left ventricular ejection fraction <50%) or other primary electrical disorder or arrhythmogenic cardiomyopathy.

6. Absence of reversible metabolic or pharmacologic/toxicologic conditions that may cause similar electrophysiologic findings.

[a]However, initiation of ventricular arrhythmia by short-long-short cycles (R-R cycles <1300 milliseconds) with short-coupled trigger PVCs was eligible as described previously for Brugada syndrome and early repolarization syndrome.

initiation remain elusive for now but highlight the need for further refinement of the proposed current diagnostic criteria.

It is important to recognize that VF initiation by short-coupled PVCs is not exclusively limited to SCVF but can occur in other primary electrical disorders and certain forms of structural heart disease. **Box 2** gives an overview of cardiac conditions that may present with SCVF. The electrophysiologic denominator to explain the short-coupling interval for the conditions listed in **Box 2** is arrhythmia initiation by the Purkinje system.[17–21]

Indeed, electrophysiology studies in patients with SCVF/IVF by Haïssaguerre and coworkers[13,15,22,23] confirmed the presence of trigger PVCs with a

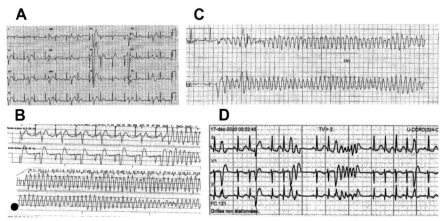

Fig. 2. Examples of SCVF. (*A–B*) ECG and telemetry tracings of a 43-year-old man with unheralded cardiac arrest at rest. (*A*) Resting ECG at the emergency department showing sinus rhythm with monomorphic bigeminal PVCs with a short-coupling interval of 240 to 280 milliseconds. (*B*) Repeat VF episode soon after arrival initiated by the same short-coupled trigger PVC. Extensive cardiac workup showed no structural heart disease and no reversible cause for the patient's arrhythmia. (*C–D*) A 36-year-old man with SCVF and electrical storm during initial presentation. (*C*) The patient initially presented to the emergency department for a witnessed unexplained syncope at rest. Spontaneous initiation of VF while still in the emergency department evolving toward electrical storm requiring intubation and transfer to the intensive care unit. VF episodes were initiated by trigger PVCs with a coupling interval of 280 milliseconds. Continuous isoproterenol perfusion eventually controlled the ventricular arrhythmia. (*D*) ECG during weaning of isoproterenol perfusion. Notice the frequent multifocal ventricular ectopy with short-coupling interval and an intermittent run of polymorphic nonsustained ventricular tachycardia. In addition to the ICD insertion, quinidine was initiated during the index hospitalization.

relatively narrow QRS (126 ± 17 milliseconds) arising from the right or left ventricular Purkinje system with a short-coupling interval of 260 to 320 milliseconds. Interestingly, sex-related differences seem to exist with regard to the ventricular origin of Purkinje trigger PVCs in SCVF/IVF and multifocal ectopic Purkinje-related premature contractions. In the study by Surget and colleagues,[13] right ventricular Purkinje trigger PVCs occurred more frequently in men (76%), whereas left ventricular Purkinje triggers in women typically originated from the left ventricle (83%).

Given the limited understanding of the molecular mechanisms of SCVF at this point, it should be recognized that the current diagnostic criteria of SCVF are likely to change in the future once increased insight into the pathophysiology will be available. Recent data from the Dutch IVF registry showed that at least a subgroup of patients with SCVF experience recurrent ventricular arrhythmia initiated by both short- and long-coupled (>350 milliseconds) PVCs.[8] Documentation of VF initiation was only available in 15% of all patients with IVF with SCVF accounting for 73% of all episodes.[8] These observations suggest that the true prevalence of SCVF is likely much higher than previously estimated and that SCVF might possibly be the major cause of IVF-related UCA.

Box 2
Differential diagnosis of cardiac conditions with ventricular fibrillation initiation by trigger premature ventricular contractions with short-coupling intervals

Primary electrical disorders

- Short-coupled ventricular fibrillation
- Brugada syndrome
- Early repolarization syndrome
- Short-QT syndrome
- Multifocal ectopic Purkinje-related premature contractions syndrome

Structural heart disease

- Acute myocarditis
- Acute ischemia/myocardial infarction (acute and subacute phase)

MOLECULAR AND GENETIC ASPECTS OF SHORT-COUPLED VENTRICULAR FIBRILLATION

Molecular and genetic mechanisms of SCVF remain still largely elusive. At present, there is no functional cellular or animal model to reproduce and study the SCVF phenotype. A positive family history of sudden unexplained cardiac death can be found in 8% to 15% of patients with SCVF, suggesting an underlying genetic substrate in at least a subset of cases.[8,9]

However, a consistent, unifying genetic substrate for SCVF has not been identified, so far, despite broad genetic testing including whole-exome sequencing.[9,24,25] The fact that the genetic substrate remains elusive for many individuals with SCVF could suggest polygenetic or combined genetic and nongenetic mechanisms underlying its pathophysiology.

The strongest data supporting a genetic contribution to certain SCVF subsets come from the Dutch IVF registry, which identified a risk haplotype (c.1–340C > T) affecting the noncoding region of the dipeptidyl-aminopeptidase–like protein 6 (DPP6) gene (7q36).[26] Cellular studies suggest that DPP6 acts as putative regulatory β-subunit of the rapidly recovering cardiac transient outward K^+ current ($I_{to,f}$) mediating the early repolarization during phase 1 of the cardiac action potential.[27,28] Functional data showed that the Dutch DPP6 variant results in a gain-of-function of the I_{to} current in Purkinje fibers.[29] The electrophysiologic properties and expression profile of cardiac ion channels predispose Purkinje cells as potential arrhythmogenic source for ventricular arrhythmia. Compared with normal ventricular cardiomyocytes, the I_{to} current of Purkinje cells is of increased amplitude and function, predisposing Purkinje cells for triggered activity.[30]

The Dutch DPP6 variant is a founder mutation and has been linked to familial IVF/SCVF in the Netherlands. Like other forms of SCVF, the DPP6 risk haplotype is not associated with ECG abnormalities or structural heart disease.[26,31,32] The Dutch DPP6 risk haplotype is characterized by a high risk of VF arrest or sudden cardiac death occurring in up to 30% of gene carriers before the age of 58 years, but late-onset forms in elderly individuals are also not uncommon.[26,31,32] To date, the DPP6-c.1–340C > T variant has not been identified outside the Netherlands.[32] Although the DPP6 haplotype is significantly enriched in Dutch patients with SCVF, it has only been confirmed in 48% of affected Dutch patients, suggesting that it is not the sole risk factor to explain the arrhythmic phenotype in this population.[8]

The recently described truncating H332R variant is another DPP6 mutation linked to IVF.[33] The truncated DPP6-H332R protein is characterized by an increased binding affinity to Kv4.3 (KCND3), one of the pore-forming α-subunits of $I_{to,f}$, resulting in a significant increase of the $I_{to,f}$ current compared with the wild-type DPP6 form.[33,34]

The functional data on DPP6 variants support the concept of SCVF as a malignant Purkinje arrhythmia and are consistent with the above-mentioned results of ablation studies in patients with SCVF/IVF.[13,22,35]

DIAGNOSIS

A comprehensive and systematic stepwise diagnostic approach is crucial to eliminate alternative causes of apparently unexplained cardiac arrest and to distinguish SCVF from other primary electrical disorders with overlapping electrophysiologic features, such as Brugada syndrome, early repolarization syndrome, or short-QT syndrome[1,36] (**Table 1**).

As discussed above, documentation of VF onset is crucial to establish the diagnosis of SCVF. Rhythm tracings from prehospital automated external defibrillators and in-hospital telemetry rhythm strips can provide valuable diagnostic information but often get lost. Repeat resting ECGs and complementary functional tests (exercise testing, pharmacologic provocation) are helpful to unmask subclinical primary electrical disorders and distinguish them from SCVF.[37–39] Routine electrophysiology studies are currently not recommended for the diagnosis and risk stratification of SCVF given the overall low-inducibility rate and poor predictive values.[40] A systematic analysis of the diagnostic strategy in different UCA cohorts identified so-called high-yield tests, including cardiac magnetic resonance, exercise treadmill testing, and sodium channel provocation.[41] The incorporation of these high-yield tests as part of a standardized approach to patients with UCA will help to establish a specific diagnosis in 43% of cases and strengthen the diagnostic certitude about IVF/SCVF.[41] Periodic clinical reassessment is recommended, as phenotype findings of inherited arrhythmia or cardiomyopathies may fluctuate and manifest over time.[39] For example, a substudy of the CASPER registry reported an alternative diagnosis in 21% of patients with an initial diagnosis of IVF over a follow-up period of 30 ± 17 months.[39]

Genetic testing in the context of IVF/SCVF remains challenging given the above-mentioned absence of a robust genetic substrate at this point. In the presence of a strong family history of IVF or unexplained cardiac death, targeted testing for known familial SCVF-related mutations is recommended.[42] In the presence of IVF, broad genetic testing may nevertheless be useful when performed by specialized cardiogenetic clinics with adequate expertise in the interpretation and management of genetic results and test-related

Table 1
Overlap between short-coupled ventricular fibrillation and other electrical disorders with primary ventricular fibrillation

	Short-Coupled VF	Early Repolarization Syndrome	Brugada Syndrome	Short QT Syndrome
J-point abnormalities on resting ECG	−	+	+	−
QTc on resting ECG	Normal; 330 milliseconds < QTc ≤ 360 milliseconds in up to 35%	Usually normal	Usually normal	≤330 milliseconds
Ventricular arrhythmia				
Morphology	Polymorphic VT/VF	Polymorphic VT/VF	Polymorphic VT/VF[a]	Polymorphic VT/VF
Initiation by short-coupled PVCs	+ (coupling interval < 330 milliseconds)	+	+	+
Electroanatomic substrate	?	Inferior RV epicardium, anterior RVOT/RV epicardium	RVOT epicardium	?
Origin of triggering PVCs	His-Purkinje system (RVOT?)	His-Purkinje system of right ventricle	RVOT and other RV sites	?
Clinical circumstances of events	Predominantly at sleep/rest	Predominantly at sleep/rest	Predominantly at sleep/rest	Predominantly at sleep/rest
Strength of genetic linkage	Rare familial forms	Rare familial forms	25%–30% of cases	Rare familial forms
Efficacy of isoproterenol for acute treatment	+	+	+	+
Efficacy of quinidine for acute treatment and chronic prevention	+	+	+	+

Abbreviations: LV, left ventricle; PVC, premature ventricular complex; QTc, corrected QT interval; RV, right ventricle; RVOT, right ventricular outflow tract; VT, ventricular tachycardia.
From Steinberg C, Laksman ZWM, Krahn AD. Idiopathic and short-coupled ventricular fibrillation. In: Zipes and Jalife's Cardiac Electrophysiology: From Cell to Bedside, Eighth Edition. Chapter 100, 1157 to 1165; with permissionFigure legends

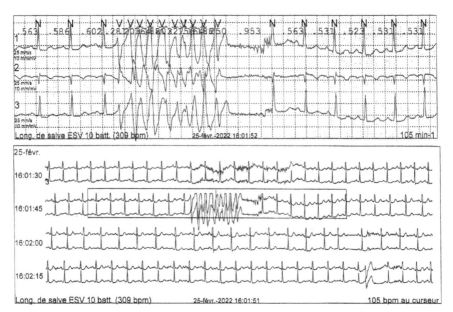

Fig. 3. SCVF diagnosed before cardiac arrest. Shown are Holter tracings of a 50-year-old female patient who was assessed for longstanding intermittent palpitations and recent episodes of unprovoked presyncope. Holter monitoring showed intermittent runs of polymorphic nonsustained ventricular tachycardia initiated by a PVC with a coupling interval of 240 to 280 milliseconds. The patient's symptoms of presyncope perfectly correlated with the runs of nonsustained polymorphic VT. Following the results of the Holter, the patient was urgently admitted. Extensive cardiac investigations, including cardiac magnetic resonance (CMR), echocardiogram, and coronary angiography, were unremarkable. A diagnosis of likely SCVF was retained, and after thorough discussion, the patient underwent insertion of a primary prevention ICD.

limitations. A broad genetic approach may reveal pathogenic or likely pathogenic variants of other otherwise subclinical primary electrical disorders or preclinical hereditary cardiomyopathies in up to 10% to 17%.[43–45]

MANAGEMENT AND FOLLOW-UP

All patients with SCVF with resuscitated aborted cardiac arrest or documented polymorphic VT/VF should receive an ICD.[46,47] A subcutaneous ICD represents an attractive alternative for patients with SCVF who are unlikely to benefit from antitachycardia pacing, and most of them will not require cardiac pacing. ICD programming for patients with SCVF should follow contemporary guidelines to avoid inappropriate shocks.[48] Device programming should typically include a single therapy zone with a high cutoff rate (>210–220 beats/min) and a long detection interval, which has been shown to be appropriate for similar inherited arrhythmia syndromes.[49]

Very few data exist on the role of primary prevention ICDs in patients with presumptive SCVF, as the diagnosis is typically established at the time of aborted cardiac arrest or recurrent VF with appropriate ICD treatment. Based on survival

data from the Dutch IVF registry, the investigators recommend a prophylactic ICD insertion in DPP6 haplotype carriers between ages 20 and 50 years.[31,32] Given the high rate of device-related complications over follow-up in this relatively young patient cohort and a limited positive predictive value of the DPP6 haplotype, this approach remains controversial.[31,50,51]

In certain cases, SCVF may be suspected by documentation of nonsustained ventricular arrhythmia with or without syncope/presyncope before a cardiac arrest (**Fig. 3**). Given the aggressive nature of SCVF, the author believes that a primary prevention ICD should be strongly recommended in these cases. Recurrent VF, including episodes of electrical storm, is common in SCVF. Appropriate ICD therapies occur in 21% to 92% of SCVF over a median follow-up of 41 to 63 months, with a median delay to the first recurrence of 4 to 12 months.[9,51–53]

Adjunct pharmacologic treatment is recommended for patients with SCVF with frequent VF recurrence, patients with electrical storm, or those who refuse ICD implantation.[47] Quinidine, a potent inhibitor of I_{to}, is the only effective oral antiarrhythmic therapy for SCVF.[47,54,55] Long-term treatment with oral quinidine has demonstrated

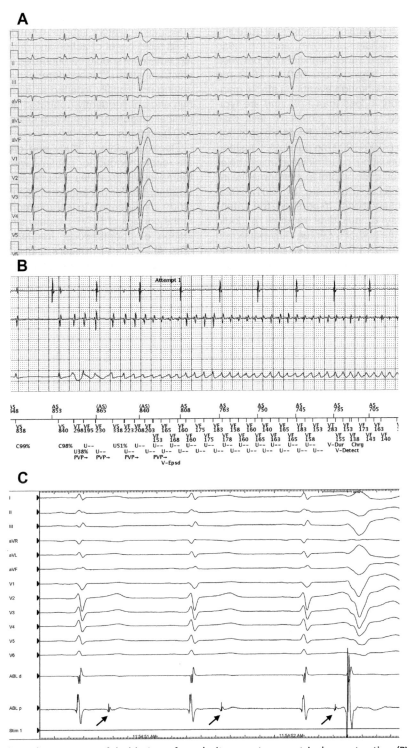

Fig. 4. Key findings from a successful ablation of a culprit premature ventricular contraction (PVC) triggering SCVF in a 49-year-old otherwise healthy man with previously unexplained cardiac arrest. Following comprehensive clinical and genetic testing without a distinct phenotype, his working diagnosis was IVF. The patient presented subsequently with electrical storm and received multiple appropriate ICD shocks. Analysis of the ICD recordings showed a significant increase in spontaneous PVCs. The coupling interval of spontaneous PVCs and VF episodes was short, ranging from 286 ± 14 milliseconds. (A) Twelve-lead electrocardiogram recording sinus rhythm with frequent monomorphic PVCs. Note the short-coupled interval of the PVC, which was also seen

freedom from recurrent VF over a mean follow-up period of 9.1 ± 5.6 years.[9,55] The optimal quinidine dose for SCVF remains unknown, and the mean daily quinidine dose varies significantly between different studies ranging from 600 to 2000 mg per day.[54–57] Breakthrough events on stable quinidine doses occur in less than 17% and are typically associated with daily doses of less than 300 mg.[9] Gastrointestinal side effects are common at higher doses (>700–1000 mg per day).[57] Instead of drug discontinuation, coadministration of cholestyramine is often quite helpful to overcome the intestinal side effects (Steinberg C., 2017-2023, unpublished observations). In addition, the potential myelotoxicity of quinidine requires periodic monitoring. At the author's center, they perform a complete blood count 3 to 4 times per year. The persistence of limited accessibility in many countries represents a major challenge of quinidine therapy.[58]

In the case of quinidine intolerance or lack of access, verapamil should be considered as alternative treatment. There are limited data suggesting reasonable efficacy of verapamil in patients with SCVF, and a combination of quinidine and verapamil can be considered in selected cases with refractory ventricular arrhythmia unsuitable for ablation.[10,59,60] Caution is advised for the coadministration of quinidine and verapamil given the significant drug interaction resulting in a reduced quinidine clearance.[61] In these cases, the quinidine dose should be reduced to minimize the risks of drug-related toxicity. Disease- and mutation-specific treatment using the combination of dalfampridine/cilostazol has been reported for SCVF related to a truncating DPP6 variant, but more data are required to establish the role of this experimental treatment for SCVF.[33]

A particular challenge is the approach to SCVF with electrical storm. Continuous perfusions of isoproterenol or oral loading with high doses of quinidine are effective therapies to terminate VF storm in patients with SCVF or early repolarization syndrome when added to standard intensive care treatment (airway protection, sedation, and mechanical circulatory support if needed).[62] Because of its rapid onset of action and greater availability, isoproterenol should be prioritized in the context of electrical storm.[63] Isoproterenol perfusions in this setting are usually initiated at rates of 1 to 5 μg/min and subsequently uptitrated according to the clinical response, targeting a sinus rate of 100 to 120 beats/min.

Electrophysiology study and catheter ablation are recommended for patients with recurrent ICD therapies/VF episodes despite adequate medical treatment or for patients with SCVF with electrical storm unresponsive to isoproterenol.[47] VF ablation in the context of SCVF typically aims for the elimination of spontaneous, frequent trigger PVCs (**Fig. 4**).[22,53,64] VF triggers and drivers predominantly arise from the Purkinje system.[15,23] However, a significant subset of patients with SCVF/IVF present additional proarrhythmic substrates in the form of focal myocardial microstructural alterations, resulting in zones of slow conduction not visible on cardiac magnetic resonance.[15,23] As it is not uncommon for trigger PVCs to arise from the epicardium, ablation strategies of VF triggers should anticipate combined endocardial and epicardial mapping of the right and left ventricle.[15,23] When performed by experienced centers, ablation of SCVF triggering PVCs is associated with encouraging short- and long-term success rates of 89% and 83%, respectively.[15,53] It should nevertheless be mentioned that these studies reflect highly selected, refractory patients referred to international specialty centers, which may limit the overall applicability of the reported ablation results.

FUTURE DIRECTIONS

The understanding of SCVF is still at a very early stage, and at this point, it remains uncertain if it is a distinct primary arrhythmia syndrome or a just a special phenotype of IVF. Large-scale international registries are required to improve the clinical characterization of patients with SCVF and the

---

repeatedly by telemetry and identical when compared with ICD recordings. (*B*) ICD tracing of a VF episode that was terminated by an appropriate shock. The VF episode was initiated by a short-coupled PVC (identical with PVC in panel A). Note that there is no preceding pause or bradycardia (ambient heart rate at 70 beats per minute). (*C*) Activation mapping at the site of earliest activation: free-wall insertion of the moderator band. The distinct, low-amplitude potential following each sinus beat with a fixed coupling interval of 212 milliseconds is a Purkinje potential arising from the moderator band (*arrow*) and precedes the PVC. Note the intermittent conduction block into the right ventricular myocardium. Ablation at the site of the Purkinje potential successfully suppressed the PVCs. (G Mellor et al., Short-Coupled Ventricular Fibrillation: Concealed Purkinje Depolarization, Journal of Cardiovascular Electrophysiology, 07 Jun 2016, 27(10):1236-1237. DOI: 10.1111/jce.12999.)

understanding of their clinical evolution. Given the absence of a robust genetic substrate, complementary broad genetic approaches, including whole-genome sequencing and/or genome-wide association studies, may shed further light into the cause of SCVF. Functional in vitro models, ideally based on human inducible pluripotent stem cells technology, may help to refine the understanding of the arrhythmogenesis and to develop tailored therapies.

CLINICS CARE POINTS

- Short-coupled ventricular arrhythmia represents a distinct phenotype accounting for at least 7% to 14% of idiopathic ventricular fibrillation cases.
- Documentation of the ventricular fibrillation onset is crucial to establish the diagnosis of short-coupled ventricular arrhythmia.
- Short-coupled ventricular arrhythmia is characterized by a high risk of ventricular fibrillation recurrence. Quinidine is highly effective and is the first-line antiarrhythmic medication.

FUNDING

Dr Steinberg is supported by the Fonds de Recherche du Québec – Santé.

REFERENCES

1. Visser M, van der Heijden JF, Doevendans PA, et al. Idiopathic ventricular fibrillation: the struggle for definition, diagnosis, and follow-up. Circulation Arrhythmia and electrophysiology 2016;9(5). https://doi.org/10.1161/CIRCEP.115.003817.
2. Survivors of out-of-hospital cardiac arrest with apparently normal heart. Need for definition and standardized clinical evaluation. Consensus statement of the joint steering committees of the unexplained cardiac arrest registry of Europe and of the idiopathic ventricular fibrillation registry of the United States. Circulation 1997;95(1):265–72.
3. Derval N, Lim HS, Haissaguerre M. Dynamic electrocardiographic recordings in patients with idiopathic ventricular fibrillation. J Electrocardiol 2013;46(5):451–5.
4. Viskin S, Zeltser D, Ish-Shalom M, et al. Is idiopathic ventricular fibrillation a short QT syndrome? Comparison of QT intervals of patients with idiopathic ventricular fibrillation and healthy controls. Heart Rhythm 2004;1(5):587–91.
5. Derval N, Simpson CS, Birnie DH, et al. Prevalence and characteristics of early repolarization in the CASPER registry: cardiac arrest survivors with preserved ejection fraction registry. J Am Coll Cardiol 2011;58(7):722–8.
6. Haissaguerre M, Derval N, Sacher F, et al. Sudden cardiac arrest associated with early repolarization. N Engl J Med 2008;358(19):2016–23.
7. Steinberg CLZ, Krahn AD. Idiopathic and short-coupled ventricular fibrillation. In: Jalife JSW, editor. Zipes and Jalife's cardiac electrophysiology - from cell to Bedside. Eighth Edition ed. Elsevier; 2020. p. 1157–65. chap 100.
8. Groeneveld SA, van der Ree MH, Mulder BA, et al. Prevalence of short-coupled ventricular fibrillation in a large cohort of Dutch patients with idiopathic ventricular fibrillation. Circulation 2022;145(18):1437–9.
9. Steinberg C, Davies B, Mellor G, et al. Short-coupled ventricular fibrillation represents a distinct phenotype among latent causes of unexplained cardiac arrest: a report from the CASPER registry. Eur Heart J 2021;42(29):2827–38.
10. Leenhardt A, Glaser E, Burguera M, et al. Short-coupled variant of torsade de pointes. A new electrocardiographic entity in the spectrum of idiopathic ventricular tachyarrhythmias. Circulation 1994;89(1):206–15.
11. Aizawa Y, Takatsuki S, Kimura T, et al. Ventricular fibrillation associated with complete right bundle branch block. Heart Rhythm 2013;10(7):1028–35.
12. Matsuo K, Kurita T, Inagaki M, et al. The circadian pattern of the development of ventricular fibrillation in patients with Brugada syndrome. Eur Heart J 1999;20(6):465–70.
13. Surget E, Cheniti G, Ramirez FD, et al. Sex differences in the origin of Purkinje ectopy-initiated idiopathic ventricular fibrillation. Heart Rhythm 2021;18(10):1647–54.
14. Viskin S, Lesh MD, Eldar M, et al. Mode of onset of malignant ventricular arrhythmias in idiopathic ventricular fibrillation. J Cardiovasc Electrophysiol 1997;8(10):1115–20.
15. Haissaguerre M, Hocini M, Cheniti G, et al. Localized structural alterations underlying a subset of unexplained sudden cardiac death. Circulation Arrhythmia and electrophysiology 2018;11(7):e006120.
16. Viskin S, Rosso R, Rogowski O, et al. The "short-coupled" variant of right ventricular outflow ventricular tachycardia: a not-so-benign form of benign ventricular tachycardia? J Cardiovasc Electrophysiol 2005;16(8):912–6.
17. Marume K, Ishibashi K, Noda T, et al. Short coupled Torsade de pointes with myocardial injury: a possible sequela of myocarditis. J Cardiol Cases 2019;19(2):62–5.
18. Rosso R, Hochstadt A, Viskin D, et al. Polymorphic ventricular tachycardia, ischaemic ventricular

fibrillation, and torsade de pointes: importance of the QT and the coupling interval in the differential diagnosis. Eur Heart J 2021;42(38):3965–75.

19. Wilde AAM, Garan H, Boyden PA. Role of the Purkinje system in heritable arrhythmias. Heart Rhythm 2019;16(7):1121–6.

20. Ghovanloo MR, Atallah J, Escudero CA, et al. Biophysical characterization of a novel SCN5A mutation associated with an atypical phenotype of atrial and ventricular arrhythmias and sudden death. Front Physiol 2020;11:610436.

21. Gao X, Ye D, Zhou W, et al. A novel functional variant residing outside the SCN5A-encoded Nav1.5 voltage-sensing domain causes multifocal ectopic Purkinje-related premature contractions. HeartRhythm Case Rep 2022;8(1):54–9.

22. Haissaguerre M, Shah DC, Jais P, et al. Role of Purkinje conducting system in triggering of idiopathic ventricular fibrillation. Lancet 2002;359(9307):677–8.

23. Haissaguerre M, Duchateau J, Dubois R, et al. Idiopathic ventricular fibrillation: role of Purkinje system and microstructural myocardial abnormalities. JACC Clin Electrophysiol 2020;6(6):591–608.

24. Visser M, Dooijes D, van der Smagt JJ, et al. Next-generation sequencing of a large gene panel in patients initially diagnosed with idiopathic ventricular fibrillation. Heart Rhythm 2017;14(7):1035–40.

25. Leinonen JT, Crotti L, Djupsjobacka A, et al. The genetics underlying idiopathic ventricular fibrillation: a special role for catecholaminergic polymorphic ventricular tachycardia? Int J Cardiol 2018;250:139–45.

26. Alders M, Koopmann TT, Christiaans I, et al. Haplotype-sharing analysis implicates chromosome 7q36 harboring DPP6 in familial idiopathic ventricular fibrillation. Am J Hum Genet 2009;84(4):468–76.

27. Niwa N, Nerbonne JM. Molecular determinants of cardiac transient outward potassium current (I(to)) expression and regulation. J Mol Cell Cardiol 2010; 48(1):12–25.

28. Radicke S, Cotella D, Graf EM, et al. Expression and function of dipeptidyl-aminopeptidase-like protein 6 as a putative beta-subunit of human cardiac transient outward current encoded by Kv4.3. J Physiol 2005;565(Pt 3):751–6.

29. Xiao L, Koopmann TT, Ordog B, et al. Unique cardiac Purkinje fiber transient outward current beta-subunit composition: a potential molecular link to idiopathic ventricular fibrillation. Circ Res 2013; 112(10):1310–22.

30. Boyden PA, Dun W, Robinson RB. Cardiac Purkinje fibers and arrhythmias; the GK moe award lecture 2015. Heart Rhythm 2016;13(5):1172–81.

31. Ten Sande JN, Postema PG, Boekholdt SM, et al. Detailed characterization of familial idiopathic ventricular fibrillation linked to the DPP6 locus. Heart Rhythm 2016;13(4):905–12.

32. Postema PG, Christiaans I, Hofman N, et al. Founder mutations in The Netherlands: familial idiopathic ventricular fibrillation and DPP6. Neth Heart J 2011;19(6):290–6.

33. Sturm AC, Kline CF, Glynn P, et al. Use of whole exome sequencing for the identification of Ito-based arrhythmia mechanism and therapy. J Am Heart Assoc 2015;4(5). https://doi.org/10.1161/JAHA.114.001762.

34. Nerbonne JM, Kass RS. Molecular physiology of cardiac repolarization. Physiol Rev 2005;85(4): 1205–53.

35. Haissaguerre M, Cheniti G, Hocini M, et al. Purkinje network and myocardial substrate at the onset of human ventricular fibrillation: implications for catheter ablation. Eur Heart J 2022;43(12):1234–47.

36. Krahn AD, Healey JS, Chauhan V, et al. Systematic assessment of patients with unexplained cardiac arrest: cardiac arrest survivors with preserved ejection fraction registry (CASPER). Circulation 2009;120(4): 278–85.

37. Somani R, Krahn AD, Healey JS, et al. Procainamide infusion in the evaluation of unexplained cardiac arrest: from the cardiac arrest survivors with preserved ejection fraction registry (CASPER). Heart Rhythm 2014;11(6):1047–54.

38. Krahn AD, Healey JS, Chauhan VS, et al. Epinephrine infusion in the evaluation of unexplained cardiac arrest and familial sudden death: from the cardiac arrest survivors with preserved Ejection Fraction Registry. Circulation Arrhythmia and electrophysiology 2012;5(5):933–40.

39. Vittoria Matassini M, Krahn AD, Gardner M, et al. Evolution of clinical diagnosis in patients presenting with unexplained cardiac arrest or syncope due to polymorphic ventricular tachycardia. Heart Rhythm 2014;11(2):274–81.

40. Champagne J, Geelen P, Philippon F, et al. Recurrent cardiac events in patients with idiopathic ventricular fibrillation, excluding patients with the Brugada syndrome. BMC Med 2005;3:1.

41. Alqarawi W, Dewidar O, Tadros R, et al. Defining idiopathic ventricular fibrillation: a systematic review of diagnostic testing yield in apparently unexplained cardiac arrest. Heart Rhythm 2021;18(7):1178–85.

42. Stiles MK, Wilde AAM, Abrams DJ, et al. 2020 APHRS/HRS expert consensus statement on the investigation of decedents with sudden unexplained death and patients with sudden cardiac arrest, and of their families. Heart Rhythm 2021;18(1):e1–50.

43. Mellor G, Laksman ZWM, Tadros R, et al. Genetic testing in the evaluation of unexplained cardiac arrest: from the CASPER (cardiac arrest survivors with preserved ejection fraction registry). Circ Cardiovasc Genet 2017;10(3). https://doi.org/10.1161/CIRCGENETICS.116.001686.

44. Lahrouchi N, Raju H, Lodder EM, et al. Utility of postmortem genetic testing in cases of sudden

arrhythmic death syndrome. J Am Coll Cardiol 2017; 69(17):2134–45.

45. Grondin S, Davies B, Cadrin-Tourigny J, et al. Importance of genetic testing in unexplained cardiac arrest. Eur Heart J 2022;43(32):3071–81.

46. Al-Khatib SM, Stevenson WG, Ackerman MJ, et al. 2017 AHA/ACC/HRS guideline for management of patients with ventricular arrhythmias and the prevention of sudden cardiac death: Executive summary: a report of the American college of cardiology/American heart association task force on clinical practice guidelines and the heart rhythm society. Heart Rhythm 2018;15(10):e190–252.

47. Zeppenfeld K, Tfelt-Hansen J, de Riva M, et al. 2022 ESC Guidelines for the management of patients with ventricular arrhythmias and the prevention of sudden cardiac death. Eur Heart J 2022;43(40): 3997–4126.

48. Wilkoff BL, Fauchier L, Stiles MK, et al. 2015 HRS/ EHRA/APHRS/SOLAECE expert consensus statement on optimal implantable cardioverter-defibrillator programming and testing. Heart Rhythm 2016;13(2): e50–86.

49. Sacher F, Probst V, Maury P, et al. Outcome after implantation of a cardioverter-defibrillator in patients with Brugada syndrome: a multicenter study-part 2. Circulation 2013;128(16):1739–47.

50. Olde Nordkamp LR, Postema PG, Knops RE, et al. Implantable cardioverter-defibrillator harm in young patients with inherited arrhythmia syndromes: a systematic review and meta-analysis of inappropriate shocks and complications. Heart Rhythm 2016; 13(2):443–54.

51. Blom LJ, Visser M, Christiaans I, et al. Incidence and predictors of implantable cardioverter-defibrillator therapy and its complications in idiopathic ventricular fibrillation patients. Europace 2019;21(10): 1519–26.

52. Conte G, Belhassen B, Lambiase P, et al. Out-of-hospital cardiac arrest due to idiopathic ventricular fibrillation in patients with normal electrocardiograms: results from a multicentre long-term registry. Europace 2019;21(11):1670–7.

53. Knecht S, Sacher F, Wright M, et al. Long-term follow-up of idiopathic ventricular fibrillation ablation: a multicenter study. J Am Coll Cardiol 2009;54(6): 522–8.

54. Malhi N, Cheung CC, Deif B, et al. Challenge and impact of quinidine access in sudden death syndromes: a national experience. JACC Clin Electrophysiol 2019;5(3):376–82.

55. Belhassen B, Glick A, Viskin S. Excellent long-term reproducibility of the electrophysiologic efficacy of quinidine in patients with idiopathic ventricular fibrillation and Brugada syndrome. Pacing and clinical electrophysiology : PACE (Pacing Clin Electrophysiol) 2009;32(3):294–301.

56. Mazzanti A, Maragna R, Vacanti G, et al. Hydroquinidine prevents life-threatening arrhythmic events in patients with short QT syndrome. J Am Coll Cardiol 2017;70(24):3010–5.

57. Andorin A, Gourraud JB, Mansourati J, et al. The QUIDAM study: hydroquinidine therapy for the management of Brugada syndrome patients at high arrhythmic risk. Heart Rhythm 2017;14(8):1147–54.

58. Viskin S, Wilde AA, Guevara-Valdivia ME, et al. Quinidine, a life-saving medication for Brugada syndrome, is inaccessible in many countries. J Am Coll Cardiol 2013;61(23):2383–7.

59. Li COY, Franciosi S, Deyell MW, et al. Intermediate-coupled premature ventricular complexes and ventricular tachycardia during exercise recovery. HeartRhythm Case Rep 2021;7(2):127–30.

60. Kataoka N, Nagase S, Okawa K, et al. Multifocal Purkinje-related premature contractions and electrical storm suppressed by quinidine and verapamil in a case with short-coupled ventricular fibrillation. J Cardiol Cases 2022;25(6):338–42.

61. Edwards DJ, Lavoie R, Beckman H, et al. The effect of coadministration of verapamil on the pharmacokinetics and metabolism of quinidine. Clin Pharmacol Ther 1987;41(1):68–73.

62. Haissaguerre M, Sacher F, Nogami A, et al. Characteristics of recurrent ventricular fibrillation associated with inferolateral early repolarization role of drug therapy. J Am Coll Cardiol 2009;53(7):612–9.

63. Laksman Z, Barichello S, Roston TM, et al. Acute management of ventricular arrhythmia in patients with suspected inherited heart rhythm disorders. JACC Clin Electrophysiol 2019;5(3):267–83.

64. Mellor G, Steinberg C, Laksman Z, et al. Short-coupled ventricular fibrillation. J Cardiovasc Electrophysiol 2016;27(10):1236–7.

The Novel Familial ST-Depression Syndrome – Current Knowledge and Perspectives

Alex Hørby Christensen, MD, PhD[a,b,c],*, Henning Bundgaard, MD, DMSc[a,c]

KEYWORDS

- Arrhythmia • Sudden cardiac death • Atrial fibrillation • Polymorphic ventricular tachycardia
- Electrocardiography

KEY POINTS

- Familial ST-depression syndrome is an autosomal dominantly inherited cardiac disease characterized by constant, nonischemic ST-segment depressions in multiple leads.
- The diagnosis is based on proposed diagnostic criteria encompassing ECG features and familial occurrence.
- Its clinical presentation includes supraventricular arrhythmias, polymorphic ventricular tachycardia, sudden cardiac death, and left ventricular systolic dysfunction.

INTRODUCTION

More than a century after its discovery, the electrocardiogram (ECG) retains its position as a cornerstone in the clinical management of patients presenting with cardiac symptoms. Indeed, triaging of patients with acute chest pain is exclusively based on the presence of specific electrocardiographic patterns and clinical care for patients presenting with arrhythmic symptoms greatly relies on findings on the standard 12-lead ECG.

Despite the long history of the ECG, and many years of scientific exploration using this diagnostic modality, a new phenotype was described in 2018; familial ST-depression syndrome (FSTD). The disease is characterized by the familial occurrence of persistent, nonischemic concave ST-depressions in multiple leads[1–3] and the clinical presentation may include arrhythmias (including sudden cardiac death, SCD), and left ventricular systolic dysfunction. Thereby, FSTD joins the spectrum of inherited cardiac diseases that are diagnosed based on specific electrocardiographic patterns such as the long QT syndrome,[4,5] catecholaminergic polymorphic ventricular tachycardia,[6] Brugada syndrome,[7] progressive cardiac conduction disorder,[8] short QT syndrome,[9,10] and early repolarization syndrome.[11] These phenotypes may be highly variable in their presentation which may span from individuals diagnosed due to incidental ECG findings, to previous healthy individuals suffering SCD as their first disease manifestation. This very variable presentation, even within families, underlines the crucial role of identifying at-risk individuals and proper risk stratification.

The aim of the current review is to provide an up-to-date overview of the existing knowledge on the epidemiologic, clinical, and genetic aspects of familial ST-depression syndrome.

[a] The Unit for Inherited Cardiac Diseases, Department of Cardiology, The Heart Centre, Copenhagen University Hospital - Rigshospitalet, Blegdamsvej 9, Copenhagen OE DK-2100, Denmark; [b] Department of Cardiology, Copenhagen University Hospital - Herlev-Gentofte Hospital, Borgmester Ib Juuls Vej 1, Herlev DK-2730, Denmark; [c] Department of Clinical Medicine, University of Copenhagen, Blegdamsvej 3B, 2200 Copenhagen N, Denmark
* Corresponding author. Department of Cardiology, Copenhagen University Hospital - Herlev-Gentofte Hospital, Borgmester Ib Juuls Vej 1, Herlev DK-2730, Denmark.
E-mail address: alexhc@dadlnet.dk

Card Electrophysiol Clin 15 (2023) 343–348
https://doi.org/10.1016/j.ccep.2023.04.008

EPIDEMIOLOGY

The prevalence of FTSD is currently unknown, but the disease is likely rare, and less prevalent than the typical estimates for hypertrophic cardiomyopathy (1:500), long QT syndrome (1:2500), arrhythmogenic right ventricular cardiomyopathy (1:5000), and catecholaminergic polymorphic ventricular tachycardia (1:10,000; likely lower in Denmark).[12] We have currently identified 54 Danish patients from 19 families with FSTD originating predominantly from the eastern and central parts of Denmark. However, the initial FSTD report[1] also included patients from the United Kingdom and the Netherlands, which together with sporadic case descriptions we have received from other countries, underlies that FSTD likely exists in many countries and is probably underdiagnosed due to unawareness of the condition. We are currently working on an initiative to screen large ECG datasets to provide reliable prevalence estimates of the ECG phenotype.

DIAGNOSIS

Diagnostic criteria have been proposed (**Table 1**) to facilitate proper identification and handling of patients suspected of having FSTD. The diagnosis is predominantly based on constant concave-shaped ST-depressions in multiple leads (**Fig. 1**) unexplained by factors such as ischemic heart disease, significant valvular heart disease, myocardial hypertrophy, presence of bundle branch blocks, hypertension, digoxin treatment, electrolyte abnormalities, and so forth. The first patients we identified[1] had very pronounced ST-segment abnormalities in more than half the leads, but the identification of additional families led to the observation that in some families, in particular younger, asymptomatic relatives, the ECG phenotype was less pronounced which led to updated proposed diagnostic criteria.[3] The ECG phenotype must be persistent over time, be proven hereditary, and show accentuation during exercise. Indeed, we have evaluated suspected FSTD cases where we eventually rejected the diagnosis, with the main causes for discarding the diagnosis being observations of transient normalization of the ECG phenotype and/or lack of proven inheritance of the ECG pattern. Another interesting finding is that our initial data suggest that the ECG phenotypes present in childhood/around puberty with initial ST-segment changes predominately in the inferior leads, while the most pronounced ST-segment depressions are in leads V4, V5, and lead II in adults.[3] The ECG phenotype seems to progress very slowly in most individuals.

ARRHYTHMIAS

The most commonly observed arrhythmias are atrial fibrillation/flutter (AF), other supraventricular arrhythmias, and polymorphic ventricular tachycardia. We have observed arrhythmias in patients with or without accompanying left ventricular systolic dysfunction, and in approximately 40% of the identified patients, closely linked to the age at evaluation and patient sex. The typical age at onset of AF is around 50 years with an overrepresentation of men. This relatively late age of AF onset is in contrast to the much earlier onset of the ECG phenotype underlining that the electrical abnormalities, as demonstrated on the standard 12 lead ECG, are clinically tolerated for decades in most patients. To date, no unique or consistent characteristics of the AF associated with FSTD have been noted: the response to pharmaceutical therapy and/or catheter ablation seems comparable to other AF patients, the AF type may be paroxysmal, persistent or permanent, very prominent left atrial dilatation is not common, and AF is generally not related to left ventricular dysfunction with or without secondary mitral regurgitation.

Prevention of ventricular arrhythmias (VA) and of sudden cardiac death is a cornerstone in the care of patients with inherited cardiac diseases. The typical type of VA we have observed in FSTD is fast polymorphic ventricular arrhythmias—sustained or nonsustained—with relatively short coupling intervals at initiation (**Fig. 2**, panel A). No QT prolongation or electrical alternans were noted prior to arrhythmia initiation. Most patients with VAs have had some degree of left ventricular systolic dysfunction with onset at age in their fifties or sixties. However, a UK patient from the initial report suffered multiple life-threatening episodes of VA at the age of 16 years; however, this patient also had a chromosomal duplication which may have contributed to the observed severe phenotype.[1] No apparent arrhythmic triggers have been identified, for example, no clear association with exercise, sleep, sudden loud acoustic stimuli, exposure to cold, fever, and so forth. In the limited number of patients who have undergone invasive electrophysiological testing data suggest the basal regions of the left ventricle as the main focus of the arrhythmic substrate.

LEFT VENTRICULAR SYSTOLIC DYSFUNCTION

Reduced left ventricular ejection fraction (LVEF), with or without accompanying clinical heart failure, has been found in up to 25% of FSTD patients with an overrepresentation of older and/or male patients. It is important to underline that the

Table 1
Proposed updated diagnostic criteria for Familial ST-depression Syndrome

Probands	Relatives
1. Unexplained concave-upward ST-depression ≥0.1 mV in at least 4 leads (V3-V6 and/or I-III) 80 ms after J point[a]	1. Unexplained concave-upward ST-depression ≥0.05 mV in at least 4 leads (V3-V6 and/or I-III) 80 ms after J point[a]
2. ST-elevation ≥0.1 mV in aVR	2. —
Common criteria for probands and relatives	
3. No episodes of normalized ECG, that is, persistent ECG pattern over time	
4. Accentuation of ST depression during exercise	
5. Autosomal dominant pattern of inheritance	

[a] A notch in the ascending part of the ST segment may be present. Criteria 3 to 5 apply to both probands and relatives.
Data from Christensen AH, Vissing CR, Pietersen A, Tfelt-Hansen J, Hartvig Lindkær Jensen T, Pehrson S, Henriksen FL, Sandgaard NCF, Iversen KK, Jensen HK, Olesen MS, Bundgaard H. Electrocardiographic Findings, Arrhythmias, and Left Ventricular Involvement in Familial ST-Depression Syndrome. Circ Arrhythm Electrophysiol. 2022;15:e010688.

reduction in systolic function is not considered tachycardia-induced, explained by a high burden of premature ventricular contractions (PVC), or viewed as a consequence of comorbidities (ischemic heart disease, hypertension, diabetes, and so forth.) and we consider it part of the late phase of the FSTD phenotype. Left ventricular hypertrophy, reduction in right ventricular ejection fraction, or late gadolinium enhancement on cardiac MRI have been uncommon findings.[1–3]

Analysis of myocardial histology in percutaneously obtained samples from the right side of the interventricular septum has not shown any pathognomonic findings. Results vary from near-normal myocardium to variable degrees of myocyte and nuclear enlargement, some amount of interstitial fibrosis, and subendocardial smooth muscle cell hyperplasia.[2,3] These findings likely reflect the fact that the samples were obtained in different phases of the disease as well as a contribution of patient-specific factors (age, sex, comorbidities, and so forth.); factors known to affect the myocardial architecture.[13,14]

CLINICAL MANAGEMENT

Optimal risk stratification and clinical management of FSTD are currently unknown, no randomized studies have been conducted, and the disease has not been included in any guidelines. Based on the observation that the ECG phenotype seems to precede the onset of arrhythmias and/or left ventricular systolic dysfunction by several decades we do not currently recommend prophylactic treatment with drugs or devices in asymptomatic individuals. Prophylactic treatment with betablockers is generally regarded as very effective in long QT syndrome,[15] although the

choice of betablocker remains controversial,[16] but ineffective, and possibly harmful, in Brugada syndrome.[17] Furthermore, the majority of the younger asymptomatic FSTD patients, have a low burden of PVCs, no exercise-induced arrhythmias, and combined with the absence of documented SCD cases among this younger age groups we do not currently recommend treatment. Along the same lines, in the absence of better alternatives, implantation of cardioverter-defibrillator (ICD) should probably follow general guidelines for non-ischemic cardiomyopathy,[12] although we would consider ICD implantation in FSTD patients with a suspected arrhythmic syncope, in particular in the presence of documented nonsustained ventricular tachycardia, a high PVC burden, or reduced LVEF.

Our initial experiences with the treatment of electrical storms in FSTD have shown disappointing results for amiodarone, betablockers, quinidine, and catheter ablations. Pacing had a very positive effect in one patient. We have not tried verapamil, mostly due to the fact, that the patients have generally had significantly reduced LVEF. Taken together, there is a considerable gap in our knowledge—and unmet need—in the optimal clinical handling of FSTD patients.

INHERITANCE AND GENETICS

An integrated part of the FSTD diagnosis is the familial occurrence of the ECG pattern. From the first 19 families with documented FSTD around 50% of tested family members have had the ECG phenotype with a roughly equal distribution of affected males and females. Furthermore, we observed both male and female transmission to offspring consistent with autosomal dominant inheritance

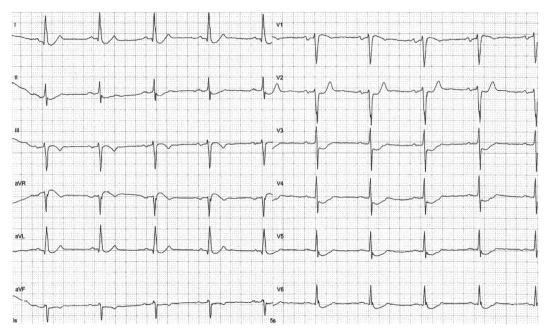

Fig. 1. Electrocardiogram from a 62-year-old male showing marked concave-shaped ST-segment depressions in leads V3-V6, I-II, aVL, and aVF and reciprocal ST-segment elevation in aVR. The patient had a history of persistent atrial fibrillation treated with betablocker, apixaban, and cardioversion. Echocardiography showed preserved left ventricular ejection fraction, no valvular heart disease, and normal coronary arteries.

with high penetrance. Based on these observations we recommend cascade screening as in other cardiogenetic diseases.

Identification of the underlying genetic cause of FSTD would be a major step forward and likely shed new light on cardiac cellular electrophysiology, as an important stepping stone for understanding the underlying molecular disease mechanisms and guiding treatment, as well as enabling identification of at-risk relatives and prenatal diagnostics. Over time we have performed Sanger sequencing of small gene panels, NGS-based large gene panels (including all known genes associated with established cardiovascular diseases), multiplex ligation-dependent probe amplification, comparative genomic hybridization

A   **B**

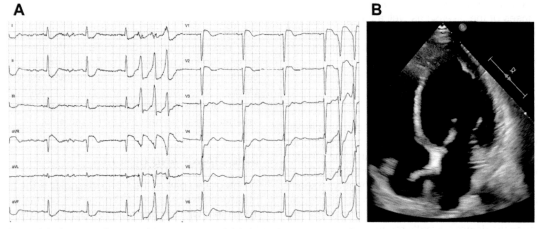

Fig. 2. (*A*) Electrocardiogram from a 71-year-old female showing runs of non-sustained polymorphic ventricular tachycardia and pronounced ST-segment changes in multiple leads. She had a history of aborted sudden cardiac death, left ventricular systolic dysfunction, and normal coronary arteries. Arrhythmia onset is characterized by relatively short-coupled trigger premature ventricular complexes. (*B*) Two-dimensional echocardiogram from the same patient with a dilated left ventricle and a left ventricular ejection fraction of 25%.

arrays, and exome sequencing with various capture kits and copy number variation analyses without any positive findings.

PERSPECTIVES

Many aspects of FSTD are still unknown and current conceptions about the disease will likely change during the next decade. Lessons learned from the understanding of for example, Brugada syndrome is that after three decades of research, the perception of the disease has changed from an idiopathic, lethal condition to now a predominantly oligogenic disease[18] with a relatively low risk of arrhythmias in the majority of patients.[19]

Establishing a reliable estimate of FSTD prevalence is an important step to evaluate the public health impact of the disease and focusing on preventive measures. Furthermore, the identification of additional families will increase our insight into disease manifestations, including ECG characteristics, incidence of arrhythmias and systolic dysfunction, arrhythmic triggers, and biomarkers, and will help optimize risk stratification. Indeed, the optimal handling of ventricular arrhythmias is largely unknown and remains a clinical challenge. Insight into the underlying genetics is also important as it will likely provide new insight into cardiac electrophysiology that is important beyond FSTD. Lastly, finding a causal genetic variant affecting for example, a structural protein, an ion channel, transcription factor, and so forth, may guide precision medicine with specific interventions, including novel drug targets.

A question we have been asked numerous times is whether FSTD should be classified as a primary arrhythmic disease or a cardiomyopathy. Based on the available data we currently consider it a mixed entity with features that support both classifications, including a characteristic ECG pattern, arrhythmias as the most common clinical presentation, but also left ventricular systolic dysfunction in the later phases. A clear distinction between primary arrhythmia syndromes and cardiomyopathies is probably often not biologically accurate as several diagnostic entities typically regarded as "electrical diseases" (eg, Brugada or long QT syndrome) may have structural and/or functional myocardial abnormalities.[20,21] Knowledge of the underlying genetics will likely also make this distinction more accurate.

In conclusion, FSTD is a novel inherited cardiac syndrome associated with arrhythmias and systolic dysfunction. The coming years will provide intriguing new insights into many unexplored aspects of the disease.

CLINICS CARE POINTS

- Clinicians should be aware of a possible genetic etiology when encountering patients with constant, unexplained ST-segment depression in multiple leads.
- Cascade screening is therefore recommended.
- Diagnosis is based on suggested diagnostic criteria.
- Treatment is currently not recommended in asymptomatic patients without documented arrhythmias or structural heart disease.
- The optimal treatment is unknown, but an ICD should be considered in patients with familial ST-depression syndrome with presumed arrhythmic syncope.

DISCLOSURES

None.

ACKNOWLEDGMENTS

The AP Møller Foundation (H. Bundgaard), The Research Foundation at Rigshospitalet (H. Bundgaard), The Independent Research Fund Denmark (0134–00363B, A.H. Christensen), The Novo Nordisk Foundation Denmark (NNF20OC0065799, A.H. Christensen), and NordForsk supported this study.

REFERENCES

1. Bundgaard H, Jøns C, Lodder EM, et al. A novel familial cardiac arrhythmia syndrome with Widespread ST-segment depression. N Engl J Med 2018;379: 1780–1.
2. Christensen AH, Nyholm BC, Vissing CR, et al. Natural history and clinical characteristics of the first 10 Danish families with familial ST-depression syndrome. J Am Coll Cardiol 2021;77:2617–9.
3. Christensen AH, Vissing CR, Pietersen A, et al. Electrocardiographic findings, arrhythmias, and left ventricular Involvement in familial ST-depression syndrome. Circ Arrhythm Electrophysiol 2022;15: e010688.
4. Jervell A, Lange-Nielsen F. Congenital deaf-mutism, functional heart disease with prolongation of the Q-T interval and sudden death. Am Heart J 1957;54: 59–68.

5. Romano C, Gemme G, Pongiglione R. Rare cardiac arrhythmias of the Pediatric age. II. Syncopal Attacks due to paroxysmal ventricular fibrillation. (Presentation of 1st case in Italian Pediatric Literature). Clin Pediatr (Bologna) 1963;45:656–83.

6. Coumel P, Fidelle J, Lucet V, et al. Catecholaminergic-induced severe ventricular arrhythmias with Adams-Stokes syndrome in children: report of four cases. Br Heart J 1978;40(supplement):28–37.

7. Brugada P, Brugada J. Right bundle branch block, persistent ST segment elevation and sudden cardiac death: a distinct clinical and electrocardiographic syndrome. A multicenter report. J Am Coll Cardiol 1992;20:1391–6.

8. Schott JJ, Alshinawi C, Kyndt F, et al. Cardiac conduction defects associate with mutations in SCN5A. Nat Genet 1999;23:20–1.

9. Gaita F, Giustetto C, Bianchi F, et al. Short QT Syndrome: a familial cause of sudden death. Circulation 2003;108:965–70.

10. Gussak I, Brugada P, Brugada J, et al. Idiopathic short QT interval: a new clinical syndrome? Cardiology 2000;94:99–102.

11. Kalla H, Yan GX, Marinchak R. Ventricular fibrillation in a patient with prominent J (Osborn) waves and ST segment elevation in the inferior electrocardiographic leads: a Brugada syndrome variant? J Cardiovasc Electrophysiol 2000;11:95–8.

12. Zeppenfeld K, Tfelt-Hansen J, de Riva M, et al. ESC Guidelines for the management of patients with ventricular arrhythmias and the prevention of sudden cardiac death. Eur Heart J 2022;43:3997–4126.

13. Nakou ES, Parthenakis FI, Kallergis EM, et al. Healthy aging and myocardium: a complicated process with various effects in cardiac structure and physiology. Int J Cardiol 2016;209:167–75.

14. Keller KM, Howlett SE. Sex Differences in the Biology and Pathology of the aging heart. Can J Cardiol 2016;32:1065–73.

15. Villain E, Denjoy I, Lupoglazoff JM, et al. Low incidence of cardiac events with beta-blocking therapy in children with long QT syndrome. Eur Heart J 2004; 25:1405–11.

16. Abu-Zeitone A, Peterson DR, Polonsky B, et al. Efficacy of different beta-blockers in the treatment of long QT syndrome. J Am Coll Cardiol 2014;64: 1352–8.

17. Brodie OT, Michowitz Y, Belhassen B. Pharmacological therapy in Brugada syndrome. Arrhythmia Electrophysiol Rev 2018;7:135–42.

18. Barc J, Tadros R, Glinge C, et al. Genome-wide association analyses identify new Brugada syndrome risk loci and highlight a new mechanism of sodium channel regulation in disease susceptibility. Nat Genet 2022;54:232–9.

19. Honarbakhsh S, Providencia R, Garcia-Hernandez J, et al. Brugada syndrome risk Investigators. A primary prevention clinical risk Score Model for patients with Brugada syndrome (BRUGADA-RISK). JACC Clin Electrophysiol 2021;7: 210–22.

20. Frustaci A, Priori SG, Pieroni M, et al. Cardiac histological substrate in patients with clinical phenotype of Brugada syndrome. Circulation 2005;112:3680–7.

21. Leren IS, Hasselberg NE, Saberniak J, et al. Cardiac Mechanical Alterations and Genotype specific Differences in Subjects with long QT syndrome. JACC Cardiovasc Imaging 2015;8:501–10.

Prevention of Sudden Death and Management of Ventricular Arrhythmias in Arrhythmogenic Cardiomyopathy

Alessandro Trancuccio, MD[a,b,1], Deni Kukavica, MD, PhD[a,b,1], Andrea Sugamiele, BS[a], Andrea Mazzanti, MD, PhD[a,b], Silvia G. Priori, MD, PhD[a,b],*

KEYWORDS

- Arrhythmogenic cardiomyopathy • Sudden cardiac death • Implantable cardioverter defibrillator
- Ventricular arrhythmias • Heart failure

KEY POINTS

- Stratification of SCD risk is a key clinical challenge in the management of patients with ACM.
- This review presents the state-of-the-art approaches to prevent the occurrence of SCD in patients with ACM.
- Refinement of current risk stratification models is critical to facilitate shared decision making regarding ICD implantation.

INTRODUCTION

Arrhythmogenic cardiomyopathy (ACM) is an umbrella term for a group of inherited diseases of the cardiac muscle characterized by progressive fibro-fatty replacement of the myocardium.[1] As suggested by the name, the disease confers electrical instability to the heart and increases the risk of the development of life-threatening arrhythmias (LAE), representing one of the leading causes of sudden cardiac death (SCD), especially in young athletes.[2,3] In the light of the recent data from a meta-analysis which included 5485 patients affected by ACM and found that patients with ACM suffer SCD at a rate of 3.57 (95% CI: 0.56–8.27) per 1000 person years,[4] the issue of prevention of SCD in this population assumes a particular relevance.

In this review, the authors review the current knowledge of the disease, highlighting the state-of-the-art approaches to the prevention of the occurrence of SCD.

ARRHYTHMOGENIC CARDIOMYOPATHY: AN OVERVIEW
Epidemiology

Most authors estimate the disease prevalence to be between 1:1000 and 1:5,000.[5,6] However, due to a number of issues, such as the age- and sex-

Funding: Ricerca Corrente funding scheme of the Italian Ministry of Health and Italian Ministry of Research and Dipartimenti di Eccellenza 2018 to 2022 grant to the Molecular Medicine Department (University of Pavia).
[a] Department of Molecular Medicine, University of Pavia, Pavia, Italy; [b] Molecular Cardiology, IRCCS Istituti Clinici Scientifici Maugeri, Pavia, Italy
[1] Contributed equally as first authors.
* Corresponding author. Molecular Cardiology – IRCCS ICS Maugeri, Via S. Maugeri, 10, Pavia 27100, Italy.
E-mail address: silvia.priori@icsmaugeri.it

Card Electrophysiol Clin 15 (2023) 349–365
https://doi.org/10.1016/j.ccep.2023.04.004

dependent penetrance typical of the disease,[7] a substantial decline in rates of autopsy[8] that contribute significantly to the diagnosis and the fact that the diagnostic criteria[9] have been specific for the right ventricular form of the disease,[10,11] epidemiologic data remain incomplete and underestimate the prevalence of the disease.

Genetic Architecture of Arrhythmogenic Cardiomyopathy

In parallel with the paradigm shifts which brought about changes in the nomenclature, the genetic architecture of ACM has changed profoundly over the years. Most recent data from the literature suggest that among the five genes encoding for desmosomal proteins (PKP2 encoding for plakophilin-2, DSP encoding for desmoplakin, DSG2 encoding for desmoglein-2, DSC2 encoding for desmocollin, and JUP encoding for plakoglobin), PKP2 variants are the most prevalent.[12,13] However, as most cohorts have been diagnosed using the 2010 Task Force Criteria which favor the right ventricular form of the disease and considering that variants in PKP2 are associated with a right-dominant phenotype caution ought to be exercised when interpreting these data.

In addition to desmosomal variants, a range of non-desmosomal gene variants have been associated with ACM. However, recent evidence-based reappraisal found that in addition to the abovementioned five desmosomal genes, variants on only three other genes ought to be considered as disease-causing: TMEM43 encoding for transmembrane protein 43, DES encoding for desmin, and PLN encoding for phospholamban.[14] Even though these three genes do not code for desmosomal proteins, the disease-causing variants on these genes alter the expression of desmosomal proteins as shown using immunohistochemistry on heart samples from patients with TMEM43-related,[15] DES-related,[16] and PLN-related[17,18] ACM. These data are supported by studies from PLN p.R14del cardiomyopathy that show that the absence of desmosomal protein alterations translates into a phenotype of dilated cardiomyopathy and not ACM phenotype.[18] Put together, evidence suggests that the ACM, despite notable clinicopathological differences,[19] may truly be a disease of different genes converging on the desmosome.

Disease Definition and Diagnosis

Over the years, the definition of ACM has become increasingly more inclusive with a wide variety of heterogeneous clinical entities included.

Currently, the diagnosis of ACM is made using the 2010 updated Task Force Criteria,[9] which are multiparametric and multidisciplinary, requiring expertise in electrophysiology, genetics, and cardiac imaging. Evidence suggesting that only 7% to 15% of patients carriers of a pathogenic DSP gene variant, typically associated with left-dominant ACM,[20] meet the diagnostic criteria[21,22] adding to the growing understanding that 2010 updated Task Force Criteria, are limited in the recognition of left-dominant forms of ACM, leading to their underdiagnosis. To address this, a novel set of criteria called "Padua criteria"[23] have been recently proposed but these remain yet to be validated.

Clinical Presentation and Course of Arrhythmogenic Cardiomyopathy

Patients with ACM present to medical attention, for a wide variety of reasons that shall be treated in this paragraph, on average during the fourth decade of life[7] without major gender differences.[24,25] In athletes, the clinical presentation is anticipated by a decade,[26] whereas pediatric cases remain exceedingly rare but are associated with a more malignant disease.[27,28]

Clinical presentation is heterogeneous and represents a spectrum ranging from SCD to incidental diagnosis in asymptomatic individuals. As suggested by preclinical[29] and clinical studies,[30] SCD may occur in the absence of overt disease. Importantly, a third of patients come to medical attention for arrhythmia-related symptoms, such as syncopal spells or hemodynamically stable monomorphic ventricular tachycardia (MMVT).[7] Relevantly, MMVT seems to be typical of a more advanced stage of the disease, as evidenced by older age[31] and transmural scar[32] in these patients. A peculiar presentation of ACM, which seems to be particularly associated to *DSP* gene variants, is acute myocarditis, and a finding of a particularly high burden of late gadolinium enhancement at cardiac magnetic resonance ought to raise the suspicion of ACM.[20,33] Another clinically relevant disease presentation is atrial fibrillation (AFib) in young individuals,[7] which could be supported by identification of a number of pathogenic desmosomal variants in a large cohort of patients with early-onset AFib.[34] Last, the signs and symptoms of heart failure (HF) at presentation are infrequent and only 3% of patients presented in New York Heart Association (NYHA) class III.[35]

Evidently, patients with ACM present at different stages of the disease, rendering the management complex. Over the lifetime of an individual affected by ACM, the arrhythmic risk is persistently present, but tends to be more accentuated between the third and fifth decade of life when it is estimated to be in the order of 4% per year.[7] Conceptually, four stages of ACM have been proposed (concealed disease, clinically overt disease, right ventricular failure, and lastly biventricular failure),[36,37] but uniform structural disease progression is rare, and seems to be genotype-dependent, as shown by markedly higher rates of HF development at follow-up in *DSP* gene variant carriers as compared with *PKP2* gene variant carriers,[38] confirmed in geographically and ethnically different cohorts.[39]

TREATMENT

The treatment of ACM is based on (1) lifestyle interventions; (2) pharmacologic treatment using class II and class III antiarrhythmic drugs for the control of arrhythmic symptoms and using drugs approved for the treatment of HF; (3) surgical treatment using ablation or cardiac denervation; and last, (4) the judicious use of implantable cardioverter defibrillator (ICD).[6] Importantly, no pharmacologic or surgical treatment has proven to be effective in preventing or reducing SCD in ACM,[7] in contrast to other inherited arrhythmia syndromes.[40]

In terms of lifestyle changes, restriction from high-intensity exercise seems to be the most important preventive tool.[6] In their seminal 2003 work, Corrado and colleagues demonstrated that patients with ACM who participate in sports have a fivefold increased risk of experiencing sudden death compared with nonathletes.[41] Later works demonstrated that high-intensity exercise is associated with both increased arrhythmic risk[7,42,43] and development of HF,[43] providing an evidence-based rationale for exercise restriction.[6]

The cornerstone of treatment aimed at both suppressing ventricular arrhythmias (VA) and treating HF are beta-blockers (BBs), despite the absence of solid clinical evidence to support this indication.[6] In fact, Marcus and colleagues found that BBs were not significantly associated with VA, and more recently our group demonstrated that the use of BB was not associated with a significant reduction in LAE rates,[7] a finding later confirmed by Cappelletto and colleagues.[44] Relevantly, a state-of-the-art statistical analysis based on marginal structural models was used to reanalyze the data presented by Cappelletto and colleagues, demonstrating that BB use was associated with reduction of major VA, but not with a significant improvement in survival.[45]

Similarly, the use of anti-arrhythmic drugs (AAD) is largely based on data from small observational studies.[6] Regarding sotalol, arguably the most studied compound, it has been shown to prevent the inducibility of VA[46] but was not associated with a reduction in clinically relevant arrhythmias.[46,47] Similar discrepancies have been reported for amiodarone with some groups failing to identify a reduction in clinical VAs,[44,46] whereas others have found a significant antiarrhythmic effect.[47] More recently, historic hesitancy regarding the use of flecainide has been cast[48] away, as the Scheinman group has shown that addition of flecainide on the top of BB therapy in patients who experienced a failure of catheter ablation[49] was associated with an excellent recurrence control, finding later corroborated by the Salpêtrière group.[50] In analogy with what has been reported for BB, no evidence regarding the survival benefit of AAD of any class exists.[7]

HF drugs are used according to the current European Society of Cardiology guidelines.[51] Evidence from retrospective studies suggested that renin-angiotensin-aldosterone system blockade was associated with slower disease progression both in terms of tricuspid annular systolic plane excursion reduction and RV dimension dilatation.[52] Recently, to provide a prospectively collected, the evidence-based approach for the use of HF agents, a double-blind randomized study with the aim of recruiting 120 patients from 19 centers in France to evaluate the efficacy of spironolactone, started in September 2021[53] (NCT03593317). Last, heart transplantation represents a curative strategy for patients with ACM, but the elevated arrhythmic burden limits the pretransplant use of inotropes, whereas the pathologic RV remodeling limits the use of mechanical support, such as LVAD.[54]

Catheter ablation represents a viable option for patients with ACM who suffer recurrent, symptomatic ventricular tachycardia (VT), and/or ICD shocks despite optimal pharmacologic treatment.[6] However, in the absence of survival benefit data, ablation cannot be considered an alternative to ICD therapy. In accordance with the degenerative nature of the disease, which typically progresses from epicardium to endocardium, different studies[55–57] and a recently published meta-analysis including 298 patients with ACM[58] all found that endo-epicardial ablation was associated with a reduction of risk of VT recurrence as compared with endocardial-only ablation without significant differences in acute complications. Another surgical approach which has been suggested is the use of bilateral cardiac sympathetic denervation (BCSD). In a small cohort ($n = 8$) of symptomatic patients who failed catheter ablation, BCSD was associated with a reduction, but not abolishment, of ICD shocks or sustained VT over 1.9 ± 0.9 years of follow-up.[59]

In this challenging clinical scenario, where different pharmacologic or surgical treatments have been shown to reduce the arrhythmic burden but not to confer a tangible survival benefit at follow-up, the use of ICD remains the only remaining therapeutic option to prevent SCD in patients with ACM.[4,60,61] Regarding the selection of the device, the high rate of ATP termination (92%)[62] favors the use of traditional transvenous ICD with pacing capability.[6] On the other hand, the use of subcutaneous ICD as compared with transvenous ICD was associated with lower rates of lead dysfunction, tricuspid valve and device infections, no differences in terms of appropriate shock rates, and a modest trend toward increased risk of inappropriate shocks.[63,64] Considering the young age of patients and the remarkable arrhythmic burden that they suffer, the lack of data corroborating survival benefit for any other therapy, physical and psychological impact of ICD implantation[65] and its economic costs,[66] and the long period in which ICD-related complications may develop,[67] incurring additional health care costs,[64,68] the appropriate and timely selection of patients who would benefit most from ICD therapy represents the paramount issue and are dealt in the next section of this review.

PREVENTION OF SUDDEN CARDIAC DEATH: THE IMPORTANCE OF RISK STRATIFICATION
General Considerations

The identification of subjects affected by ACM at risk of LAEs is a crucial moment in the management, and it requires an attentive, patient-centered, multiparametric evaluation, which is best achieved in tertiary expert centers specialized in inherited arrhythmia syndromes.

Unlike other cardiomyopathies, such as hypertrophic cardiomyopathy (HCM),[69,70] or channelopathies, such as long QT syndrome (LQTS),[71,72] where a direct relationship between the severity of the phenotype and the arrhythmic risk has been shown; in ACM, this may not necessarily hold true. Although this has been a source of controversy,[73] the evidence from both preclinical[29] and clinical studies[30] suggest that ACM may manifest with LAEs even in the absence of clinical onset of electrocardiographic and structural changes (**Fig. 1**).

As ACM is a progressive degenerative disease, periodic reevaluation of an individual's risk is recommended. A recent multicentric study showed that the arrhythmic risk and its predictors were dynamic and that periodic risk reassessment was associated with a significant improvement in the accuracy of risk stratification.[74]

Methodological Considerations for Approaching Risk Stratification

Many studies from various research groups have explored risk factors for arrhythmias in patients with ACM, and recently, two meta-analyses have summarized such results.[4,75] Unfortunately, no consensus has been reached regarding the best way to stratify the arrhythmic risk in ACM. Individual studies have tested and occasionally validated in multivariable analyses, which have not always been adequately powered, a large set of different factors with varying results.

The head-to-head comparison of ACM with other inherited arrhythmia syndromes, such as LQTS and Brugada syndrome (BrS), allows us to understand how at least three factors may explain discrepancies between different studies and the resultant difficulty in identifying unique risk factors in ACM.

Differences in the inclusion criteria used for different studies have contributed to some of the methodological issues in risk stratification that the field faces today. The adoption of the currently used 2010 Task Force Criteria[9] translated into profound changes in the study populations, such that studies performed with different diagnostic criteria cannot be compared reliably. Specifically, patients with an overt phenotype have a significantly higher proportion of events with up to 10% of patients with definite ACM-suffering LAEs,[75] whereas on the other hand, 3.7% of all genotype positive-phenotype-negative individuals suffer LAE.[75] Similarly, the variable inclusion of patients with a

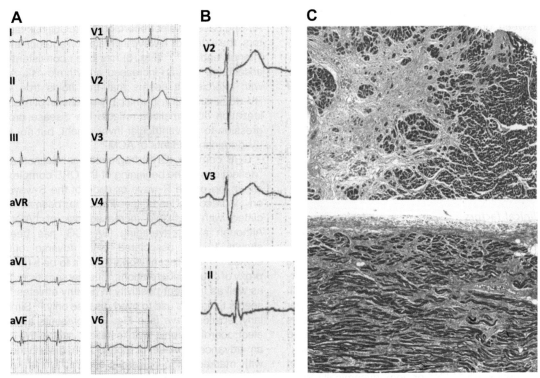

Fig. 1. Sudden cardiac death as the first clinical manifestation of ACM. The figure illustrates the case of an 18-year-old man, without cardiological history, victim of sudden cardiac death during physical exercise. The analysis of previous ECG tracings performed for routine checkups showed sinus rhythm, in the absence of T-wave inversion suggestive of ACM (*A*), and minimal QRS fragmentation in right precordial/inferior leads (*B*). Autoptic examination using Masson's trichrome stain (*C*) demonstrated the presence of subacute biventricular inflammation, with multiple foci of intramural fibrotic substitution in both ventricles, chronic interstitial lymphocytic infiltration, and disarray at the level of the anterior wall of LV. Postmortem genetic testing identified a pathogenic truncating variant on the *DSP* gene.

history of LAE ("secondary prevention") and patients without a history of LAE ("primary prevention") represents another important source of heterogeneity. It is thus clear how variable inclusion criteria can profoundly modify the event rates observed and therefore the risk factors identified.

Importantly, the heterogeneity of the study endpoints used, ranging from SCD and its surrogates such as LAEs[7] to composite outcomes including sustained MMVTs and appropriate ICD interventions,[13] has similarly contributed to differences in event rates and risk factors identified. In contrast to LQTS and BrS, diseases in which the occurrence of sustained ventricular arrhythmias almost invariably represents a surrogate for SCD, in ACM the occurrence of sustained MMVTs may be hemodynamically well tolerated.[7] On the one hand, the inclusion of appropriate ICD shock as an endpoint may be criticized as the definition of "appropriate" is not always clear-cut, as device programming and pharmacologic therapy are heterogeneous, and as it may be argued that,

logically, it represents circularity. On the other hand, the restriction of endpoints to SCD or its equivalents ("hard endpoints") may not be feasible in all contemporary cohorts for a variety of reasons, including high rates of ICD implantation. We advocate for the use of "hard" endpoints, whenever possible, with the inclusion of only those arrhythmic events for which it can be reasonably assumed that they would have been fatal without external intervention, such as hemodynamically nontolerated arrhythmias and/or arrhythmias with a cycle length less than 250 ms. The best way to handle outcomes in ICD carriers still remains an issue of considerable debate and partially contributes to the abovementioned heterogeneity induced by variable inclusion of patients in "primary" and "secondary" prevention.

Finally, at odds with LQTS and BrS, the sheer number of risk factors studied is significantly larger and these risk factors are dynamic, owing to the progressive nature of the disease. It is intuitive to understand how the heterogeneity in the inclusion of a variable proportion of risk factors between one study and another constitutes a further element of variability which makes cross-validations difficult.

Risk Stratification Factors for Life-Threatening Arrhythmias

Different risk factors have been identified and can be classified into (1) clinical factors, (2) electrocardiographic parameters, (3) multimodality imaging parameters, (4) parameters deriving from invasive testing (eg, electrophysiological study), (5) genetic background, and (6) biomarkers.

Clinical factors

In analogy to other inherited arrhythmia syndromes such as HCM,[76] LQTS,[71] BrS,[77] catecholaminergic polymorphic ventricular tachycardia (CPVT),[78] patients with ACM who survived a cardiac arrest should be considered at high risk with an estimated rate of LAE in excess of 10% per year.[60] Accordingly, ICD implantation in patients in secondary prevention is universally recognized as a class I recommendation for ICD implantation.[6]

In patients in primary prevention, history of syncopal spells[4,7,75,79] or hemodynamically tolerated sustained MMVT[4,7,75,79] (Fig. 2) imparts a two- to fourfold increased risk of LAE, and ICD implantation should be considered.[6]

Male gender has been consistently associated[4,7,80–83] to a 1.5- to 3-fold increased risk. Relevantly, elevated serum testosterone levels were independently associated with major arrhythmic events in male patients, whereas estradiol levels were protective in female patients.[84] Moreover, elevated testosterone levels worsened, whereas normal premenopausal estradiol levels decreased, apoptosis and lipogenesis in human-induced pluripotent stem cell-derived cardiomyocytes (iPSC-CMs) from a patient with a *PKP2* mutation.[84]

Intense physical activity is a modifiable risk factor with a strong negative prognostic value in ACM,[7,85,86] but some nuance exists. In classical ACM, evidence from both clinical[7] and preclinical studies converges on the detrimental role of exercise. At the cellular level, exercise worsens the Ca^{2+} mishandling[87] and results in DNA damage with excess oxidant production[88]; and at the tissue level, results in contractile deficit and increased apoptosis.[89] Interestingly, Smith and colleagues did not identify a significant association between severe VA and exercise in patients with left ventricle (LV)-dominant ACM carriers of *DSP* mutations,[20] and insights from a murine model of *DSP* haploinsufficiency suggested that unexpectedly, exercise restored transcript levels of the majority of dysregulated genes in cardiac myocytes.[90]

Electrocardiographic parameters

Among baseline electrocardiogram (ECG) risk factors, the extent of T-wave inversion on anterior and inferior leads[4,83,85] (Fig. 3) has been consistently associated with an increased arrhythmic risk. As with exercise, it seems that this holds true in RV-dominant ACM, in which the extension of repolarization abnormalities reflects the disease progression to a biventricular involvement, but not in LV-dominant variants of ACM.[91]

QRS complex (QRS) fragmentation, defined as "deflections at the beginning of the QRS complex, either top of the R-wave or nadir of the S-wave, on ≥ 2 precordial leads" (see Fig. 3) has been associated with a sixfold increased risk of LAEs.[4] Although signal averaging (SA-ECG) has been shown to be associated with adverse outcomes[25,92] and recent works found it to be a good proxy of structural alterations,[93] its low sensitivity,[94] as well as frequent positivity in healthy athletes,[95] seems to limit its use to overt disease only.[93] Similarly, epsilon wave (see Fig. 3) represents a late electrocardiographic manifestation, suggestive of an advanced phase of conduction disturbance with marked endo-epicardial scarring[96] and has been shown to contribute only marginally to the diagnosis with high interobserver variability,[97] which likely explains its inclusion as a risk factor in a handful of studies.[91,98]

Periodic registration of 24-hour Holter ECG is useful in documenting episodes of nonsustained VT (VTns) (Fig. 4), the prognostic role of which has been well demonstrated in individual studies[83,99–101] as well as meta-analyses.[4,75] Daily premature ventricular contraction (PVC) burden (expressed as ln[PVCs count/24h]) was shown to be associated with an increased arrhythmia risk at follow-up and included in 2019 arrhythmogenic right ventricular cardiomyopathy (ARVC) risk calculator,[102,103] even though meta-analyses failed to confirm this association.[4,75] To further complicate the picture, a recent multicenter study on 408 patients revealed that both PVC and VTns burden declined over the course of 5 years of follow-up (−1200 PVCs per day and −14% VTns, respectively), both when considered at baseline and when included as time-varying covariates.[74] Whether these changes in the arrhythmic burden are a part of the natural history of the disease, daily variations in PVC burden, or they represent the result of initiating pharmacologic therapy or selection bias remains to be elucidated.

Finally, AFib can be found in 10% to 30% of patients with ACM[104,105] and data from a large cohort of 301 patients with ACM[7] demonstrated that AFib was a strong predictor of LAEs at follow-up.

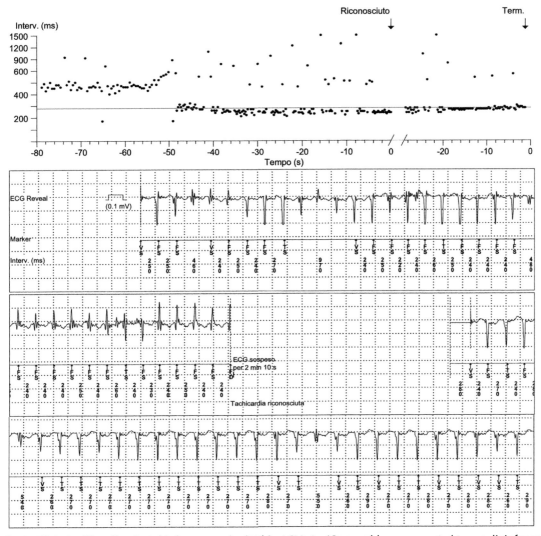

Fig. 2. Clinical utility of implantable loop recorder (ILR) in ACM. An 18-year-old man presented to our clinic for an episode of palpitations associated with vertigo during physical exercise. During the visit at our clinic, a definitive diagnosis of ARVC was made based on repolarization abnormalities, arrhythmia burden, and the identification of a pathogenic *PKP2* gene variant. Therapeutic options were discussed and an indication for an implantable defibrillator (ICD) implantation was made, which the patient refused. To correlate symptoms with the arrhythmia burden, an ILR was proposed, which the patient accepted. One year after the implantation of ILR, a second episode of palpitations associated with vertigo occurred during physical exertion, with documentation of a rapid tachycardia (mean frequency 250 bpm), lasting 3 minutes. Following this episode, interpreted as sustained ventricular tachycardia, the patient accepted an indication for an ICD.

Imaging

In right-dominant, classical ACM forms, RV undergoes a progressive dilatation, in the order of 0.3 to 0.5 mm per year, and progressive dysfunction, with the reduction of RV fractional area change by 0.6% to 0.7% per year.[106,107] In this context, documentation of RV dysfunction seems to be a robust risk factor for LAE, as evaluated by standard 2D echocardiography[108,109] (**Fig. 5**), tissue Doppler imaging,[110] or cardiac MRI.[111] These findings were confirmed by meta-analyses,[4,75] seem to remain

predictive over the course of follow-up,[74] and have been included in the 2019 ARVC risk calculator.[102,103]

Interestingly, although the reduction of RV function seems to be a risk factor useful in predicting LAEs in all forms of ACM,[91] reduction of LV ejection fraction seems to be particularly important for LV-dominant forms, and in particular, patients with *DSP* gene variants.[20,91] Other predictors related to cardiac function, such as strain, have been proposed to help diagnosis,[112] identify patients at risk

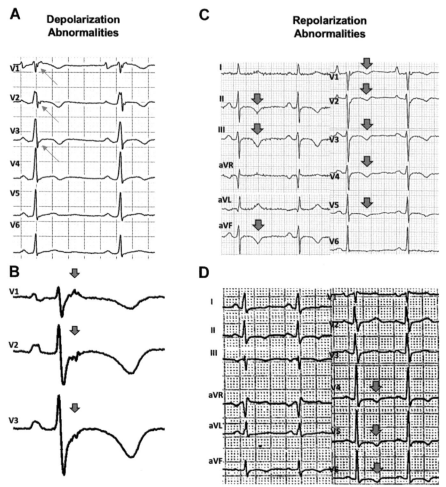

Fig. 3. Electrocardiographic abnormalities typical of arrhythmogenic cardiomyopathy (ACM). The figure shows typical depolarization (*A, B*) and repolarization (*C, D*) abnormalities documented in patients with ACM and correlated to an increased arrhythmic risk (see text for details). (*A*) QRS complex fragmentation in the right precordial leads (*blue arrows*) in a typical RV-dominant ACM case, caused by truncating variant in *PKP2* gene. (*B*) Documentation of epsilon wave in the right precordial leads (*blue arrows*), a peculiar ECG sign suggestive of an advanced phase of the disease, in a patient with *PKP2*-related ACM and severe biventricular dysfunction, which led to cardiac transplant. (*C*) T-wave inversion extending beyond V3 (*blue arrows*) in a patient harboring a *DSG2* pathogenic variant, a marker of biventricular involvement. (*D*) T-wave inversion confined to infero-lateral leads (*blue arrows*), typical of LV-dominant forms of ACM caused by *DSP* mutations.

of structural progression[113] and arrhythmia, but now, although reduced RV strain (see **Fig. 5**) and LV strain were found to be associated to sustained VA, they do not seem to have incremental value over RV ejection fraction (EF) and LV EF.[111]

In addition to the morpho-functional parameters, the presence of late gadolinium enhancement (LGE) has been extensively studied in ACM. LGE burden seems to follow a genotype-specific distribution,[19] and a large burden of it (eg, >20%[114]), even in the context of acute myocarditis,[33] ought to raise suspicion of the diagnosis of ACM. Elegant works have shown that LV LGE burden correlated with low QRS voltages on the peripheral leads and

extension of T-wave inversions on the precordial leads (**Fig. 6**),[114] suggesting that these electrocardiographic factors are proxies of the underlying pathologic process. Unsurprisingly, LV LGE has been shown to be a potent predictor of arrhythmic risk,[115] also in a recent meta-analysis.[116]

Invasive tests: electrophysiological study

Several studies studied the role for electroanatomical mapping in risk stratification of patients with ACM.[117,118] Santangeli and colleagues[117] found that the presence of delayed and fragmented electrograms, but not the extent of electroanatomic scars, was a strong predictor of

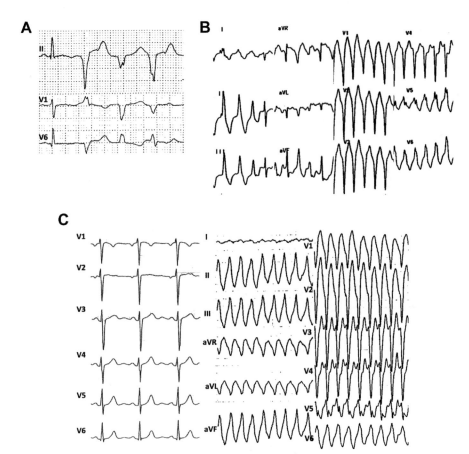

Fig. 4. Arrhythmias during exercise stress test (EST) and 24-hour Holter ECG. Arrhythmias in ACM are documented at 24-hour Holter ECG, which frequently demonstrates a modest arrhythmic burden of the disease, and the use of 12-lead ECG Holter such as in (*A*), permits the evaluation of arrhythmia morphology (*A*). Exercise stress testing is an invaluable tool for eliciting arrhythmias in patients with ACM, which frequently organize into brief runs of non-sustained ventricular tachycardia (*B*), and more rarely and threateningly may organize into sustained ventricular tachycardia even in the presence of a normal baseline ECG (*C*).

events at follow-up. These data support the concept that not all scars in ACM have the same role: some fibrofatty scars (with fragmented and delayed electrograms) are arrhythmogenic, whereas dense scars (without slow and fragmented conduction areas) are not, regardless of their extension.

Some studies supported the testing of vulnerability to LAE during programmed electrical stimulation (PES) as a predictor of arrhythmic outcomes,[99,119,120] whereas others reported low predictive value.[117,121] Its use is currently supported by the 2022 ESC Guidelines to guide ICD implant in symptomatic patients with moderate right or left ventricular dysfunction.[6] Recent data by Gasperetti and colleagues[120] demonstrated that inducible VT predicted clinical sustained VA during the 5-year follow-up with a sensitivity and specificity of 75.7% and 67.5%, respectively. However, the proportion of ICD carriers was more than

doubled in the PVS positive group than in PVS negative, and when ICD shock was not included as an endpoint, no significant differences between those with and without a positive PVS were observed (18.2% vs 11.9%, $P = .132$).

Genetic/familial information

Although the genetic background shapes the phenotype of ACM, its prognostic value remains undefined. A recent study by Protonotarios and colleagues showed that the 2019 ARVC risk score calculator performed well in patients with *PKP2* gene mutations, whereas its performance in other genotypes was modest.[91] At present, it is fair to state that in ACM, unlike other arrhythmogenic syndromes,[72,78] the genotype does not represent an independent predictor of outcome. An exception to this generalization is represented by multiple variants on genes encoding for desmosomal proteins and founder mutations such as the

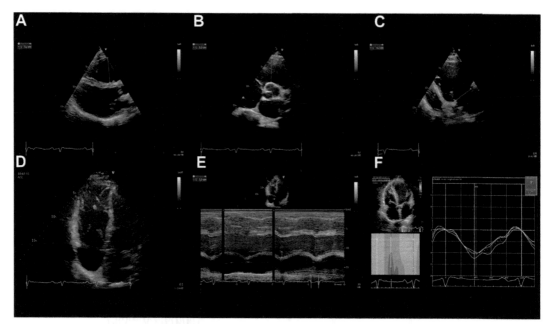

Fig. 5. Echocardiographic abnormalities in advanced-stage ACM. Typical echocardiographic abnormalities can be seen on an echocardiogram of this 55 year-old man, affected by biventricular ACM in an advanced stage. Right ventricle is severely dilated, as shown in the parasternal long axis view (*A*, where it measures 52 mm), in the parasternal short axis view (*B*, where it measures 51 mm), in the modified parasternal long axis view for the RV inflow tract (*C*, where it measures 42 mm), and in the apical four-chamber view (*D*). In addition to severe RV dilatation, notable reduction of RV function can be appreciated, with TAPSE measuring 15 mm (*E*) and RV strain amounting to −10% (*F*).

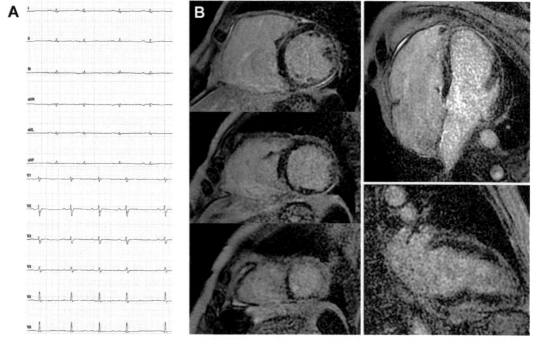

Fig. 6. Correlation between electrocardiographic abnormalities and cardiac magnetic resonance findings. Low QRS voltages on the peripheral leads and extension of T-wave inversions on the precordial leads (*A*) correlate strongly with the extension of late gadolinium enhancement at cardiac MRI. In this case, LGE can be appreciated in the subepicardial segments of the lateral and inferior wall of the left ventricle in its entirety, as shown on the three short axis segments, and on the four-chamber and two-chamber short axis images (*B*).

Newfoundland p.S358 L on *TMEM43*[122] or the Dutch p.Arg14del on *PLN*, for which a mutation-specific prediction model has been developed.[123]

Biomarkers

A novel frontier of risk prediction in ACM is represented by biomarkers. Bridging integrator 1 was the first biomarker to be shown to correlate with functional status and predict future VA occurrence in a small cohort of ACM patients.[124] Following this first demonstration, a plethora of biomarkers have been tested in ACM. High plasma testosterone levels were strongly predictive of arrhythmic events in a recent work by Ren and colleagues.[125] Most recently, high plasma levels of acylation-stimulating protein (ASP), a protein involved in lipogenesis, have been shown to correlate with structural and functional remodeling, and high levels of ASP seemed to be predictive of both arrhythmic and HF events.[126]

Risk Prediction Scores

In inherited arrhythmia syndromes, different risk factors have often been combined into risk prediction models, which have been developed[70,72,127] with the threefold aim to estimate an individual patient's arrhythmic risk, standardize the risk stratification approach, and support an eventual shared physician–patient decision about using an ICD.

In 2019, 15 centers from Europe and North America jointly made the first systematic attempt to develop a risk score for the prediction of the 5-year risk of sustained VA in patients with definite ACM and no history of sustained VA/SCD.[83] After the selection of prespecified predictors based on a meta-analysis including 45 studies,[75] the final model included male sex, age, syncope, non sustained ventricular tachycardia (NSVT), 24-hour PVC count, T-wave inversion in anterior and inferior leads, and RV EF as risk stratifiers[83] with good concordance between predicted and observed risks was observed (C-index 0.77). Recently, the model was also validated externally in a large international multicenter cohort of 429 individuals from 29 centers in North America and Europe, confirming reproducibility and accuracy in an independent patient population (C-index 0.70).[13] In the same study, the authors demonstrated[13] that the risk calculator outperformed risk stratification approaches recommended in the three published consensus documents,[128–130] suggesting that the model could be a useful tool to help physician in the hard decision-making regarding ICD implantation in the primary prevention of SCD in ACM.

Although the 2019 ARVC risk calculator represents a major step forward, some limitations of the model have to be recognized. First, as appropriate ICD shocks accounted for the majority of the outcomes, the model suffers from overestimation of the true risk of SCD, a limitation which is due to the intrinsic composition of modern ACM populations, including a high rate of ICD implants. Second, as already mentioned, the model has been developed in cohorts heavily enriched in right-dominant forms and consequently the model performed best on patients with *PKP2* gene variants, but its utility was limited in gene-elusive patients.[91]

SUMMARY

Arrhythmogenic cardiomyopathy is a rare, complex, progressive disease which requires expertise in arrhythmology, imaging, and HF. Despite the availability of different therapeutic approaches, published evidence suggests that ICD therapy is the only lifesaving treatment in patients with ACM.[4,60,61] Appropriate and timely selection of patients who would benefit most from ICD implantation represents the key clinical challenge in the management of patients with ACM.

Despite quantum leaps in disease understanding, heterogeneity among studies, partly imputable also to the historical and contemporary issues with the diagnostic criteria, has led to the appearance of a myriad of clinical features, electrocardiographic parameters, imaging markers, electrophysiological study, genetic information, and biomarkers, all of which have been proposed as risk stratifiers for patients with ACM. Recently, risk score prediction models, incorporating some of the aforementioned risk factors, have been developed and validated, and their utility remains limited to patients with right-dominant forms of ACM. A further refinement of the aforementioned risk stratification models, which are essential for facilitating the shared decision-making regarding the judicious use of an ICD in a process that places the patient at the forefront, is needed.

CLINICS CARE POINTS

- Diagnosis of ACM is made using multiparametric and multidisciplinary 2010 Updated Task Force Criteria, but they are limited in the recognition of left-dominant forms of arrhythmogenic cardiomyopathy.

- Genetic analysis should be proposed in all patients with a suspected diagnosis of arrhythmogenic cardiomyopathy.

- Over the lifetime of an individual affected by arrhythmogenic cardiomyopathy, the arrhythmic risk tends to be more accentuated between the third and fifth decade of life when it is estimated to be in the order of 4% per year.
- Unlike other cardiomyopathies, such as hypertrophic cardiomyopathy, or channelopathies, such as Long QT Syndrome, where a direct relationship between the severity of the phenotype and the arrhythmic risk has been shown, in arrhythmogenic cardiomyopathy this may not necessarily hold true.
- No pharmacological or surgical treatment has proven to be effective in preventing or reducing sudden cardiac death in arrhythmogenic cardiomyopathy.
- Published evidence suggests that implantable cardioverter defibrillator therapy is the only lifesaving treatment in patients with arrhythmogenic cardiomyopathy.
- Appropriate and timely selection of patients who would benefit most from implantable cardioverter defibrillator implantation represents the key clinical challenge in the management of patients with arrhythmogenic cardiomyopathy.
- Risk score prediction models have been developed and validated, but their utility remains limited to patients with right-dominant forms of arrhythmogenic cardiomyopathy.

DISCLOSURE

Authors declared no conflict of interest.

REFERENCES

1. Marcus FI, Fontaine GH, Guiraudon G, et al. Right ventricular dysplasia: a report of 24 adult cases. Circulation 1982;65:384–98.
2. Finocchiaro G, Papadakis M, Robertus J-L, et al. Etiology of sudden death in sports: insights from a United Kingdom regional registry. J Am Coll Cardiol 2016;67:2108–15.
3. Maron BJ, Haas TS, Ahluwalia A, et al. Demographics and epidemiology of sudden deaths in young competitive athletes: from the United States national registry. Am J Med 2016;129:1170–7.
4. Agbaedeng TA, Roberts KA, Colley L, et al. Incidence and predictors of sudden cardiac death in arrhythmogenic right ventricular cardiomyopathy: a pooled analysis. Europace 2022;24:1665–74.
5. McKenna WJ, Judge DP. Epidemiology of the inherited cardiomyopathies. Nat Rev Cardiol 2021; 18:22–36.
6. Zeppenfeld K, Tfelt-Hansen J, de Riva M, et al. 2022 ESC Guidelines for the management of patients with ventricular arrhythmias and the prevention of sudden cardiac death. Eur Heart J 2022; 43:3997–4126.
7. Mazzanti A, Ng K, Faragli A, et al. Arrhythmogenic right ventricular cardiomyopathy: clinical course and predictors of arrhythmic risk. J Am Coll Cardiol 2016;68:2540–50.
8. Basso C, Aguilera B, Banner J, et al. Guidelines for autopsy investigation of sudden cardiac death: 2017 update from the Association for European Cardiovascular Pathology. Virchows Arch 2017; 471:691–705.
9. Marcus FI, McKenna WJ, Sherrill D, et al. Diagnosis of arrhythmogenic right ventricular cardiomyopathy/dysplasia: proposed modification of the task force criteria. Circulation 2010;121:1533–41.
10. Corrado D, van Tintelen PJ, McKenna WJ, et al. Arrhythmogenic right ventricular cardiomyopathy: evaluation of the current diagnostic criteria and differential diagnosis. Eur Heart J 2020;41: 1414–29.
11. Kukavica D, Trancuccio A, Arnò C, et al. Desmoplakin cardiomyopathy and arrhythmogenic right ventricular cardiomyopathy: two distinct forms of cardiomyopathy? Minerva Cardiol Angiol 2022;70: 217–37.
12. Krahn AD, Wilde AAM, Calkins H, et al. Arrhythmogenic right ventricular cardiomyopathy. JACC Clin Electrophysiol 2022;8:533–53.
13. Jordà P, Bosman LP, Gasperetti A, et al. Arrhythmic risk prediction in arrhythmogenic right ventricular cardiomyopathy: external validation of the arrhythmogenic right ventricular cardiomyopathy risk calculator. Eur Heart J 2022;43:3041–52.
14. James CA, Jongbloed JDH, Hershberger RE, et al. An international evidence based reappraisal of genes associated with arrhythmogenic right ventricular cardiomyopathy (ARVC) using the ClinGen framework. Circ Genomic Precis Med 2021;14(3): e003273.
15. Christensen AH, Andersen CB, Tybjaerg-Hansen A, et al. Mutation analysis and evaluation of the cardiac localization of TMEM43 in arrhythmogenic right ventricular cardiomyopathy. Clin Genet 2011;80: 256–64.
16. Bermúdez-Jiménez FJ, Carriel V, Brodehl A, et al. Novel desmin mutation p.Glu401Asp impairs filament formation, disrupts cell membrane integrity, and causes severe arrhythmogenic left ventricular cardiomyopathy/dysplasia. Circulation 2018;137: 1595–610.
17. van der Zwaag PA, van Rijsingen IAW, Asimaki A, et al. Phospholamban R14del mutation in patients diagnosed with dilated cardiomyopathy or arrhythmogenic right ventricular cardiomyopathy: evidence

supporting the concept of arrhythmogenic cardiomyopathy. Eur J Heart Fail 2012;14:1199–207.

18. Te Rijdt WP, Asimaki A, Jongbloed JDH, et al. Distinct molecular signature of phospholamban p.Arg14del arrhythmogenic cardiomyopathy. Cardiovasc Pathol 2019;40:2–6.

19. Chen L, Song J, Chen X, et al. A novel genotype-based clinicopathology classification of arrhythmogenic cardiomyopathy provides novel insights into disease progression. Eur Heart J 2019;40: 1690–703.

20. Smith ED, Lakdawala NK, Papoutsidakis N, et al. Desmoplakin cardiomyopathy, a fibrotic and inflammatory form of cardiomyopathy distinct from typical dilated or arrhythmogenic right ventricular cardiomyopathy. Circulation 2020;141: 1872–84.

21. Grondin S, Wazirian A-C, Jorda P, et al. Missense variants in the spectrin repeat domain of DSP are associated with arrhythmogenic cardiomyopathy: a family report and systematic review. Am J Med Genet 2020;182:2359–68.

22. Casella M, Gasperetti A, Sicuso R, et al. Characteristics of patients with arrhythmogenic left ventricular cardiomyopathy: combining genetic and histopathologic findings. Circ Arrhythm Electrophysiol 2020;13:e009005.

23. Corrado D, Perazzolo Marra M, Zorzi A, et al. Diagnosis of arrhythmogenic cardiomyopathy: the Padua criteria. Int J Cardiol 2020;319:106–14.

24. Groeneweg JA, Bhonsale A, James CA, et al. Clinical presentation, long-term follow-up, and outcomes of 1001 arrhythmogenic right ventricular dysplasia/cardiomyopathy patients and family members. Circ Cardiovasc Genet 2015;8:437–46.

25. Choudhary N, Tompkins C, Polonsky B, et al. Clinical presentation and outcomes by sex in arrhythmogenic right ventricular cardiomyopathy: findings from the North American ARVC registry. J Cardiovasc Electrophysiol 2016;27:555–62.

26. Ruwald AC, Marcus F, Estes NA 3rd, et al. Association of competitive and recreational sport participation with cardiac events in patients with arrhythmogenic right ventricular cardiomyopathy: results from the North American multidisciplinary study of arrhythmogenic right ventricular cardiomyopath. Eur Heart J 2015;36(27):1735–43.

27. Roudijk RW, Verheul L, Bosman LP, et al. Clinical characteristics and follow-up of pediatric-onset arrhythmogenic right ventricular cardiomyopathy. JACC Clin Electrophysiol 2022;8:306–18.

28. Smedsrud MK, Chivulescu M, Forså MI, et al. Highly malignant disease in childhood-onset arrhythmogenic right ventricular cardiomyopathy. Eur Heart J 2022;43:4694–703.

29. Gomes J, Finlay M, Ahmed AK, et al. Electrophysiological abnormalities precede overt structural

changes in arrhythmogenic right ventricular cardiomyopathy due to mutations in desmoplakin-A combined murine and human study. Eur Heart J 2012; 33:1942–53.

30. Isbister JC, Nowak N, Yeates L, et al. Concealed cardiomyopathy in autopsy-inconclusive cases of sudden cardiac death and implications for families. J Am Coll Cardiol 2022;80:2057–68.

31. Bhonsale A, Groeneweg JA, James CA, et al. Impact of genotype on clinical course in arrhythmogenic right ventricular dysplasia/cardiomyopathy-associated mutation carriers. Eur Heart J 2015;36:847–55.

32. Lin C-Y, Lin Y-J, Li C-H, et al. Heterogeneous distribution of substrates between the endocardium and epicardium promotes ventricular fibrillation in arrhythmogenic right ventricular dysplasia/cardiomyopathy. Europace 2018;20:501–11.

33. Ammirati E, Raimondi F, Piriou N, et al. Acute myocarditis associated with desmosomal gene variants. JACC Heart Fail 2022;10:714–27.

34. Yoneda ZT, Anderson KC, Quintana JA, et al. Early-onset atrial fibrillation and the prevalence of rare variants in cardiomyopathy and arrhythmia genes. JAMA Cardiol 2021;6:1371–9.

35. Kimura Y, Noda T, Otsuka Y, et al. Potentially lethal ventricular arrhythmias and heart failure in arrhythmogenic right ventricular cardiomyopathy: what are the differences between men and women? JACC Clin Electrophysiol 2016;2:546–55.

36. Basso C, Corrado D, Marcus FI, et al. Arrhythmogenic right ventricular cardiomyopathy. Lancet 2009;373:1289–300.

37. Corrado D, Basso C, Judge DP. Arrhythmogenic cardiomyopathy. Circ Res 2017;121:784–802.

38. Lopez-Ayala JM, Pastor-Quirante F, Gonzalez-Carrillo J, et al. Genetics of myocarditis in arrhythmogenic right ventricular dysplasia. Heart Rhythm 2015;12:766–73.

39. Chen S, Chen L, Saguner AM, et al. Novel risk prediction model to determine adverse heart failure outcomes in arrhythmogenic right ventricular cardiomyopathy. J Am Heart Assoc 2022;11:e024634.

40. Moss AJ, Zareba W, Hall WJ, et al. Effectiveness and limitations of beta-blocker therapy in congenital long-QT syndrome. Circulation 2000;101: 616–23.

41. Corrado D, Basso C, Rizzoli G, et al. Does sports activity enhance the risk of sudden death in adolescents and young adults? J Am Coll Cardiol 2003;42:1959–63.

42. Wang W, Tichnell C, Murray BA, et al. Exercise restriction is protective for genotype-positive family members of arrhythmogenic right ventricular cardiomyopathy patients. Europace 2020;22:1270–8.

43. James CA, Bhonsale A, Tichnell C, et al. Exercise increases age-related penetrance and arrhythmic risk in arrhythmogenic right ventricular dysplasia/

cardiomyopathy-associated desmosomal mutation carriers. J Am Coll Cardiol 2013;62(14):1290–7.

44. Cappelletto C, Gregorio C, Barbati G, et al. Antiarrhythmic therapy and risk of cumulative ventricular arrhythmias in arrhythmogenic right ventricle cardiomyopathy. Int J Cardiol 2021;334:58–64.

45. Gregorio C, Cappelletto C, Romani S, et al. Using marginal structural joint models to estimate the effect of a time-varying treatment on recurrent events and survival: an application on arrhythmogenic cardiomyopathy. Biom J 2022;64:1374–88.

46. Wichter T, Borggrefe M, Haverkamp W, et al. Efficacy of antiarrhythmic drugs in patients with arrhythmogenic right ventricular disease. Results in patients with inducible and noninducible ventricular tachycardia. Circulation 1992;86:29–37.

47. Marcus GM, Glidden DV, Polonsky B, et al. Efficacy of antiarrhythmic drugs in arrhythmogenic right ventricular cardiomyopathy: a report from the North American ARVC Registry. J Am Coll Cardiol 2009;54:609–15.

48. Ruskin JN. The cardiac arrhythmia suppression trial (CAST). N Engl J Med 1989;321:386–8.

49. Ermakov S, Gerstenfeld EP, Svetlichnaya Y, et al. Use of flecainide in combination antiarrhythmic therapy in patients with arrhythmogenic right ventricular cardiomyopathy. Heart Rhythm 2017;14:564–9.

50. Rolland T, Badenco N, Maupain C, et al. Safety and efficacy of flecainide associated with beta-blockers in arrhythmogenic right ventricular cardiomyopathy. Europace 2022;24:278–84.

51. McDonagh TA, Metra M, Adamo M, et al. 2021 ESC Guidelines for the diagnosis and treatment of acute and chronic heart failure. Eur Heart J 2021;42:3599–726.

52. Tu B, Wu L, Zheng L, et al. Angiotensin-converting enzyme inhibitors/angiotensin receptor blockers: anti-arrhythmic drug for arrhythmogenic right ventricular cardiomyopathy. Front Cardiovasc Med 2021;8:769138.

53. Morel E, Manati AW, Nony P, et al. Blockade of the renin-angiotensin-aldosterone system in patients with arrhythmogenic right ventricular dysplasia: a double-blind, multicenter, prospective, randomized, genotype-driven study (BRAVE study). Clin Cardiol 2018;41:300–6.

54. Scheel PJ 3rd, Giuliano K, Tichnell C, et al. Heart transplantation strategies in arrhythmogenic right ventricular cardiomyopathy: a tertiary ARVC centre experience. ESC Hear Fail 2022;9:1008–17.

55. Santangeli P, Zado ES, Supple GE, et al. Long-term outcome with catheter ablation of ventricular tachycardia in patients with arrhythmogenic right ventricular cardiomyopathy. Circ Arrhythm Electrophysiol 2015;8:1413–21.

56. Mahida S, Venlet J, Saguner AM, et al. Ablation compared with drug therapy for recurrent ventricular tachycardia in arrhythmogenic right ventricular cardiomyopathy: results from a multicenter study. Heart Rhythm 2019;16:536–43.

57. Berruezo A, Fernández-Armenta J, Mont L, et al. Combined endocardial and epicardial catheter ablation in arrhythmogenic right ventricular dysplasia incorporating scar dechanneling technique. Circ Arrhythm Electrophysiol 2012;5:111–21.

58. Romero J, Cerrud-Rodriguez RC, Di Biase L, et al. Combined endocardial-epicardial versus endocardial catheter ablation alone for ventricular tachycardia in structural heart disease: a systematic review and meta-analysis. JACC Clin Electrophysiol 2019;5:13–24.

59. Assis FR, Krishnan A, Zhou X, et al. Cardiac sympathectomy for refractory ventricular tachycardia in arrhythmogenic right ventricular cardiomyopathy. Heart Rhythm 2019;16:1003–10.

60. Corrado D, Leoni L, Link MS, et al. Implantable cardioverter-defibrillator therapy for prevention of sudden death in patients with arrhythmogenic right ventricular cardiomyopathy/dysplasia. Circulation 2003;108:3084–91.

61. Hodgkinson KA, Parfrey PS, Bassett AS, et al. The impact of implantable cardioverter-defibrillator therapy on survival in autosomal-dominant arrhythmogenic right ventricular cardiomyopathy (ARVD5). J Am Coll Cardiol 2005;45:400–8.

62. Link MS, Laidlaw D, Polonsky B, et al. Ventricular arrhythmias in the North American multidisciplinary study of ARVC: predictors, characteristics, and treatment. J Am Coll Cardiol 2014;64:119–25.

63. Wang W, Gasperetti A, Sears SF, et al. Subcutaneous and transvenous defibrillators in arrhythmogenic right ventricular cardiomyopathy: a comparison of clinical and quality-of-life outcomes. JACC Clin Electrophysiol 2023;9(3):394–402.

64. Piot O, Defaye P, Lortet-Tieulent J, et al. Healthcare costs in implantable cardioverter-defibrillator recipients: a real-life cohort study on 19,408 patients from the French national healthcare database. Int J Cardiol 2022;348:39–44.

65. Sears SFJ, Conti JB. Quality of life and psychological functioning of icd patients. Heart 2002;87:488–93.

66. García-Pérez L, Pinilla-Domínguez P, García-Quintana A, et al. Economic evaluations of implantable cardioverter defibrillators: a systematic review. Eur J Health Econ 2015;16:879–93.

67. Christensen AH, Platonov PG, Svensson A, et al. Complications of implantable cardioverter-defibrillator treatment in arrhythmogenic right ventricular cardiomyopathy. Europace 2022;24:306–12.

68. van Barreveld M, Verstraelen TE, Buskens E, et al. Hospital utilisation and the costs associated with complications of ICD implantation in a contemporary primary prevention cohort. Neth Heart J 2022. https://doi.org/10.1007/s12471-022-01733-4.

69. Spirito P, Bellone P, Harris KM, et al. Magnitude of left ventricular hypertrophy and risk of sudden death in hypertrophic cardiomyopathy. N Engl J Med 2000;342:1778–85.

70. O'Mahony C, Jichi F, Pavlou M, et al. A novel clinical risk prediction model for sudden cardiac death in hypertrophic cardiomyopathy (HCM risk-SCD). Eur Heart J 2014;35:2010–20.

71. Mazzanti A, Maragna R, Vacanti G, et al. Interplay between genetic substrate, QTc duration, and arrhythmia risk in patients with long QT syndrome. J Am Coll Cardiol 2018;71:1663–71.

72. Mazzanti A, Trancuccio A, Kukavica D, et al. Independent validation and clinical implications of the risk prediction model for long QT syndrome (1-2-3-LQTS-Risk). Europace 2021;24(4):614–9.

73. Zorzi A, Rigato I, Pilichou K, et al. Phenotypic expression is a prerequisite for malignant arrhythmic events and sudden cardiac death in arrhythmogenic right ventricular cardiomyopathy. Europace 2016;18:1086–94.

74. Carrick RT, Te Riele ASJM, Gasperetti A, et al. Longitudinal prediction of ventricular arrhythmic risk in patients with arrhythmogenic right ventricular cardiomyopathy. Circ Arrhythm Electrophysiol 2022; 15:e011207.

75. Bosman LP, Sammani A, James CA, et al. Predicting arrhythmic risk in arrhythmogenic right ventricular cardiomyopathy: a systematic review and meta-analysis. Heart Rhythm 2018;15:1097–107.

76. Elliott PM, Sharma S, Varnava A, et al. Survival after cardiac arrest or sustained ventricular tachycardia in patients with hypertrophic cardiomyopathy. J Am Coll Cardiol 1999;33:1596–601.

77. Probst V, Veltmann C, Eckardt L, et al. Long-term prognosis of patients diagnosed with Brugada syndrome: results from the FINGER Brugada syndrome registry. Circulation 2010;121:635–43.

78. Mazzanti A, Kukavica D, Trancuccio A, et al. Outcomes of patients with catecholaminergic polymorphic ventricular tachycardia treated with β-blockers. JAMA Cardiol 2022;7:504–12.

79. Wang W, Cadrin-Tourigny J, Bhonsale A, et al. Arrhythmic outcome of arrhythmogenic right ventricular cardiomyopathy patients without implantable defibrillators. J Cardiovasc Electrophysiol 2018;29:1396–402.

80. Bhonsale A, James CA, Tichnell C, et al. Risk stratification in arrhythmogenic right ventricular dysplasia/cardiomyopathy-associated desmosomal mutation carriers. Circ Arrhythm Electrophysiol 2013;6:569–78.

81. Orgeron GM, James CA, Te Riele A, et al. Implantable cardioverter-defibrillator therapy in arrhythmogenic right ventricular dysplasia/cardiomyopathy: predictors of appropriate therapy, outcomes, and complications. J Am Heart Assoc 2017;6:e006242.

82. Lin C-Y, Chung F-P, Lin Y-J, et al. Gender differences in patients with arrhythmogenic right ventricular dysplasia/cardiomyopathy: clinical manifestations, electrophysiological properties, substrate characteristics, and prognosis of radiofrequency catheter ablation. Int J Cardiol 2017;227:930–7.

83. Cadrin-Tourigny J, Bosman LP, Nozza A, et al. A new prediction model for ventricular arrhythmias in arrhythmogenic right ventricular cardiomyopathy. Eur Heart J 2019;40:1850–8.

84. Akdis D, Saguner AM, Shah K, et al. Sex hormones affect outcome in arrhythmogenic right ventricular cardiomyopathy/dysplasia: from a stem cell derived cardiomyocyte-based model to clinical biomarkers of disease outcome. Eur Heart J 2017;38:1498–508.

85. Lie ØH, Rootwelt-Norberg C, Dejgaard LA, et al. Prediction of life-threatening ventricular arrhythmia in patients with arrhythmogenic cardiomyopathy: a primary prevention cohort study. JACC Cardiovasc Imaging 2018;11:1377–86.

86. Maupain C, Badenco N, Pousset F, et al. Risk stratification in arrhythmogenic right ventricular cardiomyopathy/dysplasia without an implantable cardioverter-defibrillator. JACC Clin Electrophysiol 2018;4:757–68.

87. van Opbergen CJM, Bagwan N, Maurya SR, et al. Exercise causes arrhythmogenic remodeling of intracellular calcium dynamics in plakophilin-2-deficient hearts. Circulation 2022;145:1480–96.

88. Pérez-Hernández M, van Opbergen CJM, Bagwan N, et al. Loss of Nuclear envelope integrity and increased oxidant production cause DNA damage in adult hearts deficient in PKP2: a molecular substrate of ARVC. Circulation 2022;146:851–67.

89. Cerrone M, Marrón-Liñares GM, van Opbergen CJM, et al. Role of plakophilin-2 expression on exercise-related progression of arrhythmogenic right ventricular cardiomyopathy: a translational study. Eur Heart J 2022;43:1251–64.

90. Cheedipudi SM, Hu J, Fan S, et al. Exercise restores dysregulated gene expression in a mouse model of arrhythmogenic cardiomyopathy. Cardiovasc Res 2020;116:1199–213.

91. Protonotarios A, Bariani R, Cappelletto C, et al. Importance of genotype for risk stratification in arrhythmogenic right ventricular cardiomyopathy using the 2019 ARVC risk calculator. Eur Heart J 2022;43:3053–67.

92. Liao Y-C, Lin Y-J, Chung F-P, et al. Risk stratification of arrhythmogenic right ventricular cardiomyopathy based on signal averaged electrocardiograms. Int J Cardiol 2014;174:628–33.

93. Pearman CM, Lee D, Davies B, et al. Incremental value of the signal-averaged ECG for diagnosing arrhythmogenic cardiomyopathy. Heart Rhythm 2023;20:224–30.

94. Nava A, Folino AF, Bauce B, et al. Signal-averaged electrocardiogram in patients with arrhythmogenic right ventricular cardiomyopathy and ventricular arrhythmias. Eur Heart J 2000;21:58–65.

95. Jongman JK, Zaidi A, Muggenthaler M, et al. Relationship between echocardiographic right-ventricular dimensions and signal-averaged electrocardiogram abnormalities in endurance athletes. Europace 2015;17:1441–8.

96. Tanawuttiwat T, Te Riele ASJM, Philips B, et al. Electroanatomic correlates of depolarization abnormalities in arrhythmogenic right ventricular dysplasia/cardiomyopathy. J Cardiovasc Electrophysiol 2016; 27:443–52.

97. Platonov PG, Calkins H, Hauer RN, et al. High interobserver variability in the assessment of epsilon waves: implications for diagnosis of arrhythmogenic right ventricular cardiomyopathy/dysplasia. Heart Rhythm 2016;13:208–16.

98. Kikuchi N, Yumino D, Shiga T, et al. Long-term prognostic role of the diagnostic criteria for arrhythmogenic right ventricular cardiomyopathy/dysplasia. JACC Clin Electrophysiol 2016;2:107–15.

99. Bhonsale A, James CA, Tichnell C, et al. Incidence and predictors of implantable cardioverter-defibrillator therapy in patients with arrhythmogenic right ventricular dysplasia/cardiomyopathy undergoing implantable cardioverter-defibrillator implantation for primary prevention. J Am Coll Cardiol 2011;58:1485–96.

100. Cappelletto C, Stolfo D, De Luca A, et al. Lifelong arrhythmic risk stratification in arrhythmogenic right ventricular cardiomyopathy: distribution of events and impact of periodical reassessment. Europace 2018;20:f20–9.

101. Aquaro GD, Pingitore A, Di Bella G, et al. Prognostic role of cardiac magnetic resonance in arrhythmogenic right ventricular cardiomyopathy. Am J Cardiol 2018;122:1745–53.

102. Cadrin-Tourigny J, Bosman LP, Nozza A, et al. A new prediction model for ventricular arrhythmias in arrhythmogenic right ventricular cardiomyopathy. Eur Heart J 2022;43:e1–9.

103. Cadrin-Tourigny J, Bosman LP, Wang W, et al. Sudden cardiac death prediction in arrhythmogenic right ventricular cardiomyopathy: a multinational collaboration. Circ Arrhythm Electrophysiol 2021; 14:e008509.

104. Baturova MA, Haugaa KH, Jensen HK, et al. Atrial fibrillation as a clinical characteristic of arrhythmogenic right ventricular cardiomyopathy: experience from the Nordic ARVC Registry. Int J Cardiol 2020; 298:39–43.

105. Bourfiss M, Te Riele ASJM, Mast TP, et al. Influence of genotype on structural atrial abnormalities and atrial fibrillation or flutter in arrhythmogenic right ventricular dysplasia/cardiomyopathy. J Cardiovasc Electrophysiol 2016;27:1420–8.

106. Chivulescu M, Lie ØH, Popescu BA, et al. High penetrance and similar disease progression in probands and in family members with arrhythmogenic cardiomyopathy. Eur Heart J 2020;41: 1401–10.

107. Mast TP, James CA, Calkins H, et al. Evaluation of structural progression in arrhythmogenic right ventricular dysplasia/cardiomyopathy. JAMA Cardiol 2017;2:293–302.

108. Saguner AM, Vecchiati A, Baldinger SH, et al. Different prognostic value of functional right ventricular parameters in arrhythmogenic right ventricular cardiomyopathy/dysplasia. Circ Cardiovasc Imaging 2014;7:230–9.

109. Woźniak O, Borowiec K, Konka M, et al. Implantable cardiac defibrillator events in patients with arrhythmogenic right ventricular cardiomyopathy. Heart 2022;108:22–8.

110. Hosseini S, Erhart L, Anwer S, et al. Tissue Doppler echocardiography and outcome in arrhythmogenic right ventricular cardiomyopathy. Int J Cardiol 2022;368:86–93.

111. Bourfiss M, Prakken NHJ, James CA, et al. Prognostic value of strain by feature-tracking cardiac magnetic resonance in arrhythmogenic right ventricular cardiomyopathy. Eur Heart J Cardiovasc Imaging 2022;24:98–107.

112. Pieles GE, Grosse-Wortmann L, Hader M, et al. Association of echocardiographic parameters of right ventricular remodeling and myocardial performance with modified task force criteria in adolescents with arrhythmogenic right ventricular cardiomyopathy. Circ Cardiovasc Imaging 2019; 12:e007693.

113. Malik N, Win S, James CA, et al. Right ventricular strain predicts structural disease progression in patients with arrhythmogenic right ventricular cardiomyopathy. J Am Heart Assoc 2020;9:e015016.

114. Cipriani A, Bauce B, De Lazzari M, et al. Arrhythmogenic right ventricular cardiomyopathy: characterization of left ventricular phenotype and differential diagnosis with dilated cardiomyopathy. J Am Heart Assoc 2020;9:e014628.

115. Aquaro GD, De Luca A, Cappelletto C, et al. Prognostic value of magnetic resonance phenotype in patients with arrhythmogenic right ventricular cardiomyopathy. J Am Coll Cardiol 2020;75:2753–65.

116. Liu Y, Yu J, Liu J, et al. Prognostic value of late gadolinium enhancement in arrhythmogenic right ventricular cardiomyopathy: a meta-analysis. Clin Radiol 2021;76:628.e9-15.

117. Santangeli P, Dello Russo A, Pieroni M, et al. Fragmented and delayed electrograms within fibrofatty scar predict arrhythmic events in arrhythmogenic right ventricular cardiomyopathy: results from a prospective risk stratification study. Heart Rhythm 2012;9:1200–6.

118. Migliore F, Zorzi A, Silvano M, et al. Prognostic value of endocardial voltage mapping in patients with arrhythmogenic right ventricular cardiomyopathy/dysplasia. Circ Arrhythm Electrophysiol 2013;6: 167–76.

119. Saguner AM, Medeiros-Domingo A, Schwyzer MA, et al. Usefulness of inducible ventricular tachycardia to predict long-term adverse outcomes in arrhythmogenic right ventricular cardiomyopathy. Am J Cardiol 2013;111:250–7.

120. Gasperetti A, Carrick RT, Costa S, et al. Programmed ventricular stimulation as an additional primary prevention risk stratification tool in arrhythmogenic right ventricular cardiomyopathy: a multinational study. Circulation 2022;146:1434–43.

121. Corrado D, Calkins H, Fau - Link MS, et al. Prophylactic implantable defibrillator in patients with arrhythmogenic right ventricular cardiomyopathy/dysplasia and no prior ventricular fibrillation or sustained ventricular tachycardia. Circulation 2010; 122(12):1144–52.

122. Hodgkinson KA, Howes AJ, Boland P, et al. Long-term clinical outcome of arrhythmogenic right ventricular cardiomyopathy in individuals with a p.S358L mutation in TMEM43 following implantable cardioverter defibrillator therapy. Circ Arrhythm Electrophysiol 2016;9:e003589.

123. Verstraelen TE, van Lint FHM, Bosman LP, et al. Prediction of ventricular arrhythmia in phospholamban p.Arg14del mutation carriers-reaching the frontiers of individual risk prediction. Eur Heart J 2021;42:2842–50.

124. Hong T-T, Cogswell R, James CA, et al. Plasma BIN1 correlates with heart failure and predicts arrhythmia in patients with arrhythmogenic right ventricular cardiomyopathy. Heart Rhythm 2012;9: 961–7.

125. Ren J, Chen L, Zhang N, et al. Plasma testosterone and arrhythmic events in male patients with arrhythmogenic right ventricular cardiomyopathy. ESC Hear Fail 2020;7:1547–59.

126. Ren J, Chen L, Chen X, et al. Acylation-stimulating protein and heart failure progression in arrhythmogenic right ventricular cardiomyopathy. ESC Hear Fail 2023;10:492–501.

127. Wahbi K, Ben Yaou R, Gandjbakhch E, et al. Development and validation of a new risk prediction score for life-threatening ventricular Tachyarrhythmias in laminopathies. Circulation 2019;140: 293–302.

128. Al-Khatib SM, Stevenson WG, Ackerman MJ, et al. 2017 AHA/ACC/HRS guideline for management of patients with ventricular arrhythmias and the prevention of sudden cardiac death: executive summary: a report of the American college of Cardiology/American heart association task force on clinical practice Gu. Heart Rhythm 2018;15: e190–252.

129. Corrado D, Wichter T, Link MS, et al. Treatment of arrhythmogenic right ventricular cardiomyopathy/dysplasia: an international task force consensus statement. Circulation 2015;132:441–53.

130. Towbin JA, McKenna WJ, Abrams DJ, et al. 2019 HRS expert consensus statement on evaluation, risk stratification, and management of arrhythmogenic cardiomyopathy. Heart Rhythm 2019;16: e301–72.

Sudden Death Risk Assessment in Hypertrophic Cardiomyopathy Across the Lifespan
Reconciling the American and European Approaches

Ahmad Al Samarraie, MD[a,b], Adrian Petzl, MD[a,b],
Julia Cadrin-Tourigny, MD, PhD[a,b], Rafik Tadros, MD, PhD[a,b],*

KEYWORDS

- Hypertrophic cardiomyopathy • Sudden cardiac death • Implantable cardioverter-defibrillator
- Risk stratification • Risk score

KEY POINTS

- Hypertrophic cardiomyopathy (HCM) is the most common inherited cardiac disease, with sudden cardiac death (SCD) being its most feared complication.
- Implantable cardioverter-defibrillators (ICD) are the most effective treatment for the primary prevention of SCD, however, ICD indications differ between leading societies of cardiology.
- The European Society of Cardiology recommends the use of a risk calculator developed in 2014, the HCM Risk-SCD, for risk stratification of SCD.
- The American Heart Association and American College of Cardiology rely on stand-alone risk factors updated in 2020 for indications of prophylactic ICD implantation.
- Recently, two risk stratification models, HCM Risk-Kids and PRIMaCY, were developed and validated in the pediatric population.

INTRODUCTION

Hypertrophic cardiomyopathy (HCM) is the most common inherited cardiac disease, with a prevalence of 0.2% in the general population.[1] Although relatively rare, sudden cardiac death (SCD) is the most devastating and often unpredictable complication of HCM, with an overall incidence of 0.5% to 1% per year in the general HCM population.[2–7] Since the modern description of HCM by Teare in 1958 followed by Braunwald in 1964[8,9], no treatment has been as effective as implantable cardioverter-defibrillators (ICD) for the primary prevention of SCD.[10–14] Risk stratification to guide decision-making for ICD use is thus paramount in HCM. The approach to risk stratification and the indications for an ICD, however, differ between international guidelines. The European Society of Cardiology (ESC) recommends the use of a risk calculator, while the American Heart Association (AHA) and American College of Cardiology (ACC) rely on stand-alone risk factors.[15,16] The present review addresses the most current literature on the risk stratification of SCD in HCM, contrasting

a Cardiovascular Genetics Centre, Montreal Heart Institute, 5000 Bélanger, Montreal, Quebec H1T 1C8, Canada; b Faculty of Medicine, Université de Montréal, 2900 Edouard Montpetit, Montreal, Quebec H3T 1J4, Canada
* Corresponding author. Montreal Heart Institute, 5000 Bélanger, Montreal, Quebec H1T 1C8, Canada.
E-mail address: rafik.tadros@umontreal.ca

Card Electrophysiol Clin 15 (2023) 367–378
https://doi.org/10.1016/j.ccep.2023.04.010

the ESC and AHA/ACC guidelines and providing guidance for ICD use across the lifespan.

TRADITIONAL STAND-ALONE RISK FACTORS

In 2003, the ACC in collaboration with the ESC established a set of major risk factors for SCD in HCM.[17] These included.

- Personal history of cardiac arrest secondary to ventricular fibrillation (VF) or sustained ventricular tachycardia (VT);
- Family history of SCD;
- Maximal left ventricle wall thickness (LVWT) ≥30 mm;
- Unexplained syncope;
- Non-sustained ventricular tachycardia (NSVT);
- Abnormal blood pressure response during exertion.

Other factors such as left ventricular outflow tract (LVOT) obstruction with a peak gradient ≥30 mmHg and high-risk genetic mutations were listed as potential risk modifiers.

A personal history of cardiac arrest in the context of a malignant ventricular arrhythmia confers the highest risk for subsequent episodes, up to 10% per year.[18] An ICD is therefore indicated for secondary prevention. For all other major risk factors, the presence of any of them warrants a strong consideration for ICD implantation for primary prevention according to the ACC/ESC expert consensus document published in 2003.[17]

Optimization. To improve the assessment of SCD, the AHA, and ACC published in 2011 new guidelines for the management of HCM.[19] The approach to risk stratification used the same established risk factors, with some changes.

- All major risk factors remain unchanged except for abnormal blood pressure response during exertion, which was downgraded to a possible risk factor, thus making it a class IIa indication *(is reasonable)* for SCD risk assessment.
- Potential risk modifiers have been updated as well and constitute a class IIb indication *(might be considered)* for SCD risk assessment. They are as follows: late-gadolinium enhancement (LGE) on cardiac magnetic resonance (CMR) imaging, double and compound mutations, LV apical aneurysm, and marked LVOT obstruction.

Fig. 1 compares HCM risk factors included in both approaches. The 2011 AHA/ACC guidelines put greater emphasis on a positive family history of SCD, severe LVWT, and recent syncope presumed

to be caused by arrhythmia. These three clinical markers constitute class IIa indications for ICD implantation. On the other hand, NSVT identified on Holter or abnormal blood pressure response during exertion are also class IIa indications, but only in the presence of other risk modifiers. Otherwise, these two conditions constitute class IIb indications for ICD implantation.[19–21]

Limitations. For both 2003 and 2011 risk stratification models, O'Mahony et al. highlighted several limitations.[22] First, all major risk factors are weighed equally without accounting for their potential individual effect size.

Second, both algorithms treat clinical markers in a dichotomous way, when they are thought to be correlated with a continuous increase in risk.[23,24] Indeed, Elliott et al. demonstrated that most SCD occur in patients with LVWT less than 30 mm. Patients with LVWT below this threshold could thus potentially benefit from an ICD implantation.[23] As for NSVT, several studies revealed that faster, longer and repetitive runs of NSVT were more likely to be associated with malignant ventricular arrhythmias.[25,26]

Third, both algorithms rely on relative risks to estimate SCD, not absolute ones, which could possibly lead to inconsistent ICD use since patients with the same absolute risk of SCD could be managed differently.[22]

Fourth, both approaches are furthermore limited by low positive predictive values (PPV) of their clinical markers due in part to the low prevalence of SCD in HCM.[3,27,28] Thus, discriminating between high-risk and low-risk patients becomes challenging as evidenced by an area under the curve (AUC) of 0.63 and 0.61 at one year along with an AUC of 0.64 and 0.63 at five years for the 2003 and 2011 guidelines respectively.[22] However, these risk factors have high negative predictive values (NPV) of at least 90%, which suggests that their absence is usually reassuring.[29] Indeed, only about 3% of SCD cases in HCM occur in low-risk patients who do not have any of the established risk factors.[27]

EUROPEAN APPROACH: THE HCM RISK-SCD

In an attempt to overcome challenges generated by traditional stand-alone risk factor approaches, the ESC proposed a risk calculator to stratify patients based on established and new clinical markers. This model is based on a 2014 retrospective multicentre cohort study by O'Mahony et al. that included 3675 patients with HCM followed for a median of 5.7 years.[30] The cohort characteristics, main findings and validation results are summarised in **Table 1**.

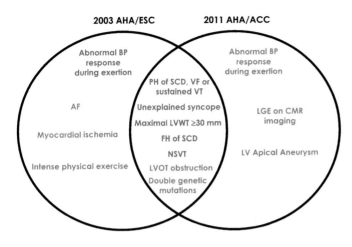

Fig. 1. Comparison Between HCM Risk Factors Included in the 2003 AHA/ESC and the 2011 AHA/ACC Guidelines. ACC, American College of Cardiology; AF, atrial fibrillation; AHA, American Heart Association; BP, blood pressure; CMR, cardiac magnetic resonance; ESC, European Society of Cardiology; FH, family history; HCM, hypertrophic cardiomyopathy; LGE, late gadolinium enhancement; LV, left ventricle; LVOT, left ventricle outflow tract; LVWT, left ventricle wall thickness; NSVT, non-sustained ventricular tachycardia; PH, personal history; SCD, sudden cardiac death; VF, ventricular fibrillation; VT, ventricular tachycardia. *Red text*, major risk factors; *Blue text*, possible risk factors.

During the study period, 198 patients (5%) reached the primary endpoint of SCD or equivalent events (see **Table 1** for the breakdown of events). The risk stratification algorithm includes the following variables: age, left atrial (LA) diameter, maximal left ventricle outflow tract gradient (LVOTG), maximal LVWT, NSVT, family history of SCD, and unexplained syncope. A 5-year risk of SCD can subsequently be calculated. **Table 2** describes all variables included in this risk calculator. The online version of this model can be accessed at https://doc2do.com/hcm/webHCM.html.

Moderate discriminative ability with a C-index of 0.70 was shown. Similar results were obtained when dividing the study cohort into a derivation and validation cohorts. The risk calculator was later validated in external cohorts, as reviewed in two recent meta-analyses.[31,32]

Based on European guidelines, ICD implantation is recommended for secondary prevention and should be considered for primary prevention when the 5-year risk of SCD is ≥6%. It may be considered with an absolute risk of 4-<6% and is generally not indicated with a 5-year risk of <4%.[15]

Table 1
The HCM Risk-SCD study, O'Mahony et al., 2014

Studied Population	3675 Patients Derived from 6 Centers in the UK, Spain, Italy, and Greece		
Baseline characteristics	Age, years		48 ± 17
	Male		2349 (64%)
	FH of SCD		886 (24%)
	NSVT		634 (17%)
	Unexplained syncope		507 (14%)
	Maximal LVWT, mm		20 ± 5
	Maximal LVOTG, mmHg		12 (5–49)
	LA diameter, mm		44 ± 8
	Septal myectomy		34 (1%)
	Alcohol septal ablation		10 (0.3%)
Follow-up	Enrolment period		1972–2011
	Median follow-up, years		5.7
	Primary endpoints	SCD events	198 (5%)
		SCD	118 (60%)
		Appropriate ICD shocks	53 (27%)
		Aborted SCD	27 (14%)
C-statistic	Derivation cohort		0.70
	Validation cohort (secondary model)		0.67
	Using conventional risk factors		0.54

Abbreviations: FH, family history; HCM, hypertrophic cardiomyopathy; ICD, implantable cardioverter-defibrillator; LA, left atrial; LVOTG, left ventricle outflow tract gradient; LVWT, left ventricle wall thickness; NSVT, non-sustained ventricular tachycardia; SCD, sudden cardiac death.

Table 2
Risk factors included in the HCM Risk-SCD risk calculator

		Description	Variable Type
Variables	Age	Age at evaluation[33]	Continuous
	FH of SCD	SCD in ≥1 first degree-relatives <40 years of age or SCD in first degree-relatives with confirmed HCM at any age[34,35]	Dichotomous
	NSVT	Identified on 24-hour Holter and defined as: ≥3 consecutive beats, ≥120 bpm, and <30 s in duration[20,25,26]	Dichotomous
	Unexplained syncope	PH of syncope likely to be caused by ventricular arrhythmia[33–36]	Dichotomous
	Maximal LVWT	Determined with echocardiography in parasternal long axis[23,24]	Continuous
	Maximal LVOTG	Determined with echocardiography from the apical five chamber view at rest or during physiological provocation (Valsalva, exercise, standing)[34,35,37]	Continuous
	LA diameter	Determined with echocardiography in parasternal long axis[33]	Continuous

Abbreviations: bpm, beats per minute; FH, family history; HCM, hypertrophic cardiomyopathy; LA, left atrial; LV, left ventricle; LVOTG, left ventricle outflow tract gradient; LVWT, left ventricle wall thickness; NSVT, non-sustained ventricular tachycardia; PH, personal history; s, seconds; SCD, sudden cardiac death.

Limitations. First, the HCM Risk-SCD calculator has been criticized for its limited sensitivity and moderate discriminative ability.[32] Maron et al. reported its tendency to misclassify patients at high risk of SCD, as evidenced by their study in which 60% of patients who reached the primary endpoint of SCD or equivalent events had scores <4% that would not constitute an indication for ICD.[38]

Second, LA diameter is integrated into the formula, but recent echocardiographic guidelines have suggested LA volume to be the most accurate measure of LA size.[39–41] Nevertheless, Mills et al. recently demonstrated that using LA diameter predicted from measured LA volume correlates well with the risk of SCD using measured LA diameter.[42] The coefficient of determination was excellent ($r^2 = 0.96$). The conversion formula is as follows:

$$\text{Predicted LAd} = 28 + 0.16 \times \text{measured LAv}$$

where LAd = left atrial diameter, mm; LAv = left atrial volume, mL.

Third, the ESC risk stratification algorithm omits extensive LGE by CMR imaging. This factor can be an independent SCD risk marker, even in patients considered at low risk based on conventional HCM risk factors.[43–51] ESC guidelines state that LGE is a possible predictor of SCD, but available data at the time of publication were insufficient to support its inclusion in the risk calculator.[15]

Other notable omissions not depicted by the European algorithm are LV apical aneurysms[52,53] and systolic dysfunction.[54] The latter is not considered in the stratification process, but rather simply linked to heart failure that could be associated with HCM.[15] As for aneurysms, ESC guidelines mention that a positive association between aneurysms and SCD is limited to small series of selected patients.[15]

NOVEL STAND-ALONE RISK FACTORS

Recently, the new 2020 AHA/ACC guidelines for the diagnosis and treatment of HCM updated the 2011 risk factors and indications for prophylactic ICD implantation.

The presence of LV apical aneurysms, HCM with systolic dysfunction, and extended LGE on CMR

Table 3
Stand-alone risk factors for SCD in HCM based on the 2020 AHA/ACC guidelines

Major risk factors	PH of SCD, VF, or sustained VT	Most significant risk factor. ICD indicated for secondary prevention[17,19]
	Maximal LVWT	LVWT $\geq$30 mm in any LV segment[23,24]
	FH of SCD	SCD in $\geq$1 first-degree relatives $\leq$50 years of age[55–57]
	Unexplained syncope	$\geq$1 episode of syncope likely due to arrhythmia in the previous 6 months[30,33,55,58]
	Systolic dysfunction	Defined as LVEF <50%[59–61]
	LV apical aneurysm	Any aneurysm, independent of its size[52,62]
Risk modifiers	NSVT	Identified on 24 or 48-hour Holter. Major risk factor in younger patients with HCM[27,44,53]
	Extensive LGE on CMR imaging	Represents extensive myocardial scarring or fibrosis susceptible to malignant arrhythmias[43,54,63,64]

Abbreviations: CMR, cardiac magnetic resonance; FH, family history; HCM, hypertrophic cardiomyopathy; ICD, implantable cardioverter-defibrillator; LGE, late gadolinium enhancement; LV, left ventricle; LVEF, left ventricle ejection fraction; LVWT, left ventricle wall thickness; NSVT, non-sustained ventricular tachycardia; PH, personal history; SCD, sudden cardiac death; VF, ventricular fibrillation; VT, ventricular tachycardia.

imaging are novel clinical markers that are now part of the American risk stratification approach.[16] **Table 3** presents and describes all included risk factors. Due to its relatively recent publication, only two studies have validated the new HCM algorithm.[65,66] Both studies will be described in detail in the next section comparing the American and European approaches.

Apical aneurysms infrequently complicate HCM with a prevalence of about 2.2% in the general HCM population. This late finding carries a significantly increased risk of cardiovascular complications, including SCD, with an event rate of up to 10.5% per year in the largest series to date.[67]

Systolic dysfunction is a relatively common complication of HCM, with a prevalence of approximately 8% based on data from the SHaRe Registry.[59] Studies have observed an appropriate ICD intervention rate of about 10% annually, which is similar to the rate reported for secondary prevention.[10,60] End-stage HCM is furthermore associated with other significant complications, including thromboembolic events, and terminal heart failure requiring left ventricle assist device implantation or cardiac transplantation, and all-cause death.[59]

LGE on CMR imaging is believed to represent myocardial scarring resulting from repeated episodes of silent and recurrent microvascular ischemia. This scarring becomes the substrate for potentially life-threatening ventricular arrhythmias.[68,69] Multiple studies have demonstrated that the presence of LGE is associated with an increase in the ventricular arrhythmia risk. Chan

et al. have demonstrated that extensive myocardial fibrosis ($\geq$15% of total LV weight) is associated with a two-fold increase in SCD or appropriate ICD interventions in low-risk patients, with an estimated incidence of 6% at 5 years.[43] Furthermore, a recent meta-analysis has revealed that the mere presence of LGE, independent of its size, is associated with a significant increase in the incidence of SCD or aborted SCD as compared with patients without LGE (odds ratio (OR) 2.52, p = 0.001).[70]

PRACTICAL GUIDANCE FOR IMPLANTABLE CARDIOVERTER-DEFIBRILLATORS INDICATIONS IN HYPERTROPHIC CARDIOMYOPATHY

To address SCD, the most devastating complication of HCM, two leading medical communities of cardiology, the AHA/ACC and the ESC, have both proposed algorithms. **Fig. 2** compares clinical markers included in both risk stratification methods.

Two studies have compared the individual performance of both approaches.[65,66] A first study by Dong et al. examined a Chinese cohort of 511 patients with HCM.[65] The primary endpoint was a composite of SCD or equivalent events (appropriate ICD discharge or resuscitation after cardiac arrest). During a median follow-up time of 4.7 ± 1.7 years, 15 patients reached the primary endpoint. The recent American algorithm performed somewhat better than its European counterpart, as evidenced by a numerically higher AUC (0.71 vs.

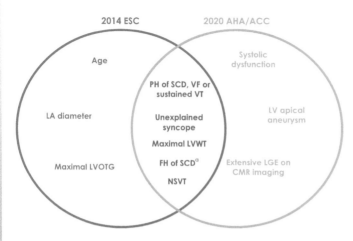

Fig. 2. Comparison Between HCM Risk Factors Included in the 2014 ESC and the 2020 AHA/ACC Guidelines. ACC, American College of Cardiology; AHA, American Heart Association; CMR, cardiac magnetic resonance; ESC, European Society of Cardiology; FH, family history; HCM, hypertrophic cardiomyopathy; LA, left atrium; LGE, late gadolinium enhancement; LV, left ventricle; LVOTG, left ventricle outflow tract gradient; LVWT, left ventricle wall thickness; NSVT, non-sustained ventricular tachycardia; PH, personal history; SCD, sudden cardiac death; VF, ventricular fibrillation; VT, ventricular tachycardia. *Red text* = established traditional risk factors. [a]Note that the definitions of FH of SCD differs in the 2014 ESC and the 2020 AHA/ACC guidelines.

0.68). Nevertheless, both approaches tend to misclassify some high-risk patients suffering SCD into low-risk categories, as evidenced by the relatively low NPV of both algorithms.[65] It is noteworthy nonetheless that the risk stratification method recommended by the AHA/ACC had a slightly better sensitivity.[65]

A second study by Zegkos et al. obtained similar findings with the American approach having a higher NPV, higher sensitivity, but lower specificity than the HCM Risk-SCD calculator.[66] Both studies demonstrate that risk stratification using novel stand-alone risk factors seem to provide a more effective protection to HCM patients at the expense, however, of a higher number of ICD implantations. **Table 4** compares ICD indications according to both medical communities.

SPECIFIC POPULATIONS

Pediatric HCM. HCM is the leading cause of SCD in the pediatric population.[71,72] Recently, two risk stratification models were developed and validated: HCM Risk-Kids[73] and PRIMaCY.[74]

HCM Risk-Kids is an algorithm developed in 2019 and is similar to the HCM Risk-SCD calculator.[73] It predicts the risk of SCD at five years in children aged 16 years or younger with HCM based on five risk factors: maximal LVWT, LA diameter, unexplained syncope, NSVT, and maximal LVOTG. The model exhibited a moderate discriminative ability with a C-statistic of 0.69 and was later validated in an external cohort.[74] The cohort characteristics, main findings, and validation results are summarised in **Table 5**. The online version of this model is available at https://hcmriskkids.org.

PRIMaCY is another risk calculator developed in 2020 that predicts the risk of SCD at five years in children aged 18 years or younger with HCM.[74] Included variables are: age at diagnosis, NSVT, unexplained syncope, septal and LV posterior wall diameters, LA diameter, and maximal LVOTG. The model displayed a good discriminative capacity with a C-statistic of 0.75 and was validated using an external cohort. The cohort characteristics, main findings, and validation results are summarised in **Table 6**. The online version of this risk calculator is available at https://primacycalculator.com.

Fig. 3 compares risk factors included in both algorithms.

Late-onset HCM. Maron et al. studied a cohort of 428 patients with HCM aged 60 years or older and followed them for 5.8 ± 4.8 years.[53] During the study period, 149 patients (35%) died, mostly from non-HCM related causes. Only five of them died suddenly. Older patients with HCM seem to be at low risk for malignant ventricular arrhythmias. Therefore, this study suggests that aggressive prophylactic ICD implantation is generally not recommended in the older population.

ESC guidelines include age at diagnosis in their clinical algorithm as opposed to the American approach. However, no studies have compared both risk stratification methods' performance in older patients. Furthermore, NSVT[20] and LVWT[24] appear to be more significant in younger patients, but no studies have assessed if there were age-independent risk factors.

Septal reduction therapy. Septal reduction therapy (SRT) consists of ventricular septal myectomy or alcohol septal ablation (ASA). An intervention is indicated in patients with LVOTG ≥50 mmHg exhibiting severe symptoms (New York Heart Association (NYHA) functional class III-IV) refractory to medical therapy in addition to those with recurrent exertional syncope.[15,16]

Table 4
ICD indications based on the 2014 ESC and the 2020 AHA/ACC guidelines

Level of ICD Recommendation	ESC 2014 Guidelines	AHA/ACC 2020 Guidelines
I Recommended	PH of SCD, VF or sustained VT	
IIa Should be considered	HCM Risk-SCD ≥6%	Maximal LVWT ≥30 mm FH of SCD Systolic dysfunction LV apical aneurysm Unexplained syncope
IIb May be considered	HCM Risk-SCD ≥4-<6% HCM Risk-SCD <4% + other factors[a]	NSVT Extensive LGE on CMR imaging

Abbreviations: ACC, American College of Cardiology; AHA, American Heart Association; CMR, cardiac magnetic resonance; ESC, European Society of Cardiology; FH, family history; HCM, hypertrophic cardiomyopathy; ICD, implantable cardioverter-defibrillator; LGE, late gadolinium enhancement; LV, left ventricle; LVWT, left ventricle wall thickness; NSVT, non-sustained ventricular tachycardia; PH, personal history; SCD, sudden cardiac death; VF, ventricular fibrillation; VT, ventricular tachycardia.

[a] Other factors such as multiple young SCD in a family or abnormal blood pressure response during exercise can be of potential importance even with a risk <4%. In these cases, ICD can be considered on an individual basis. Clinical judgment and a shared decision with the patient are recommended.

Few studies have addressed SCD risk following an SRT. McLeod et al. examined a cohort of 125 patients extracted from the Mayo Clinic HCM Database and reported that septal myectomy was associated with a significant decrease in the incidence of appropriate ICD discharges and risk for SCD, with an average annualized rate of 0.24% compared with 4.3% per year in the non-myectomy group (p = 0.004).[76] Another study assessed a cohort of 644 patients who underwent ASA and established their annual SCD risk to be less than 1%.[77]

Table 5
The HCM Risk-Kids study, Norrish et al., 2019

Studied Population	1024 Patients Aged ≤16 Years Derived from 39 Centers in 17 Countries	
Baseline characteristics[a]	Age, median, years	11 (7–14)
	Boys	699 (68.3%)
	FH of HCM (n = 1006)	534 (53.1%)
	FH of SCD (n = 1020)	130 (12.8%)
	NSVT (n = 856)	55 (6.4%)
	Unexplained syncope (n = 1023)	102 (9.9%)
	Maximal LVWT, mm (n = 997)	17.1 ± 7.4
	Maximal LVOTG, mmHg (n = 871)	9 (6–22)
	LA diameter, mm (n = 712)	33.4 ± 8.5
Follow-up	Enrolment period	1970–2017
	Median follow-up, years	5.3
	Primary endpoints SCD events	89 (8.7%)
	SCD	39 (43.8%)
	Appropriate ICD shocks	24 (27.0%)
	Aborted SCD	16 (18.0%)
	Sustained VT with HD instability	10 (11.2%)
C-statistic	Derivation cohort	0.69
	External cohort[75]	0.71

Abbreviations: FH, family history; HCM, hypertrophic cardiomyopathy; HD, hemodynamic; ICD, implantable cardioverter-defibrillator; LA, left atrial; LVOTG, left ventricle outflow tract gradient; LVWT, left ventricle wall thickness; NSVT, non-sustained ventricular tachycardia; SCD, sudden cardiac death; VT, ventricular tachycardia

[a] Total of 1024 patients unless otherwise indicated

Table 6 The PRIMaCY study, Miron et al., 2020			
Studied Population	**572 Patients Aged ≤18 Years Derived from 39 Centers in 17 Countries**		
Baseline characteristics[a]	Age at diagnosis, years		9.8 (2.1–13.9)
	Boys		394 (68.9%)
	FH of HCM (n = 550)		264 (48.0%)
	FH of SCD		105 (18.4%)
	NSVT		18 (3.1%)
	Unexplained syncope		17 (3.0%)
	Maximal LVOTG, mmHg (n = 401)		13 (0.0–46.0)
	LA diameter, z score (n = 453)		1.1 (0.1–2.1)
	Interventricular septal diameter, z score		9.5 (5.0–16.8)
	LV posterior wall diameter, z score (n = 566)		2.4 (0.3–5.0)
Follow-up	Enrolment period		1987–2018
	Follow-up, years		5
	Primary endpoints	SCD events	53 (9.3%)
		Resuscitated SCD	25 (47.2%)
		SCD	14 (26.4%)
		Aborted SCD	14 (26.4%)
C-statistic (clinical model)	Derivation cohort		0.75
	Validation cohort		0.71

Abbreviations: FH, family history; HCM, hypertrophic cardiomyopathy; LA, left atrial; LV, left ventricle; LVOTG, left ventricle outflow tract gradient; NSVT, non-sustained ventricular tachycardia; SCD, sudden cardiac death;
[a] Total of 572 patients unless otherwise indicated

As for SCD assessment, Liebregts et al. recently validated the HCM Risk-SCD in a cohort of 844 patients with a prior history of ASA. A moderate discriminative ability was obtained with a C-statistic of 0.61.[78] No other study has assessed adult or pediatric risk stratification models following SRT.

CURRENT RECOMMENDATIONS AND UNMET NEEDS

Since the first published guidelines on HCM SCD risk stratification in 2003, great progress has been made in SCD risk assessment. Both the European risk calculator and recently updated American stand-alone risk factors are highly effective methods.

We recommend employing both approaches in clinical practice. Patients that qualify for an ICD based on both algorithms should have a device implanted prophylactically while low-risk patients are not offered an ICD. For patients with contradictory recommendations, we suggest clearly explaining to the patient the uncertainty of the situation and a shared decision can be undertaken afterwards.

Despite their effectiveness, both algorithms still exhibit low sensitivities, such that some high-risk patients are still misclassified into a low-risk

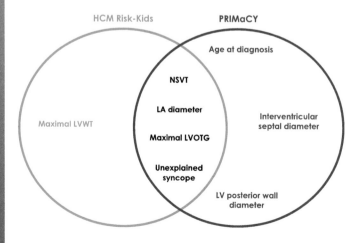

Fig. 3. Comparison Between HCM Risk Factors Included in Pediatric Risk Prediction Models (HCM Risk-Kids and PRIMaCY). HCM, hypertrophic cardiomyopathy; LA, left atrium; LV, left ventricle; LVOTG, left ventricle outflow tract gradient; LVWT, left ventricle wall thickness; NSVT, non-sustained ventricular tachycardia.

category. They also display low PPV such that numerous ICDs are implanted in low-risk patients.

Contemporary approaches also need to be validated in patients with a prior history of SRT. To this day, only one study has validated a risk stratification algorithm in a cohort of patients who underwent ASA.[78] Improvements are therefore needed to optimize current algorithms or develop new ones.

CLINICS CARE POINTS

- The HCM Risk-SCD prediction model is central to the European guidelines on SCD stratification in HCM, while the American guidelines rely on stand-alone risk factors.
- Both algorithms are effective and should be used in clinical practice. In case of discrepancy, clinical judgment and a shared decision with the patient are recommended.
- For the pediatric population, two recent risk scores have been developed and validated: HCM Risk-Kids and PRIMaCY.
- Older patients (>60 yo) are generally at low risk for SCD and prophylactic ICD implantation is rarely indicated.
- For quick access, below are the online versions of all discussed risk calculators:
   o HCM Risk-SCD: https://doc2do.com/hcm/webHCM.html
   o HCM Risk-Kids: https://hcmriskkids.org
   o PRIMaCY: https://primacycalculator.com

FUNDING SOURCES

R. Tadros is the principal investigator of the HiRO-HCM registry and Biobank supported by the Canadian Institutes of Health Research, Canada (CIHR), and currently holds the Canada Research Chair in Translational Cardiovascular Genetics.

DISCLOSURES

The authors have no conflicts of interest to disclose.

REFERENCES

1. Maron BJ, Gardin JM, Flack JM, Gidding SS, Kurosaki TT, Bild DE. Prevalence of hypertrophic cardiomyopathy in a general population of young adults. Echocardiographic analysis of 4111 subjects in the CARDIA Study. Coronary Artery Risk Development in (Young) Adults. Circulation 1995;92:785–9.

2. Maron BJ. Hypertrophic cardiomyopathy: a systematic review. JAMA 2002;287:1308–20.

3. Maron BJ, Casey SA, Poliac LC, Gohman TE, Almquist AK, Aeppli DM. Clinical course of hypertrophic cardiomyopathy in a regional United States cohort. JAMA 1999;281:650–5.

4. Maron BJ, Casey SA, Hauser RG, Aeppli DM. Clinical course of hypertrophic cardiomyopathy with survival to advanced age. J Am Coll Cardiol 2003;42: 882–8.

5. Winkel BG, Holst AG, Theilade J, et al. Nationwide study of sudden cardiac death in persons aged 1-35 years. Eur Heart J 2011;32:983–90.

6. Spirito P, Autore C, Formisano F, et al. Risk of sudden death and outcome in patients with hypertrophic cardiomyopathy with benign presentation and without risk factors. Am J Cardiol 2014;113:1550–5.

7. Elliott PM, Gimeno JR, Thaman R, et al. Historical trends in reported survival rates in patients with hypertrophic cardiomyopathy. Heart 2006;92:785–91.

8. Teare D. Asymmetrical hypertrophy of the heart in young adults. Br Heart J 1958;20:1–18.

9. Braunwald E, Lambrew C, Rockoff D, Ross J, Morrow AG. Idiopathic hypertrophic cardiomyopathy subaortic stenosis. I. Description of the disease based on the analysis of 64 patients. Circulation 1964;30(Suppl 4):3–119.

10. Maron BJ, Shen W-K, Link MS, et al. Efficacy of implantable cardioverter-defibrillators for the prevention of sudden death in patients with hypertrophic cardiomyopathy. N Engl J Med 2000;342:365–73.

11. Maron BJ, Spirito P, Shen W-K, et al. Implantable cardioverter-defibrillators and prevention of sudden cardiac death in hypertrophic cardiomyopathy. JAMA 2007;298:405–12.

12. Maron BJ, Spirito P, Ackerman MJ, et al. Prevention of sudden cardiac death with implantable cardioverter-defibrillators in children and adolescents with hypertrophic cardiomyopathy. J Am Coll Cardiol 2013;61:1527–35.

13. Maron BJ, Maron MS. Contemporary strategies for risk stratification and prevention of sudden death with the implantable defibrillator in hypertrophic cardiomyopathy. Heart Rhythm 2016;13:1115–65.

14. Maron BJ. Clinical course and management of hypertrophic cardiomyopathy. N Engl J Med 2018; 379:655–68.

15. Authors/Task Force m, Elliott PM, Anastasakis A, et al. ESC guidelines on diagnosis and management of hypertrophic cardiomyopathy: the Task Force for the Diagnosis and Management of Hypertrophic Cardiomyopathy of the European Society of Cardiology (ESC). Eur Heart J 2014;35:2733–79.

16. Ommen SR, Mital S, Burke MA, et al. AHA/ACC guideline for the diagnosis and treatment of patients

with hypertrophic cardiomyopathy: a report of the American College of Cardiology/American Heart Association Joint Committee on Clinical Practice Guidelines. Circulation 2020;142:e558–631.

17. Maron BJ, McKenna WJ, Danielson GK, et al. American College of Cardiology/European Society of Cardiology clinical expert consensus document on hypertrophic cardiomyopathy. A report of the American College of Cardiology Foundation Task Force on Clinical Expert Consensus Documents and the European Society of Cardiology Committee for Practice Guidelines. J Am Coll Cardiol 2003;42: 1687–713.

18. Maron BJ, Spirito P, Shen WK, et al. Implantable cardioverter-defibrillators and prevention of sudden cardiac death in hypertrophic cardiomyopathy. JAMA 2007;298:405–12.

19. Gersh BJ, Maron BJ, Bonow RO, et al. ACCF/AHA guideline for the diagnosis and treatment of hypertrophic cardiomyopathy: a report of the American College of Cardiology Foundation/American Heart Association Task Force on Practice Guidelines. Circulation 2011;124:e783–831.

20. Monserrat L, Elliott PM, Gimeno JR, Sharma S, Penas-Lado M, McKenna WJ. Non-sustained ventricular tachycardia in hypertrophic cardiomyopathy: an independent marker of sudden death risk in young patients. J Am Coll Cardiol 2003;42:873–9.

21. Maron BJ. Contemporary insights and strategies for risk stratification and prevention of sudden death in hypertrophic cardiomyopathy. Circulation 2010;121: 445–56.

22. O'Mahony C, Tome-Esteban M, Lambiase PD, et al. A validation study of the 2003 American College of Cardiology/European Society of Cardiology and 2011 American College of Cardiology Foundation/American Heart Association risk stratification and treatment algorithms for sudden cardiac death in patients with hypertrophic cardiomyopathy. Heart 2013;99:534–41.

23. Elliott PM, Gimeno B Jr, Mahon NG, Poloniecki JD, McKenna WJ. Relation between severity of left-ventricular hypertrophy and prognosis in patients with hypertrophic cardiomyopathy. Lancet 2001; 357:420–4.

24. Spirito P, Bellone P, Harris KM, Bernabo P, Bruzzi P, Maron BJ. Magnitude of left ventricular hypertrophy and risk of sudden death in hypertrophic cardiomyopathy. N Engl J Med 2000;342:1778–85.

25. Francia P, Santini D, Musumeci B, et al. Clinical impact of nonsustained ventricular tachycardia recorded by the implantable cardioverter-defibrillator in patients with hypertrophic cardiomyopathy. Journal of cardiovascular electrophysiology 2014;25:1180–7.

26. Wang W, Lian Z, Rowin EJ, Maron BJ, Maron MS, Link MS. Prognostic Implications of Nonsustained Ventricular Tachycardia in High-Risk Patients With Hypertrophic Cardiomyopathy. Circ Arrhythm Electrophysiol 2017;10:e004604.

27. Elliott PM, Poloniecki J, Dickie S, et al. Sudden death in hypertrophic cardiomyopathy: identification of high risk patients. J Am Coll Cardiol 2000;36: 2212–8.

28. Spirito P, Maron BJ. Relation between extent of left ventricular hypertrophy and occurrence of sudden cardiac death in hypertrophic cardiomyopathy. J Am Coll Cardiol 1990;15:1521–6.

29. Spirito P, Seidman CE, McKenna WJ, Maron BJ. The management of hypertrophic cardiomyopathy. N Engl J Med 1997;336:775–85.

30. O'Mahony C, Jichi F, Pavlou M, et al. A novel clinical risk prediction model for sudden cardiac death in hypertrophic cardiomyopathy (HCM Risk-SCD). Eur Heart J 2014;35:2010–20.

31. O'Mahony C, Akhtar MM, Anastasiou Z, et al. Effectiveness of the 2014 European Society of Cardiology guideline on sudden cardiac death in hypertrophic cardiomyopathy: a systematic review and meta-analysis. Heart 2019;105:623e631.

32. Wang J, Zhang Z, Li Y, et al. Variable and limited predictive value of the European society of cardiology hypertrophic cardiomyopathy sudden death risk model: a meta-analysis. Can J Cardiol 2019;35:1791–9.

33. Spirito P, Autore C, Rapezzi C, et al. Syncope and risk of sudden death in hypertrophic cardiomyopathy. Circulation 2009;119:1703–10.

34. Maki S, Ikeda H, Muro A, et al. Predictors of sudden cardiac death in hypertrophic cardiomyopathy. Am J Cardiol 1998;82:774–8.

35. Elliott PM, Gimeno JR, Tome MT, et al. Left ventricular outflow tract obstruction and sudden death risk in patients with hypertrophic cardiomyopathy. Eur Heart J 2006;27:1933–41.

36. Kofflard MJM, Ten Cate FJ, van der Lee C, van Domburg RT. Hypertrophic cardiomyopathy in a large community-based population: clinical outcome and identification of risk factors for sudden cardiac death and clinical deterioration. J Am Coll Cardiol 2003;41: 987–93.

37. Maron MS, Olivotto I, Betocchi S, et al. Effect of left ventricular outflow tract obstruction on clinical outcome in hypertrophic cardiomyopathy. N Engl J Med 2003;348:295–303.

38. Maron BJ, Casey SA, Chan RH, et al. Independent assessment of the European Society of Cardiology sudden death risk model for hypertrophic cardiomyopathy. Am J Cardiol 2015;116:757–64.

39. Lemire F, Tajik AJ, Hagler DJ. Asymmetric left atrial enlargement; an echocardiographic observation. Chest 1976;69:779–81.

40. Badano LP, Pezzutto N, Marinigh R, et al. How many patients would be misclassified using M-mode and two-dimensional estimates of left atrial size instead of left atrial volume? A three-dimensional

echocardiographic study. J Cardiovasc Med 2008; 9:476–84.

41. Lang RM, Badano LP, Mor-Avi V, et al. Recommendations for cardiac chamber quantification by echocardiography in adults: an update from the American society of echocardiography and the European association of, cardiovascular imaging. Eur Heart J Cardiovasc Imaging 2016;17:412.

42. Mills H, Espersen K, Jurlander R, Iversen K, Bundgaard H, Raja AA. Prevention of sudden cardiac death in hypertrophic cardiomyopathy: Risk assessment using left atrial diameter predicted from left atrial volume. Clin Cardiol 2020;43:581–6.

43. Chan RH, Maron BJ, Olivotto I, et al. Prognostic value of quantitative contrast-enhanced cardiovascular magnetic resonance for the evaluation of sudden death risk in patients with hypertrophic cardiomyopathy. Circulation 2014;130:484e495.

44. Maron BJ, Rowin EJ, Casey SA, et al. Hypertrophic cardiomyopathy associated with low cardiovascular mortality with contemporary management strategies. J Am Coll Cardiol 2015;65:1915e1928.

45. O'Hanlon R, Grasso A, Roughton M, et al. Prognostic significance of myocardial fibrosis in hypertrophic cardiomyopathy. J Am Coll Cardiol 2010; 56:867e874.

46. Bruder O, Wagner A, Jensen CJ, et al. Myocardial scar visualized by cardiovascular magnetic resonance imaging predicts major adverse events in patients with hypertrophic cardiomyopathy. J Am Coll Cardiol 2010;56:875e887.

47. Green JJ, Berger JS, Kramer CM, Salerno M. Prognostic value of late gadolinium enhancement in clinical outcomes for hypertrophic cardiomyopathy. JACC Cardiovasc Imaging 2012;5:370e377.

48. Olivotto I, Maron BJ, Appelbaum E, et al. Spectrum and clinical significance of systolic function and myocardial fibrosis assessed by cardiovascular magnetic resonance in hypertrophic cardiomyopathy. Am J Cardiol 2010;106:261e267.

49. Spirito P, Autore C, Formisano F, et al. Risk of sudden death and outcome in patients with hypertrophic cardiomyopathy with benign presentation and without risk factors. Am J Cardiol 2014;113: 1550e1555.

50. Vriesendorp PA, Schinkel AF, Van Cleemput J, et al. Implantable cardioverter-defibrillators in hypertrophic cardiomyopathy: patient outcomes, rate of appropriate and inappropriate interventions, and complications. Am Heart J 2013;166:496–502.

51. Maron BJ, Rowin EJ, Casey SA, et al. Hypertrophic cardiomyopathy in children, adolescents, and young adults associated with low cardiovascular mortality with contemporary management strategies. Circulation 2016;133:62–73.

52. Ichida M, Nishimura Y, Kario K. Clinical significance of left ventricular apical aneurysms in hypertrophic

cardiomyopathy patients: the role of diagnostic electrocardiography. J Cardiol 2014;64:265–72.

53. Maron BJ, Rowin EJ, Casey SA, et al. Risk stratification and outcome of patients with hypertrophic cardiomyopathy ≥60 years of age. Circulation 2013; 127:585–93.

54. Moon JC, McKenna WJ, McCrohon JA, et al. Toward clinical risk assessment in hypertrophic cardiomyopathy with gadolinium cardiovascular magnetic resonance. J Am Coll Cardiol 2003;41:1561–7.

55. Maron MS, Rowin EJ, Wessler BS, et al. Enhanced American College of Cardiology/American Heart Association strategy for prevention of sudden cardiac death in high-risk patients with hypertrophic cardiomyopathy. JAMA Cardiol 2019;4:644–57.

56. Bos JM, Maron BJ, Ackerman MJ, et al. Role of family history of sudden death in risk stratification and prevention of sudden death with implantable defibrillators in hypertrophic cardiomyopathy. Am J Cardiol 2010;106:1481–6.

57. Dimitrow PP, Chojnowska L, Rudzinski T, et al. Sudden death in hypertrophic cardiomyopathy: old risk factors re-assessed in a new model of maximalized follow-up. Eur Heart J 2010;31:3084–93.

58. O'Mahony C, Jichi F, Ommen SR, et al. International external validation study of the 2014 European Society of Cardiology guidelines on sudden cardiac death prevention in hypertrophic cardiomyopathy (EVIDENCE-HCM). Circulation 2018;137:1015–23.

59. Marstrand P, Han L, Day SM, et al. Hypertrophic cardiomyopathy with left ventricular systolic dysfunction: insights from the SHaRe registry. Circulation 2020;141:1371–83.

60. Harris KM, Spirito P, Maron MS, et al. Prevalence, clinical profile, and significance of left ventricular remodeling in the end-stage phase of hypertrophic cardiomyopathy. Circulation 2006;114:216e225.

61. Ismail TF, Jabbour A, Gulati A, et al. Role of late gadolinium enhancement cardiovascular magnetic resonance in the risk stratification of hypertrophic cardiomyopathy. Heart 2014;100:1851–8.

62. Rowin EJ, Maron BJ, Haas TS, et al. Hypertrophic Cardiomyopathy With Left Ventricular Apical Aneurysm: Implications for Risk Stratification and Management. J Am Coll Cardiol 2017;69:761–73.

63. Weng Z, Yao J, Chan RH, et al. Prognostic value of LGE-CMR in HCM: a meta-analysis. J Am Coll Cardiol Img 2016;9:1392–402.

64. Mentias A, Raeisi-Giglou P, Smedira NG, et al. Late gadolinium enhancement in patients with hypertrophic cardiomyopathy and preserved systolic function. J Am Coll Cardiol 2018;72:857–70.

65. Dong Y, Yang W, Chen C, et al. Validation of the 2020 AHA/ACC Risk Stratification for Sudden Cardiac Death in Chinese Patients With Hypertrophic Cardiomyopathy. Frontiers in cardiovascular medicine 2021;8:691653.

66. Zegkos T, Tziomalos G, Parcharidou D, et al. Validation of the new American College of Cardiology/ American Heart Association Guidelines for the risk stratification of sudden cardiac death in a large Mediterranean cohort with Hypertrophic Cardiomyopathy. Hellenic J Cardiol HJC 2022;63:15–21.

67. Maron MS, Finley JJ, Bos JM, et al. Prevalence, clinical significance, and natural history of left ventricular apical aneurysms in hypertrophic cardiomyopathy. Circulation 2008;118:1541–9.

68. Basso C, Thiene G, Corrado D, Buja G, Melacini P, Nava A. Hypertrophic cardiomyopathy and sudden death in the young: pathologic evidence of myocardial ischemia. Hum Pathol 2000;3:988–98.

69. Shirani J, Pick R, Roberts WC, Maron BJ. Morphology and significance of the left ventricular collagen network in young patients with hypertrophic cardiomyopathy and sudden cardiac death. J Am Coll Cardiol 2000;35:36–44.

70. Briasoulis A, Mallikethi-Reddy S, Palla M, Alesh I, Afonso L. Myocardial fibrosis on cardiac magnetic resonance and cardiac outcomes in hypertrophic cardiomyopathy: a meta-analysis. Heart 2015;101: 1406–11.

71. Colan SD, Lipshultz SE, Lowe AM, et al. Epidemiology and cause-specific outcome of hypertrophic cardiomyopathy in children: findings from the Pediatric Cardiomyopathy Registry. Circulation 2007; 115:773–81.

72. Alexander PMA, Nugent AW, Daubeney PEF, et al. National Australian Childhood Cardiomyopathy Study. Long-term outcomes of hypertrophic cardiomyopathy diagnosed during childhood: results from a national population-based study. Circulation 2018;138:29–36.

73. Norrish G, Ding T, Field E, et al. Development of a Novel Risk Prediction Model for Sudden Cardiac Death in Childhood Hypertrophic Cardiomyopathy (HCM Risk-Kids). JAMA Cardiology 2019;4:918–27.

74. Miron A, Lafreniere-Roula M, Steve Fan CP, et al. A Validated Model for Sudden Cardiac Death Risk Prediction in Pediatric Hypertrophic Cardiomyopathy. Circulation 2020;142:217–29.

75. Norrish G, Qu C, Field E, et al. External validation of the HCM Risk-Kids model for predicting sudden cardiac death in childhood hypertrophic cardiomyopathy. European journal of preventive cardiology 2022; 29:678–86.

76. McLeod CJ, Ommen SR, Ackerman MJ, et al. Surgical septal myectomy decreases the risk for appropriate implantable cardioverter defibrillator discharge in obstructive hypertrophic cardiomyopathy. Eur Heart J 2007;28:2583–8.

77. Kuhn H, Lawrenz T, Lieder F, et al. Survival after transcoronary ablation of septal hypertrophy in hypertrophic obstructive cardiomyopathy (TASH): a 10 year experience. Clin Res Cardiol 2008;97:234–43.

78. Liebregts M, Faber L, Jensen MK, et al. Validation of the HCM Risk-SCD model in patients with hypertrophic cardiomyopathy following alcohol septal ablation. Europace 2018;20:f198–203.

Impact of Cardiac Magnetic Resonance to Arrhythmic Risk Stratification in Nonischemic Cardiomyopathy

Andrea Di Marco, MD, PhD[a,b,c,*], Eduard Claver, MD[a,b], Ignasi Anguera, MD, PhD[a,b]

KEYWORDS

- Cardiac magnetic resonance • Late gadolinium enhancement • Extracellular volume fraction
- Ventricular arrhythmias • Sudden cardiac death

KEY POINTS

- Left ventricular ejection-based arrhythmic risk stratification is inadequate and unable to identify both true high-risk patients and true low-risk cases.
- Late gadolinium enhancement (LGE) detects myocardial scar, the main substrate of ventricular arrhythmias. A great wealth of evidence supports LGE as an independent and strong predictor of ventricular arrhythmias and sudden death.
- Other cardiac magnetic resonance parameters, especially those related to diffuse fibrosis, may have incremental prognostic value on the top of LGE.

INTRODUCTION

Risk stratification for ventricular arrhythmias (VAs) and sudden cardiac death (SCD) in nonischemic cardiomyopathy (NICM) is a key unresolved issue. Poor risk stratification is probably the main reason for the failure of large clinical trials of primary prevention implantable cardioverter defibrillator (ICD) in NICM.[1–3] Traditionally, risk stratification has been based mainly on left ventricular ejection fraction (LVEF), which is a powerful predictor of global prognosis but is neither highly sensitive nor specific for VA and SCD.[4] Cardiac magnetic resonance (CMR) provides detailed and unique tissue characterization and is emerging as a fundamental tool to improve the arrhythmic risk stratification in NICM. In this review, the authors analyze the available evidence regarding the predictive ability of different CMR parameters and suggest future directions for medical research in this field. The authors focus on studies specifically evaluating predictors of VA and SCD in NICM avoiding, if possible, reports assessing mixed endpoints combining VA and heart failure (HF) events or SCD and non-sudden death.

NONISCHEMIC CARDIOMYOPATHY: DEFINITIONS AND EPIDEMIOLOGY

The classification of cardiomyopathies proposed by the European Society of Cardiology (ESC) focused on morphologic and functional phenotypes, defining dilated cardiomyopathy (DCM) as the presence of left ventricular (LV) or biventricular

The authors have no disclosures related to the present article.

a Department of Cardiology, Hospital Universitari de Bellvitge, L'Hospitalet de Llobregat, Barcelona, Spain; b Bioheart-Cardiovascular Diseases Group, Cardiovascular, Respiratory and Systemic Diseases and Cellular Aging Program, Institut d'Investigació Biomèdica de Bellvitge–IDIBELL, L'Hospitalet de Llobregat, Barcelona, Spain; c Division of Cardiovascular Sciences, School of Medical Sciences, Faculty of Biology, Medicine and Health, University of Manchester, Manchester Academic Health Science Centre, Manchester, UK

* Corresponding author. Arrhythmia Unit, Department of Cardiology, Hospital Universitari de Bellvitge, Calle feixa llarga sin número, 08907, Hospitalet de llobregat, Barcelona, Spain.

E-mail address: adimarco@bellvitgehospital.cat

cardiacEP.theclinics.com

systolic dysfunction and dilatation that are not explained by abnormal loading conditions or coronary artery disease.[5] Recently, this definition of DCM was revised, recognizing that some patients with clinically relevant myocardial disease may have mild LV impairment and very mild or even absent LV dilatation, hypokinetic non-dilated cardiomyopathy (HNDC), representing patients with LVEF less than 45% and no LV dilatation, was thus included in the DCM spectrum.[6] In view of similar considerations, many studies have adopted a pragmatical definition of NICM based solely on the presence of LV dysfunction with an LVEF less than 50%, always in the absence of abnormal loading conditions or coronary artery disease.[7] Actually, the difference between the ESC definition of DCM (including HNDC) and the pragmatical definition of NICM is minimal and refers to patients with LVEF 45% to 49% and no LV dilatation. In this review, the authors comment works which have used either the ESC definition of DCM or the pragmatical definition of NICM.

Precise and contemporary data on the prevalence of NICM are lacking. A prevalence of 1:2500 is often reported,[8] but this estimation refers to a study performed between 1975 and 1984 using medical records and M-mode echocardiography.[9] The same study, for example, underestimated the prevalence of hypertrophic cardiomyopathy by approximately 10 times. Thus, considering also the prevalence of nonischemic etiology within large HF trials, it seems reasonable to expect that the prevalence of NICM is at least 1:400.[10]

The clinical phenotype of NICM can be due to multiple etiologies, including genetic variants, drugs, toxins, hormonal abnormalities, and infectious or noninfectious myocarditis.

SUDDEN CARDIAC DEATH IN NONISCHEMIC CARDIOMYOPATHY

Accurate contemporary data about the incidence of SCD in NICM are lacking. Thanks to the advances in medical therapy, cardiovascular death and SCD have declined in the last decades in HF patients.[11] In the long-term follow-up (median 9.5 years) of the control group of the DANISH trial, death from any cause occurred in 40% of patients, and 73% of deaths were due to a cardiovascular cause[12]; SCD occurred in 10% of patients, representing 25% of all deaths and 35% of cardiovascular deaths. However, arrhythmic SCD, preventable by ICD represented only a portion of all SCD. In the long-term follow-up study of the DANISH trial cohort, SCD still occurred in 6% of patients randomized to ICD.

Thus, the cumulative incidence of SCD preventable with the ICD, at a median follow-up of 9.5 years, was of 4% which represented 10% of all deaths, 13% of cardiovascular deaths, and 40% of SCD.[12]

The progressive reduction in the incidence of SCD makes the improvement of the arrhythmic risk stratification and the identification of those with the highest risk even more necessary.

LIMITATIONS OF TRADITIONAL RISK STRATIFICATION

Traditionally, LVEF has been used as the main parameter to indicate primary prevention ICD use. This is because LVEF was the fundamental inclusion criterion of all major randomized trials of primary prevention ICDs.[1-3] However, none of those trials found a significant survival benefit from primary prevention ICD.

LVEF, while being a strong predictor of overall prognosis, is neither highly sensitive nor specific for SCD.[4] In 1994, a few years before the start of the DEFINITE and the SCD-HeFT trials, Dr Dec and Dr Fuster stated in the New England Journal of Medicine: "the left ventricular ejection fraction is also a powerful, independent predictor of prognosis [..but..] patients at greatest risk of sudden death cannot yet be prospectively identified."[13]

In those times, several cohort studies had obtained conflicting results about the association between LVEF and SCD in NICM. In some reports, LVEF was not a significant predictor, and even when an association was present, it was often weaker or less significant than the association between LVEF and HF-related death.[14-17] One report actually observed a higher sudden to non-sudden death ratio among patients with higher LVEF.[17] Moreover, the choice of the 35% cutoff for LVEF was somehow arbitrary.

Some recent studies including large multicenter NICM cohorts again could not find a significant association between LVEF ≤35% and VA/SCD.[7,18,19] Other recent reports observed a significant association between LVEF and the arrhythmic endpoint, but a major limitation should be kept in mind in these cases[20,21]: most or a relevant proportion of arrhythmic events in these reports was appropriate ICD therapies, whereas ICD implantation is essentially driven by LVEF. This fact could have artificially magnified the association between LVEF and the arrhythmic outcome by creating an observation bias.

In conclusion, the inclusion criteria of randomized trials of primary prevention ICD in NICM had a rather weak scientific basis, although selected patients were supposed to have the highest risk of death, they did not necessarily have the highest risk of SCD. The failure to select patients at high risk for SCD is probably the main reason for the negative results of those trials.

CHARACTERISTICS OF THE IDEAL PREDICTOR OF SUDDEN CARDIAC DEATH

Ideally, a clinically useful predictor of SCD should possess the following features:

1. It should be obtained with a standardized and reproducible method.
2. It should demonstrate a significant and independent association with VA and SCD, consistently in several studies from different groups and across the whole spectrum of NICM.
3. The association with VA and SCD should also be strong with hazard ratios at least greater than 2 (the higher the better).
4. It should have a specific association with VA and SCD with a stronger predictive ability for VA and SCD versus HF events and non-sudden death.
5. It should be directly related to the substrate of VA, conferring pathophysiological plausibility to its association with VA and SCD.

These characteristics can be summarized with the rule of the 5S (Standardized, Significant, Strong, Specific and Substrate) as shown in **Table 1**.

PATHOPHYSIOLOGY OF VENTRICULAR ARRHYTHMIA

In patients with prior myocardial infarction (MI) it is well established that myocardial scar is the main substrate for VA, especially with regard to sustained monomorphic ventricular tachycardia (SMVT). In fact, the scar can harbor all the elements needed to sustain a VT circuit, such as areas of conduction block and areas of slow conduction.[22] Although it took longer to understand it for NICM, most SMVT are scar-related[23] and nonischemic scars can harbor late potentials and critical VT isthmi similarly to post-MI scars.[24,25] Other mechanisms of SMVT in NICM include His-Purkinje-related VT, especially bundle branch reentry VT.[26] Focal VTs from the outflow tract or the papillary muscles, which are a frequent cause of idiopathic VT, may also occur in patients with NICM.

The pathophysiology of ventricular fibrillation (VF) outside the setting of acute myocardial ischemia is more complex and less well understood. In some cases, an SMVT can degenerate into VF. When VF is the primary rhythm, it may

Table 1 Characteristics of the ideal predictor of ventricular arrhythmia/sudden cardiac death	
Characteristics of the Ideal Predictor of SD: The Rule of the 5S	
Standardized	Measurable with standardized and reproducible method
Significant	Significant and independent association with VA and SD, consistently in several large several studies from different groups and across the whole spectrum if NICM
Strong	The association with VA and SD should also be strong, with hazard ratio at least >2 (the higher the better)
Specific	Specific association with VA and SD; association with VA and SD should be stronger that any association with heart failure endpoints or non-sudden death
Substrate	Directly related to the substrate of VA, conferring pathophysiological plausibility to its association with VA and SD

be initiated by short-coupled premature ventricular complexes (PVCs), often arising from the Purkinje network, both in patients with structural heart disease and in those with normal hearts.[27] Myocardial scar is also a contributor of the vulnerable substrate behind VF and may play a role in VF initiation and maintenance. Small series of patients with ischemic and NICM suggest that PVCs triggering VF generally arise within or in the border of the scar and often display Purkinje potentials.[28] In a series of 24 patients with apparently idiopathic VF, areas of abnormal electrograms suggesting scar were observed in 63% of patients and they colocalized with VF drivers. The ablation of these abnormal electrograms resulted in 83% rate of freedom from VA recurrence during follow-up.[29] Finally, altered neurohumoral activation, electrolytes imbalances, and the process of electrical remodeling occurring in the failing heart may have pro-arrhythmic effects; abnormal function of ion channels and altered intracellular Ca^{2+} handling can favor triggered activity, whereas the down-regulation of Connexin 43 can affect the velocity of impulse conduction.[30]

LATE GADOLINIUM ENHANCEMENT PRESENCE/ABSENCE AND THE ARRHYTHMIC RISK

CMR offers the unique opportunity to evaluate cardiac morphology and function providing at the same time detailed tissue characterization. Late gadolinium enhancement (LGE) identifies areas of localized replacement fibrosis, that is, myocardial scar. This has been confirmed histologically both in experimental models of MI[31] and patients with ischemic and NICM.[32]

The fact that only a proportion of patients with NICM display LGE (usually around 40%) has allowed evaluating the prognostic impact of the simple dichotomous variable of LGE presence versus absence.

In 2016, the authors performed a meta-analysis including 29 observational studies (for a total of 2948 patients) which had investigated the association between LGE and VA or SCD.[33] The authors observed a strong and significant association between LGE and the arrhythmic endpoint (odds ratio:[OR] 4.3, P<.001), and this association was maintained both among studies with mean LVEF less than 35% (OR 4.2, P<.001) and among those with mean LVEF greater than 35% (OR 5.2, P<.001). In addition, by restricting the analysis to studies which had reported results of multivariate Cox regression for the arrhythmic endpoint, the overall adjusted hazard ratio (HR) for LGE was 6.7 with P<.001.

In more recent years, large, often multicentric, observational cohorts including greater than 6000 patients, have confirmed that LGE presence is significantly, independently and strongly associated with VA and SCD (**Fig. 1** shows the examples of LGE− and LGE + patients with different outcomes).[7,18–21] One important aspect, observed both in the meta-analysis and these large cohorts, is the high negative predictive value of LGE absence; LGE− patients have a low arrhythmic risk, with an average annual event rate less than 2% of the composite outcome comprising SMVT, appropriate ICD shocks and often any appropriate ICD therapy. In our cohort of 1165 patients with DCM, those without LGE had a cumulative incidence of the arrhythmic endpoint of 1% after a median follow-up of 3 years.[21] A risk stratification algorithm which combined LGE and LVEF was significantly superior to LVEF with the 35% cutoff, identified true high-risk and true low-risk patients and reclassified the risk in one-third of NICM cohort.[21]

The reports included in our meta-analysis either focused on patients with severe LV dysfunction or included the whole spectrum of NICM. In the first study focusing exclusively on those with mild or moderate LV dysfunction, Halliday and colleagues showed, among 399 patients with LVEF $\geq$ 40%, that LGE increased the arrhythmic risk nine times (adjusted HR 9.3, P<.001).[34] In our recently published cohort of 1165 NICM patients, the authors confirmed these results: among patients with LVEF greater than 35%, LGE was the only independent predictor of the arrhythmic endpoint with an adjusted HR of 11.8 (P<.001).[21] The authors also observed a stronger unadjusted association between LGE and the arrhythmic endpoint among those with better LVEF as compared with patients with severe LV dysfunction.[21] These observations are particularly relevant as patients with LVEF greater than 35% have a lower risk of non-sudden death and consequently those with a high risk of SCD among them might be ideal candidates for preventive ICD.

LGE is also a predictor of HF events in NICM. However, the association with these endpoints seems less consistent and somehow weaker as compared with the association between LGE and VA or SCD. One meta-analysis reported that LGE had an OR of 2.9 (P = .02) for HF hospitalizations and an OR of 5.3 (P<.001) for SCD or aborted SCD.[35] In our cohort including 1165 patients with NICM, LGE was significantly associated with a combined HF endpoint at univariate analysis, but lost statistical significance at multivariate analysis.[21] Thus, LGE might possess the quality of being a relatively specific predictor of VA and SCD.

LATE GADOLINIUM ENHANCEMENT PRESENCE/ABSENCE AND SURVIVAL BENEFIT WITH IMPLANTABLE CARDIOVERTER DEFIBRILLATOR (INCLUDING CARDIAC RESYNCHRONIZATION THERAPY ASSOCIATED WITH AN ICD)

The CMR sub-study of the DANISH trial included 236 patients (113 LGE+).[36] There was no significant difference in the cumulative incidence of SCD between LGE+ and LGE− patients (10% vs 7%) and ICD did not provide survival benefit neither among LGE + nor among LGE− patients.

Opposite results were obtained in an observational retrospective cohort study, including patients with standard indications for prophylactic ICD[37] where 206 out of a cohort of 452 patients were not implanted with an ICD at discretion of the treating physician. Appropriate ICD therapies occurred in 40% of LGE + patients and in only 4% of LGE− ones (P<.001). After propensity score adjustment, ICD implantation was not associated with significant survival benefit, mainly due to the absence of any effect among LGE− patients. By contrast, among LGE + cases, ICD implantation was associated with a significant 57% reduction in mortality.[37]

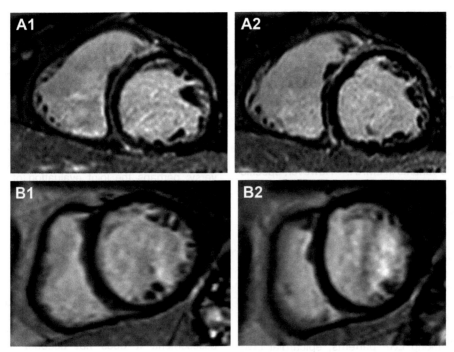

Fig. 1. Short axis views of the basal and mid-segments in LGE sequences from two NICM patients. Patient 1 (A1, A2) had extensive LGE (mid-wall septal and subepicardial), whereas patient 2 (B1, B2) had no LGE. LVEF was 40% in patient 1% and 19% in patient 2. Patient 1 had resuscitated cardiac arrest in his forties; patient 2 has never experienced any sustained VA.

Sufficiently powered randomized trials are needed to clarify whether primary prevention of ICDs improves survival among LGE + patients.

No randomized clinical trial has demonstrated a significant reduction in mortality with cardiac resynchronization therapy associated with an ICD (CRT-D) as compared with CRT pacing only (CRT-P).[3,38] One observational study, including 252 patients with NICM implanted with a CRT-P or CRT-D, performed propensity-score adjusted analysis and observed a reduction in overall mortality with CRT-D versus CRT-P only among LGE + patients.[39] The absence of LGE has also been reported as a predictor of LV reverse remodeling after CRT.[40] In a prospective registry of 218 patients with CRT-D or CRT-P (64% with NICM), the presence of LGE was the main driver of appropriate ICD therapies during follow-up, independently of echocardiographic response to CRT.[41] Therefore, it could be appropriate to implant CRT-P devices in LGE− candidates to resynchronization therapy.

LATE GADOLINIUM ENHANCEMENT EXTENT AND THE ARRHYTHMIC RISK

LGE per se is not a quantitative technique. Several strategies for LGE quantification have been proposed; however, none of them is considered the gold standard.[42]

Most of the studies evaluating the association between LGE extent and VA or SCD in NICM could not find a linear association[7,43] and observed a significant increase in the arrhythmic risk with small amount of scar, the best cutoff of LGE to predict VA or SCD was 0.71% or 2% of LV mass.

At present, considering the technical limitations intrinsic to LGE quantification and its doubtful clinical impact, the authors consider that no specific recommendation can be provided about performing LGE quantification in NICM.

A semiquantitative analysis, based on the number of segments with LGE, can avoid the technical complexities associated with LGE quantification. Guaricci and colleagues found that the number of segments with midwall LGE was significantly associated with the arrhythmic outcome and that the variable "midwall LGE in >3 segments" was an independent predictor of the arrhythmic outcome.[18] By contrast, among LGE + patients in our DCM cohort, the number of segments with LGE showed a nonsignificant trend toward an association with the arrhythmic endpoint (HR 1.1, $P = .07$).[21] Thus, the prognostic role of semiquantitative evaluation of LGE in NICM needs to be clarified.

LATE GADOLINIUM ENHANCEMENT LOCATION/PATTERN AND THE ARRHYTHMIC RISK

LGE location and pattern may be specifically associated with the etiology of NICM and, as such, they might portent different risk of VA and SCD. For example, ring-like subepicardial LGE has been reported in patients with high-risk pathogenic variants in desmosomal genes or FLNC.[44] A midwall septal pattern is usually observed in patients with pathogenic variants in LMNA.[45] However, specific variants in the same gene may be associated with a differential phenotype: for example, pathogenic variants in the Arg541 residue of LMNA are associated with epicardial or transmural LGE and high arrhythmic risk.[46]

Halliday and colleagues evaluated the arrhythmic risk associated with different LGE locations and patterns in 874 DCM patients, among LGE locations, the presence of LGE both in the septum and in the free wall was associated with the highest risk (HR 5.8, $P<.001$), whereas among LGE patterns, epicardial LGE (HR 5.5, $P<.001$) and multipattern LGE (HR 5.7, $P<.001$) were associated with the greatest risk.[43] In our cohort of 1165 DCM patients, the presence of epicardial or transmural LGE as well as the presence of LGE both in the septum and the free wall identified patients at higher risk among LGE + cases, and the discriminatory effect of these high-risk LGE features was more evident in those with LVEF greater than 35%.[21] Guaricci and colleagues, in the 1000 patients of their derivation cohort, observed that the presence of multiple LGE pattern was associated with the highest HR (HR 3.4, $P = .001$) but epicardial LGE had no significant association with the arrhythmic outcome.[18] Alba and colleagues did not find any interaction between LGE pattern or the number of patterns and the arrhythmic endpoint among 1672 NICM patients.[20]

The presence of LGE only at the right ventricular insertion points (IP) is considered to have different histologic basis (plexiform fibrosis in areas of cardiomyocytes disarray instead of replacement fibrosis)[47] and is usually seen as a benign finding not associated with higher arrhythmic risk. Actually, patients with LGE at IP were included among LGE− cases in some report.[20,21] Two recent retrospective cohorts, one with 360 patients[48] and the other with 1165 patients[49] provided very similar results: patients with LGE only at IP had a risk of VA and SCD significantly lower than LGE + patients and similar to that of LGE− ones. In addition, the presence of LGE at IP had no effect on the arrhythmic risk of LGE + patients. By contrast, another report with 600 NICM patients observed a considerable arrhythmic risk among those with LGE only at IP (cumulative incidence 17%, median follow-up 2.7 years).[19] It is uncertain whether the genetic background or the evolution of the CMR phenotype toward localized scar may have influenced the non-negligible risk of patients with LGE at IP in the last study.

In conclusion, the differential risk of specific LGE patterns or locations is another matter of controversy; perhaps the joint evaluation of the CMR phenotype and the genotype may help assessing the prognostic role of different LGE features.

LIMITATIONS OF LATE GADOLINIUM ENHANCEMENT

Contraindications to gadolinium limit the LGE assessment. LGE is not, per se, a quantitative method and this fact impacts on the different techniques developed to provide quantitative LGE assessment. It does not account for diffuse fibrosis. Although LGE is an excellent predictor of SMVT, one report suggested it has lower ability to predict VF.[50]

T1 MAPS/EXTRACELLULAR VOLUME FRACTION AND THE RISK OF VENTRICULAR ARRHYTHMIA/SUDDEN CARDIAC DEATH

CMR allows quantitative evaluation of interstitial fibrosis by means of T1 maps, obtained either before (native T1) or after gadolinium administration (post-contrast T1). In general, native T1 increases and post-contrast T1 decreases with increments in interstitial fibrosis. The extracellular volume fraction (ECV) can be calculated from native and post-contrast T1 of the myocardium and the blood, knowing the hematocrit of the patients. ECV has been validated histologically, demonstrating a good correlation with collagen volume fraction.[51] Although T1 values are influenced by field strength, vendor, and the acquisition technique, ECV has the advantage of being more reproducible.

Although the role of interstitial fibrosis as a substrate for ventricular arrhythmias is less clear than that of LGE, diffuse fibrosis may cause heterogeneous conduction slowing with pro-arrhythmic effects.[52] In a series of 51 LGE− NICM patients referred for VT ablation, post-contrast T1 values correlated with voltage abnormalities at electroanatomic mapping and lower post-contrast T1 values were associated with higher VT recurrence after ablation.[53]

There is very limited evidence about the contribution of T1 mapping and ECV to arrhythmic risk stratification. Among 58 NICM patients with ICD in primary or secondary prevention, native T1 was the only independent predictor of appropriate ICD therapies during follow-up (ECV was not reported).[54] Among 609 patients with NICM with LGE, native T1 and ECV available, ECV was the only predictor which maintained a significant association with the arrhythmic endpoint after adjustment for LGE and LVEF.[55] An optimal cutoff of ECV 30% was identified; by adding ECV $\geq$ 30% to a predictive model already including LGE and LVEF, the Harrell's C statistical of the model increased from 0.81 to 0.89, achieving an excellent predictive capacity. Importantly, ECV $\geq$ 30% discriminated the arrhythmic risk among LGE + patients: those with ECV $\geq$ 30% had considerable risk (8.5%, median follow-up 21 months), whereas those with ECV less than 30% had negligible risk (0.7%).

Further studies are needed to clarify the prognostic value of diffuse fibrosis assessment to identify the best parameter between T1 values and ECV, evaluate the incremental and potentially complementary prognostic contribution of these markers with respect to LGE, and assess their specificity with respect to the arrhythmic endpoint, considering that both native T1 and ECV have demonstrated significant associations with overall outcome (including cardiac death, heart transplant, combined endpoints mixing HF, and arrhythmic events).[56]

OTHER CARDIAC MAGNETIC RESONANCE PARAMETERS

Myocardial tissue heterogeneity may play a role in the genesis of ventricular arrhythmias, although the authors lack studies demonstrating the precise mechanisms of this pathophysiological association outside the setting of localized myocardial scar. The mean absolute deviation of the segmental pixel standard deviation (Mad-SD) at native T1 mapping has been proposed as a measure of myocardial tissue heterogeneity; among 115 NICM patients Mad-SD was an independent predictor of VA and SCD and, if combined with native T1 value, achieved a predictive ability similar to that of LGE.[57] At present, these results lack confirmation from other groups.

LV entropy has been proposed as a new LGE-CMR derived marker of myocardial tissue heterogeneity. Although the entropy of post-MI scar has been suggested as a predictor of appropriate ICD therapies,[58] no association between scar entropy and ICD therapies was observed among 44 LGE + NICM patients implanted with an ICD in primary or secondary prevention.[59]

Among 156 LGE + NICM patients, LGE interface area (the total arc length of the border between myocardium and LGE, multiplied by the slice thickness) was an independent predictor of the arrhythmic outcome.[60]

In ischemic cardiomyopathy, the amount of border zone channels, obtained from CMR with the ADAS 3D software (ADAS3D Medical, Barcelona, Spain), achieved the best predictive ability among scar-related CMR-derived parameters.[61] It is unknown if this can also apply to NICM.

Overall, the possibility of differentiating between "more arrhythmogenic" and "less arrhythmogenic" scars is very attractive; the best method to achieve this goal in NICM is yet unknown.

LV strain can be evaluated by feature tracking CMR. LV global longitudinal strain (LV-GLS) has a high correlation with LVEF[55] and lacks a direct pathophysiological link with the substrate of ventricular arrhythmias. In our cohort of 609 NICM patients GLS lost its association with the arrhythmic endpoint after adjustment for LVEF.[55] The authors believe that LV strain could be, at best, a "second-line" marker as compared with other variables directly related to LV fibrosis.

INTERACTION BETWEEN LATE GADOLINIUM ENHANCEMENT AND GENOTYPE

Among pathogenic genetic variants, a high arrhythmic risk has been associated to those localized in certain genes such as desmosomal genes, FLNC, LMNA, RBM20, and PLN.[62] A multicenter cohort including 600 NICM patients with CMR and genetic test observed that LGE was a much stronger and more significant predictor of VA/SCD than a positive genetic test; genotype+/LGE− patients had a cumulative incidence of 7%, closer to that of genotype-/LGE− patients than to that of any LGE + subgroup.[19] Small reports suggest that LGE may retain its high negative predictive value also among carriers of genetic variants in LMNA or FLNC.[63,64] However, larger studies are needed to understand whether LGE is a key prerequisite for the development of VA/SCD also in the presence of high-risk genetic variants.

CURRENT EUROPEAN SOCIETY OF CARDIOLOGY GUIDELINES

The recently published ESC guidelines for VA recognize the importance of CMR for the diagnosis and the risk stratification of NICM (class IIa). For the first time, they establish a class IIa

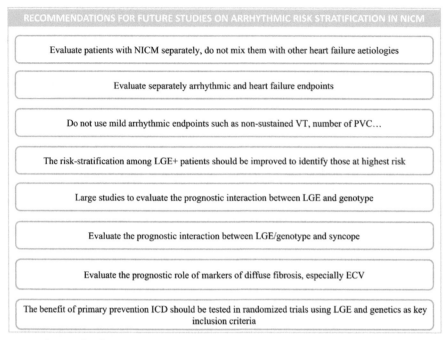

Fig. 2. Recommendations for future research in the field.

indication of primary prevention ICDs in NICM patients with LVEF greater than 35% and ≥ 2 of the following risk factors: LGE, pathogenic variants in FLNC, LMNA, PLN or RBM20, and SMVT inducibility using programmed ventricular stimulation and syncope.[65] Although recognizing that not all patients with LVEF greater than 35% are at low arrhythmic risk is an important change in paradigm, it should be acknowledged that these recommendations are highly pragmatical, the individual weight of each risk factor may be different and the prognostic value of the

combination of two or more of the aforementioned risk factors is largely unexplored. For example, patients with LVEF greater than 35%, LGE, and unexplained syncope may deserve an ICD, according to these guidelines, whereas it has been shown that a strategy of prolonged monitoring may be safe in this scenario.[66]

RECOMMENDATIONS FOR FUTURE STUDIES

Our recommendations for future studies are summarized in **Figs. 2** and **3**. Given the specificities of

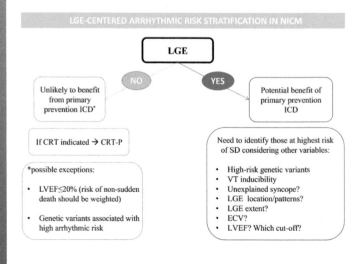

Fig. 3. Proposal of LGE-centred arrhythmic risk stratification. ECV, extracellular volume fraction; LGE, late gadolinium enhancement.

each cardiomyopathy, studies assessing the arrhythmic risk stratification should focus on NICM, excluding patients with ischemic heart disease in the same analysis. Many prior studies evaluated mixed populations, but the applicability of those results to NICM patients is very uncertain.

To improve arrhythmic risk stratification and identify ideal candidates for primary prevention ICDs, the arrhythmic endpoint should be evaluated separately from HF events, which are competing risk events limiting ICD benefit. Several studies evaluated a combined endpoint mixing arrhythmic and HF events, but in such cases, it is impossible to know the respective contribution of each predictor to each specific component of the combined endpoint.

LGE + patients have intermediate to high arrhythmic risk. This is probably the subgroup of patients where future studies should concentrate the most to try and identify those at highest risk. Further insights into the value of LGE extent, LGE location and pattern will be welcome. In addition, the prognostic interactions between LGE and genotype, the role of unexplained syncope and the incremental value of T1 mapping/ECV in LGE + cases should be investigated.

At present, there is much more evidence about the association between LGE and VA/SCD than it has ever been available for LVEF. Genetics are also increasingly recognized as fundamental contributors to arrhythmic risk stratification. Thus, the authors believe that it is time to launch clinical trials of primary prevention ICDs using LGE and genetics as main inclusion criteria.

SUMMARY

Several studies, including large multicentric cohorts for a total of greater than 9000 patients, confirm that the simple distinction between LGE presence and absence is a significant and strong predictor of the arrhythmic risk in NICM with very high negative predictive value. Moreover, the association between LGE and VA/SCD seems to be rather specific and has clear pathophysiological basis. As no other predictor is backed by a similar amount of evidence, it seems reasonable to put LGE in the center of current risk stratification for VA and SCD in NICM (**Fig. 3**).

Future studies should clarify the current matters of uncertainty (eg, the role of LGE extent, location, and pattern) and should evaluate the interactions between LGE and genetics, the role of unexplained syncope according to LGE status, and genotype as well as the potential incremental prognostic value of markers of diffuse fibrosis, especially ECV.

CLINICS CARE POINTS

- Given the amount of evidence supporting the strong, independent, and somehow specific association between late gadolinium enhancement (LGE) and ventricular arrhythmias or sudden cardiac death, it seems reasonable to have LGE in the center of current arrhythmic risk stratification in nonischemic cardiomyopathy.

- The high negative predictive value of LGE absence clearly questions the potential benefit of preventive implantable cardioverter defibrillator (ICD) in LGE− patients.

- LGE + patients have considerable arrhythmic risk but not all of them may deserve an ICD; LGE characteristics and the interaction with other risk factors may help identifying those at highest risk.

- Future studies should clarify which LGE features are associated with maximum risk and should further explore the interaction between LGE and other risk factors with special attention to genetics.

REFERENCES

1. Kadish A, Dyer A, Daubert JP, et al. Prophylactic defibrillator implantation in patients with nonischemic dilated cardiomyopathy. N Engl J Med 2004; 350:2151–8.

2. Bardy GH, Lee KL, Mark DB, et al. Amiodarone or an implantable cardioverter–defibrillator for Congestive heart failure. N Engl J Med 2005;352:225–37.

3. Kober L, Thune JJ, Nielsen JC, et al. Defibrillator implantation in patients with nonischemic systolic heart failure. N Engl J Med 2016;375:1221–30.

4. Goldberger JJ, Subacius H, Patel T, et al. Sudden cardiac death risk stratification in patients with non-ischemic dilated cardiomyopathy. J Am Coll Cardiol 2014;63:1879–89.

5. Elliott P, Andersson B, Arbustini E, et al. Classification of the cardiomyopathies: a position statement from the ESC working group on myocardial and pericardial diseases. Eur Heart J 2008;29:270–6.

6. Pinto YM, Elliot PM, Arbustini E, et al. Proposal for a revised definition of dilated cardiomyopathy, hypokinetic non-dilated cardiomyopathy, and its implications for clinical practice: a position statement of the ESC working group on myocardial and pericardial diseases. Eur Heart J 2016;37:1850–8.

7. Klem I, Klein M, Khan M, et al. Relationship of LVEF and myocardial scar to long-term mortality risk and mode of death in patients with nonischemic cardiomyopathy. Circulation 2021;143:1343–58.

8. Bozkurt B, Colvin M, Cook J, et al. Current Diagnostic and Treatment strategies for specific dilated cardiomyopathies. Circulation 2016;134:e579–646.

9. Codd MB, Sugrue DD, Gersh BJ, et al. Epidemiology of idiopathic dilated and hypertrophic cardiomyopathy: a population-based study in Olmsted County, Minnesota, 1975–1984. Circulation 1989; 80:564–72.

10. Hershberger RE, Hedges DJ, Morales A. Dilated cardiomyopathy: the complexity of a diverse genetic architecture. Nat Rev Cardiol 2013;10:531–47.

11. Moliner P, Lupon J, De Antonio M, et al. Trends in modes of death in heart failure over the last two decades: less sudden death but cancer deaths on the rise. Eur J Heart Fail 2019;21:1259–66.

12. Yafasova A, Butt JH, Elming MB, et al. Long-term follow-up of Danish. Circulation 2022;145:427–36.

13. Dec GW, Fuster V. Idiopathic dilated cardiomyopathy. N Engl J Med 1994;331:1564–75.

14. De Maria R, Gavazzi A, Caroli A, et al. Ventricular arrhythmias in dilated cardiomyopathy as an independent prognostic hallmark. Am J Cardiol 1992;69:1451–7.

15. Hofmann T, Meinertz T, Kasper W, et al. Mode of death in idiopathic dilated cardiomyopathy: a multivariate analysis of prognostic determinants. Am Heart J 1988;116:1455–63.

16. Romeo F, Pelliccia F, Cianfrocca C, et al. Predictors of sudden death in idiopathic dilated cardiomyopathy. Am J Cardiol 1989;63:138–40.

17. Gradman A, Deedwania P, Cody R, et al. Predictors of total mortality and sudden death in mild to moderate heart failure. J Am Coll Cardiol 1989;14:564–70.

18. Guaricci AI, Masci PG, Muscogiuri G, et al. CarDiac magnEtic resonance for prophylactic implantable-cardioVerter defibrillAtor ThErapy in non-ischaemic dilated CardioMyopathy: an international registry. Europace 2021;23:1072–83.

19. Mirelis JG, Escobar-Lopez L, Ochoa JP, et al. Combination of late gadolinium enhancement and genotype improves prediction of prognosis in non-ischaemic dilated cardiomyopathy. Eur J Heart Fail 2022;24:1183–96.

20. Alba AC, Gaztañaga J, Foroutan F, et al. Prognostic value of late gadolinium enhancement for the prediction of cardiovascular outcomes in dilated cardiomyopathy. Circ Cardiovasc Imaging 2020;13:e010105.

21. Di Marco A, Brown PF, Bradley J, et al. Improved risk stratification for ventricular arrhythmias and sudden death in patients with nonischemic dilated cardiomyopathy. J Am Coll Cardiol 2021;77:2890–905.

22. de Bakker JM, van Capelle FJ, Janse MJ, et al. Reentry as a cause of ventricular tachycardia in patients with chronic ischemic heart disease: electrophysiologic and anatomic correlation. Circulation 1988;77:589–606.

23. Aliot EM, Stevenson WG, Almendral-Garrote JM, et al. EHRA/HRS Expert Consensus on Catheter ablation of ventricular arrhythmias. Europace 2009;11:771–817.

24. Oloriz T, Silberbauer J, Maccabelli G, et al. Catheter ablation of ventricular arrhythmia in nonischemic cardiomyopathy: anteroseptal versus inferolateral scar sub-types. Circ Arrhythm Electrophysiol 2014;7:414–23.

25. Park J, Desjardins B, Liang JJ, et al. Association of scar distribution with epicardial electrograms and surface ventricular tachycardia QRS duration in nonischemic cardiomyopathy. J Cardiovasc Electrophysiol 2020;31:2032–40.

26. Daoud EG. Bundle branch reentry. In: Zipes D, Jalife J, editors. Cardiac electrophysiology: from cell to bedside. ed 4. Philadelphia: WB Saunders; 2004. p. 683–8.

27. Haissaguerre M, Vigmond E, Stuyvers B, et al. Ventricular arrhythmias and the His-Purkinje system. Nat Rev Cardiol 2016;13:155–66.

28. Gianni C, Burkhardt JD, Trivedi C, et al. The role of the Purkinje network in premature ventricular complex-triggered ventricular fibrillation. J Interv Card Electrophysiol 2018;52:375–83.

29. Haïssaguerre M, Hocini M, Cheniti G, et al. Localized structural Alterations underlying a subset of unexplained sudden cardiac death. Circ Arrhythm Electrophysiol 2018;11:e006120.

30. Alvarez CK, Cronin E, Baker WL, et al. Heart failure as a substrate and trigger for ventricular tachycardia. J Interv Card Electrophysiol 2019;56:229–47.

31. Kim RJ, Fieno DS, Parrish TB, et al. Relationship of MRI delayed contrast enhancement to irreversible injury, infarct age, and contractile function. Circulation 1999;100:1992–2002.

32. Iles LM, Ellims AH, Llewellyn H, et al. Histological validation of cardiac magnetic resonance analysis of regional and diffuse interstitial myocardial fibrosis. Eur Heart J Cardiovasc Imaging 2015;16:14–22.

33. Di Marco A, Anguera I, Schmitt M, et al. Late gadolinium enhancement and the risk for ventricular arrhythmias or sudden death in dilated cardiomyopathy: systematic review and meta-analysis. JACC Heart Fail 2017;5:28–38.

34. Halliday BP, Gulati A, Ali A, et al. Association between midwall late gadolinium enhancement and sudden cardiac death in patients with dilated cardiomyopathy and mild and moderate left ventricular systolic dysfunction. Circulation 2017;135:2106–15.

35. Kuruvilla S, Adenaw N, Katwal AB, et al. Late gadolinium enhancement on cardiac magnetic resonance predicts adverse cardiovascular outcomes in nonischemic cardiomyopathy: a systematic review and meta-analysis. Circ Cardiovasc Imaging 2014;7:250–8.

36. Elming MB, Hammer-Hansen S, Voges I, et al. Myocardial fibrosis and the effect of primary

prophylactic defibrillator implantation in patients with non-ischemic systolic heart failure-Danish-MRI. Am Heart J 2020;221:165–76.

37. Gutman SJ, Costello BT, Papapostolou S, et al. Reduction in mortality from implantable cardioverter-defibrillators in non-ischaemic cardiomyopathy patients is dependent on the presence of left ventricular scar. Eur Heart J 2019;40:542–50.

38. Bristow MR, Saxon LA, Boehmer J, et al. Cardiac-resynchronization therapy with or without an implantable defibrillator in advanced chronic heart failure. N Engl J Med 2004;350:2140–50.

39. Leyva F, Zegard A, Acquaye E, et al. Outcomes of cardiac resynchronization therapy with or without defibrillation in patients with nonischemic cardiomyopathy. J Am Coll Cardiol 2017;70:1216–27.

40. Leyva F, Taylor RJ, Foley PW, et al. Left ventricular midwall fibrosis as a predictor of mortality and morbidity after cardiac resynchronization therapy in patients with nonischemic cardiomyopathy. J Am Coll Cardiol 2012;60:1659–67.

41. Linhart M, Doltra A, Acosta J, et al. Ventricular arrhythmia risk is associated with myocardial scar but not with response to cardiac resynchronization therapy. Europace 2020;22:1391–400.

42. Schulz-Menger J, Bluemke DA, Bremerich J, et al. Standardized image interpretation and post-processing in cardiovascular magnetic resonance - 2020 update. J Cardiovasc Magn Reson 2020;22:19.

43. Halliday BP, Baksi AJ, Gulati A, et al. Outcome in dilated cardiomyopathy related to the extent, location, and pattern of late gadolinium enhancement. JACC Cardiovasc Imaging 2019;12:1645–55.

44. Augusto JB, Eiros R, Nakou E, et al. Dilated cardiomyopathy and arrhythmogenic left ventricular cardiomyopathy: a comprehensive genotype-imaging phenotype study. Eur Heart J Cardiovasc Imaging 2020;21:326–36.

45. Hasselberg NE, Haland TF, Saberniak J, et al. Lamin A/C cardiomyopathy: young onset, high penetrance, and frequent need for heart transplantation. Eur Heart J 2018;39:853–60.

46. Di Marco A, Ruiz-Cueto M, Salazar-Mendiguchía J, et al. Genotype-phenotype correlation of LMNA variants involving the Arg541 residue: a case report with multimodality imaging and literature review. ESC Heart Fail 2020;7:3169–73.

47. Bradlow WM, Assomull R, Kilner PJ, et al. Understanding late gadolinium enhancement in pulmonary hypertension. Circ Cardiovasc Imaging 2010;3:501–3.

48. Yi JE, Park J, Lee HJ, et al. Prognostic implications of late gadolinium enhancement at the right ventricular insertion point in patients with non-ischemic dilated cardiomyopathy. PLoS One 2018;13:e0208100.

49. Claver E, Di Marco A, Brown PF, et al. Prognostic impact of late gadolinium enhancement at the right ventricular insertion points in non-ischaemic dilated cardiomyopathy. Eur Heart J Cardiovasc Imaging 2022. https://doi.org/10.1093/ehjci/jeac109.

50. Piers SR, Everaerts K, van der Geest RJ, et al. Myocardial scar predicts monomorphic ventricular tachycardia but not polymorphic ventricular tachycardia or ventricular fibrillation in nonischemic dilated cardiomyopathy. Heart Rhythm 2015;12:2106–14.

51. Miller CA, Naish JH, Bishop P, et al. Comprehensive validation of cardiovascular magnetic resonance techniques for the assessment of myocardial extracellular volume. Circ Cardiovasc Imaging 2013;6:373–83.

52. Pogwizd SM, McKenzie JP, Cain ME. Mechanisms underlying spontaneous and induced ventricular arrhythmias in patients with idiopathic dilated cardiomyopathy. Circulation 1998;98:2404–14.

53. Muser D, Nucifora G, Castro SA, et al. Myocardial substrate characterization by CMR T1 mapping in patients with NICM and No LGE undergoing Catheter ablation of VT. JACC Clin Electrophysiol 2021;7:831–40.

54. Claridge S, Mennuni S, Jackson T, et al. Substrate-dependent risk stratification for implantable cardioverter defibrillator therapies using cardiac magnetic resonance imaging: the importance of T1 mapping in nonischemic patients. J Cardiovasc Electrophysiol 2017;28:785–95.

55. Di Marco A, Brown PF, Bradley J, et al. Extracellular volume fraction improves risk-stratification for ventricular arrhythmias and sudden death in nonischaemic cardiomyopathy. Eur Heart J Cardiovasc Imaging 2022. https://doi.org/10.1093/ehjci/jeac142.

56. Li S, Zhou D, Sirajuddin A, et al. T1 mapping and extracellular volume fraction in dilated cardiomyopathy: a prognosis study. JACC Cardiovasc Imaging 2022;15:578–90.

57. Nakamori S, Ngo LH, Rodriguez J, et al. T$_1$Mapping tissue heterogeneity provides improved risk stratification for ICDs without needing gadolinium in patients with dilated cardiomyopathy. JACC Cardiovasc Imaging 2020;13:1917–30.

58. Androulakis AFA, Zeppenfeld K, Paiman EHM, et al. Entropy as a novel measure of myocardial tissue heterogeneity for prediction of ventricular arrhythmias and mortality in post-infarct patients. JACC Clin Electrophysiol 2019;5:480–9.

59. Gould J, Porter B, Claridge S, et al. Mean entropy predicts implantable cardioverter-defibrillator therapy using cardiac magnetic resonance texture analysis of scar heterogeneity. Heart Rhythm 2019;16:1242–50.

60. Balaban G, Halliday BP, Porter B, et al. Late-gadolinium enhancement interface area and Electrophysiological simulations predict arrhythmic events in patients with nonischemic dilated cardiomyopathy. JACC Clin Electrophysiol 2021;7:238–49.

61. Jáuregui B, Soto-Iglesias D, Penela D, et al. Cardiovascular magnetic resonance determinants of ventricular arrhythmic events after myocardial infarction. Europace 2022;24:938–47.

62. Escobar-lopez L, Ochoa JP, Mirelis JG, et al. Association of genetic variants with outcomes in patients with nonischemic dilated cardiomyopathy. J Am Coll Cardiol 2021;78:1682–99.

63. Peretto G, Barison A, Forleo C, et al. Late gadolinium enhancement role in arrhythmic risk stratification of patients with LMNA cardiomyopathy: results from a long-term follow-up multicentre study. Europace 2020;22:1864–72.

64. Celeghin R, Cipriani A, Bariani R, et al. Filamin-C variant-associated cardiomyopathy: a pooled analysis of individual patient data to evaluate the clinical profile and risk of sudden cardiac death. Heart Rhythm 2022;19:235–43.

65. Zeppenfeld K, Tfelt-Hansen J, de Riva M, et al. 2022 ESC Guidelines for the management of patients with ventricular arrhythmias and the prevention of sudden cardiac death. Eur Heart J 2022;43:3997–4126.

66. Francisco-Pascual J, Rodenas-Alesina E, Rivas-Gándara N. Etiology and prognosis of patients with unexplained syncope and mid-range left ventricular dysfunction. Heart Rhythm 2021;18:597–604.

Genetic Risk Stratification in Arrhythmogenic Left Ventricular Cardiomyopathy

Yaanik B. Desai, MD*, Victoria N. Parikh, MD**

KEYWORDS

- Arrhythmia • Sudden cardiac death • Cardiomyopathy • Risk prediction • Genetics
- Precision medicine

KEY POINTS

- Variants in multiple genes are associated with an ALVC phenotype.
- In this population, an LVEF <35% is often an insensitive risk factor for malignant ventricular arrhythmias.

INTRODUCTION

Arrhythmogenic right ventricular cardiomyopathy (ARVC) was initially described as a disease characterized by right ventricular (RV) dysfunction, ventricular arrhythmia, and high risk of sudden cardiac death (SCD) in young patients.[1,2] In early diagnostic criteria—which incorporated family history, imaging, electrocardiographic patterns, arrhythmia history, and histopathology—an expert task force specifically cited the absence of left ventricular (LV) dysfunction in major criteria.[3]

However, subsequent studies showed that LV involvement is common in patients with ARVC. In a cohort of 200 patients meeting task force criteria, 84% had some degree of LV involvement (either enlargement, dysfunction, or scar) by cardiac MRI (cMRI), and 40% had LV abnormalities in the absence of RV dysfunction.[4] In 2010, the ARVC task force modified diagnostic criteria to broaden the sensitivity of diagnosis and removed the previous requirement for the absence of LV involvement.[5]

Sen-Chowdhry and colleagues proposed a distinction between "classic" ARVC with predominantly RV dysfunction and a left-dominant phenotype, which in this review, the authors refer to as arrhythmogenic LV cardiomyopathy (ALVC).[6] The investigators suggested that patients with ALVC differ from those with dilated cardiomyopathy (DCM) in that arrhythmia is an early feature, followed by the development of structural abnormalities in advanced disease—which contrasts with DCM that initially presents with structural LV disease with the development of arrhythmia later in the disease process in some patients.

In recent years, the broader term, "arrhythmogenic cardiomyopathy" (ACM) has been increasingly used as it encompasses the complete spectrum of RV and LV involvement. ARVC and ALVC thus reflect phenotypes of ACM, distinguished by the degree and time of onset of RV versus LV involvement.

In 2019, the Heart Rhythm Society (HRS) released a consensus statement that expanded the use of the term ACM to any patient with predominant atrial or ventricular arrhythmia in the absence of structural heart disease due to ischemia, hypertension, or valvular dysfunction.[7] However, the most common use of the term ACM refers to cardiomyopathies mostly of genetic etiology predisposing to ventricular arrhythmia.

Importantly, with this considerable overlap in phenotype, diseases falling under the ACM umbrella

Department of Medicine, Division of Cardiovascular Medicine, Stanford University School of Medicine, Falk CRVC, 300 Pasteur Drive, Stanford, CA 94305, USA
* Corresponding author.
** Corresponding author.
E-mail addresses: yaanik@stanford.edu (Y.B.D.); vparikh@stanford.edu (V.N.P.)

Card Electrophysiol Clin 15 (2023) 391–399
https://doi.org/10.1016/j.ccep.2023.04.005
1877-9182/23/© 2023 Elsevier Inc. All rights reserved.

are in need of more precise definitions to enable appropriate risk stratification and therapy. Genetic diagnosis, though elusive in a large portion of ACM patients, can provide highly specific insights into the mechanism of disease, risk factors for SCD, and progression to heart failure. Here, the authors review the literature on genes in which disease-causing variants have been associated with ALVC with a focus on studies that describe the risk of ventricular arrhythmia and SCD.

DESMOPLAKIN

Desmoplakin (DSP) is a constituent protein of the desmosome—a protein complex which facilitates intercellular adhesion via the intermediate filament network (**Fig. 1**). The other genes that code for constituents of the desmosome cause ARVC. The carboxy-terminus of DSP faces the intracellular side and binds to the intermediate filaments, whereas the amino-terminus binds to other proteins in the desmosome that interact with transmembrane proteins that face the intercellular

space.[8] Variants in DSP were initially observed in cardiocutaneous syndromes[9] and then in ARVC.[10]

In 2005, Norman and colleagues identified a frameshift variant in a family of patients with predominantly LV dysplasia and arrhythmia,[11] without cutaneous manifestation. The variant that they describe truncates the protein near the N-terminus, such that the rod and carboxy-terminus "tail" are lost. The investigators hypothesized that disruption of the intracellular-facing end may explain the LV predominance, as integrity of the intracellular cytoskeletal elements is important for LV function under high-pressure load.

Subsequent studies identified additional truncating variants in DSP in families with predominantly left-sided cardiomyopathy and high incidence of ventricular arrhythmia.[12] In a cohort of 27 probands with a diagnosis of ARVC—of whom 9 had a missense variant and 13 had a non-missense variant, there was more left-sided dysfunction in the patients with a non-missense variant.[13] There was no difference in the prevalence of major arrhythmia between patients with missense and

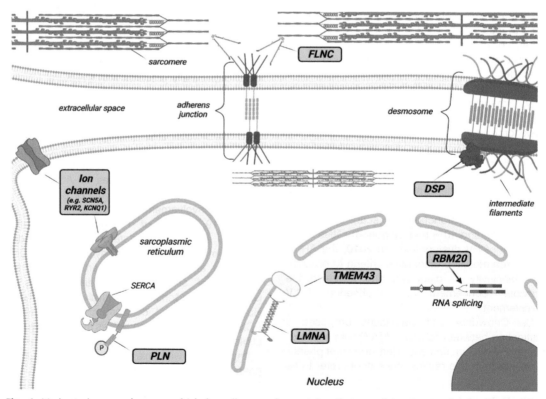

Fig. 1. Variants in several genes which broadly encode proteins that regulate structural integrity and ion handling are associated with arrhythmogenic left ventricular cardiomyopathy. The figure shows a model of two neighboring myocytes and highlights putative function of the proteins reviewed in this article. DSP, desmoplakin; FNLC, filamin C; KCNQ1, potassium voltage-gated channel subfamily Q member 1; LMNA, lamin A/C; PLN, phospholamban; RBM20, RNA-binding motif protein 20; RYR2, ryanodine receptor 2; SCN5A, sodium channel protein type 5 subunit alpha; SERCA, sarco-endoplasmic reticulum calcium ATPase; TMEM43, transmembrane protein 43. (Created with BioRender.com.)

non-missense variants, though the study may have been underpowered to detect a difference.

Smith and colleagues published a study which compared 81 patients with pathogenic variants in plakophilin-2 (PKP2) — a desmosomal gene which is the most frequently implicated in families with ARVC[14] — with 107 patients with pathogenic or likely pathogenic DSP variants.[15] There were a number of important differences between patients with PKP2 variants and those with DSP variants in this study. All of the patients with ALVC had DSP variants, and patients with DSP variants were more likely to have fibrosis denoted by late gadolinium enhancement (LGE) in the LV on cMRI. However, LGE was not predictive of the risk of ventricular arrhythmia in this study, though cMRI data were only available for approximately half of the patients with DSP variants, and the study may have been underpowered to detect a difference in outcome. Patients with DSP variants had more penetrant disease compared with patients with PKP2 variants. Rates of malignant arrhythmia were similar between both groups (28% and 30%). LV ejection fraction (LVEF) less than 55% was strongly associated with the incidence of malignant arrhythmia in patients with DSP variants, and using a cutoff of 35% would have missed over half of the patients with life-threatening arrhythmia. LV dysfunction was more predictive of malignant arrhythmia in patients with DSP variants, whereas RV dysfunction was more predictive of malignant arrhythmia in patients with PKP2 variants.

These results support the notion that DSP is most strongly associated with an ALVC phenotype and that in these patients any reduction in LVEF — not just severe reduction — predicts an increased risk of ventricular arrhythmia, which highlights the importance of genetic diagnosis in refining risk prediction.

LAMIN A/C

The lamins are a class of intermediate filament proteins which provide structural integrity to the nuclear envelope and transduce intracellular mechanical forces to the nucleus, where the signal can then serve as an input for alteration in gene expression (see **Fig. 1**).[16] Variants in lamin A/C (two splice variants of the lamin gene) have been described in skeletal diseases with cardiac manifestations (eg, Emery-Dreifuss muscular dystrophy) and in ACM[17] characterized by atrial arrhythmia, conduction disease, and ventricular arrhythmia with an increased risk of SCD.[18,19]

Van Rijsingen and colleagues studied a cohort of 269 patients with lamin (LMNA) variants from 109 families in Europe over a median follow-up of nearly 4 years.[20] Nearly 18% of the population experienced a malignant ventricular arrhythmia, which was defined as requiring cardiopulmonary resuscitation, resulting in SCD or resulting in an appropriate implantable cardioverter-defibrillator (ICD) therapy. There were four independent predictors of malignant arrhythmia: previous nonsustained ventricular tachycardia (NSVT), LVEF less than 45%, male sex and non-missense variants, which was present in 45% of the cohort. Among 97 patients with ≤1 of these risk factors, none had malignant arrhythmia during follow-up. Male sex also seemed to be associated with worse outcomes in this study. Men were more likely to have LVEF less than 45% compared with women, but gender was still an independent risk factor for malignant ventricular arrhythmia in the multivariate analysis.[21] Despite the lower LVEF in men on average, there was not a significant difference in ICD implantation in men versus women, which suggests that the increase in malignant arrhythmia was not simply due to more detection. There was a higher proportion of male probands, though the investigators note that penetrance was similar in probands and relatives. Interestingly, a smaller portion of the men had non-missense variants compared with women. The results seem to suggest that lamin cardiomyopathy leads to more malignant arrhythmia in men, though the mechanism remains unexplained.

In a study from 2016, Kumar and colleagues investigated a cohort of 122 patients with LMNA variants.[22] Patients developed atrial arrhythmia and atrioventricular (AV) block at younger median ages, followed by LV dysfunction, ventricular arrhythmia, and heart failure. Over a median follow-up period of 7 years, over 50% developed ventricular arrhythmia (from 20% at baseline). As before, this study confirmed prior results that male sex, LV dysfunction, and non- missense variants are risk factors for ventricular arrhythmia. In this study, male sex and LVEF less than 50% both led to greater than threefold increase in risk of ventricular arrhythmia. Forty-two percent of the patients had non-missense LMNA variants, which was also a risk factor for the development of ventricular arrhythmia. Of patients with sustained ventricular arrhythmia, 27% had normal LVEF, and the majority (56%) had LVEF greater than 35%. Among patients who had an ICD, half experienced an appropriate device therapy during the follow-up.

As patients with lamin A/C variants often initially present with conduction disease and atrial arrhythmias — many patients require pacemaker implantation. Some have argued that ICD implantation (rather than a pacemaker) when a pacemaker is required may be reasonable.[20] Indeed, in a small study of 41 patients with LMNA variants, Hasselberg and colleagues showed that a longer PR interval predicts ventricular arrhythmia, however, including NSVT in this definition.[23,24] Ultimately, ICD placement in a patient with an indication for a pacemaker—but in the absence of the risk factors listed above—should be an individualized patient–provider decision.

Wahbi and colleagues developed a risk prediction model for ventricular arrhythmia in 589 patients with LMNA cardiomyopathy (444 in the derivation sample and 145 in the validation sample).[25] Supporting prior findings, male sex, non-missense variants, first-degree and higher degree AV block, NSVT, and LVEF were independent predictors selected in the model. The model had an adequate performance (C-statistic of 0.776 in the derivation sample and calibration slope 0.827 and 0.800 and 1.082, respectively, in the validation sample) and is available online (https://lmna-risk-vta.fr/). A recent external validation effort of this model in a cohort of 118 patients confirmed its performance (C-statistic of 0.85) and the importance of serial reassessment in this progressive disease.[26] Of note, non-missense variants and male sex were not predictive of ventricular arrhythmia events in this cohort.

In a study from 2020, Peretto and colleagues screened a cohort of 164 patients with LMNA cardiomyopathy for cMRI data. Of the 41 patients with an available cMRI, 8 patients developed malignant arrhythmia over the study period, all of whom had LGE localized to the ventricular septum.[27] An additional 29 patients had LGE—13 localizing to the septum—but did not develop malignant ventricular arrhythmia. Although the study was small, this suggests that the absence of LGE may be reassuring against the risk of malignant arrhythmia and that septal LGE in particular may be associated with increased risk. Septal LGE was also associated with AV block in this study. Fibrosis within the AV node on autopsy of patients with LMNA cardiomyopathy[28] has previously been described and is likely a histopathologic correlate of septal LGE. Septal LGE may therefore be a marker of fibrosis leading to conduction disease in patients with LMNA cardiomyopathy and a nidus for reentry leading to ventricular arrhythmia.

FILAMIN C

Filamin C (FLNC) is an intracellular protein which crosslinks actin to the fascia adherens—a complex of proteins which anchors neighboring cells (see **Fig. 1**).[29] Variants in this gene have been identified in a class of skeletal myopathies called myofibrillar myopathy.[30] In a study published in 2016, Ortiz-Genga and colleagues identified truncating FLNC variants in 28 unrelated probands with cardiomyopathy in the absence of skeletal disease.[31] After screening family members of the probands, they identified an additional 54 carriers. Among all carriers, ventricular arrhythmia (which included NSVT) was common, affecting 82% of patients. Forty-six percent had LV dilation, and 67% had evidence of LV systolic dysfunction. Among carriers with cMRI or histopathologic data, 59% had LV fibrosis, whereas only 4% had RV fibrosis. This suggested that truncating variants in FLNC are associated with ACM with predominantly left-sided features.

In a study published in 2021, Gigli and colleagues investigated a cohort of 85 patients with truncating FLNC variants.[32] Forty-two percent of these patients were initially phenotyped as having DCM, 21% were phenotyped as having ALVC, and 3% with ARVC. On follow-up imaging, the group was heterogenous with respect to LV and RV dysfunction with predominantly left-sided dysfunction, however, with considerable overlap. During 5 years of follow-up, the incidence of SCD or major ventricular arrhythmia (defined as either sustained VT, appropriate ICD therapy, or resuscitated cardiac arrest) was 27%. Interestingly, LVEF was not a predictor of SCD and ventricular arrhythmia in this cohort (although it was a predictor of overall mortality), and most of the patients who experienced SCD or major ventricular arrhythmia had an LVEF greater than 50%.

Similarly, Akhtar and colleagues show that in a cohort of 167 European patients with truncating FLNC variants, there was no difference in incidence of malignant arrhythmia in patients with mildly-to-moderately reduced LVEF (36%–49%) and patients with severely reduced LVEF (LVEF ≤ 35%).[33]

These findings suggest that traditional guidelines, which rely on an LVEF cutoff of 35% for ICD placement, significantly underestimate risk in FLNC-associated ACM.

PHOSPHOLAMBAN

Phospholamban (PLN) is a transmembrane protein in the sarcoplasmic reticulum that modulates the sarco–endoplasmic reticulum calcium ATPase 2 (SERCA2) pump (see **Fig. 1**). PLN plays a critical role in regulating intracellular calcium and thus cardiac contraction.[34] Further, it is a key mediator of beta-adrenergic inputs on calcium handling in the cardiomyocyte. Several variants in PLN have been identified in patients with cardiomyopathy, including an arginine deletion (p.Arg14del), a

Dutch founder variant which renders "super-inhibitory" function to the PLN protein, thereby disrupting the cardiac myocytes' ability to recycle cytosolic calcium.[35]

Van der Zwaag and colleagues showed that p.Arg14del variants were equally prevalent in a cohort of 354 unrelated Dutch patients phenotyped as either DCM or ARVC.[36] Patients with DCM who carried p.Arg14del were more likely to require appropriate ICD therapy and more were more likely to have a family history of SCD than non-carriers with DCM. This study was important because it supported the notion of ACM with gene-specific phenotypic correlates.

Between 10% and 15% of patients in the Netherlands with a diagnosis of DCM carry p.Arg14del.[37] In a study of 403 Dutch carriers of this variant with mean age 44, 19% had a new malignant arrhythmia (aborted SCD, SCD, or most commonly, appropriate ICD therapy) over the median follow-up time of 3.5 years LVEF less than 45%, and the presence of prior VT (either sustained or non-sustained) was the two significant predictors of malignant arrhythmia in the multivariate model. Patients with LVEF less than 45% were four times more likely to develop malignant arrhythmia than those with LVEF $\geq$ 45%.

Again, this suggested that traditional guidelines for cardiomyopathy, which use a cutoff of 35% for ICD indication, would underestimate risk of malignant arrhythmia in patients with PLN cardiomyopathy with p.Arg14del. Indeed, when applying an LVEF cutoff of 45% rather than 35% to the cohort, sensitivity in detecting malignant arrhythmia went up to 90% from 44% (at the cost of a decrease in specificity from 87% to 65%).

More recently, Verstraelen and colleagues sought to develop a gene-specific model for the prediction of incident malignant arrhythmia.[38] The investigators studied a cohort of 679 Dutch and Spanish carriers of the p.Arg14del variant over a median of 4.3 years of follow-up. The annual rate of malignant arrhythmias was 2%, which is lower than in prior studies and potentially explained by the exclusion of patients with prior malignant arrhythmia and only 17% of probands, the remainder having been identified via cascade screening. In the multivariate model, lower LVEF, low ECG voltage, and increased daily premature ventricular contraction count were significant predictors of malignant arrhythmia. Compared with the previous model (which only considered LVEF < 45% and the presence of sustained or non-sustained ventricular arrhythmia), inclusion of these variables improved the prediction of malignant arrhythmia with a relatively low false-negative rate when using a threshold of greater than 5% 5-year event risk to justify ICD placement. The presence of LGE on cMRI was not used in the model due to insufficient data and may provide additional prognostication of risk in future studies of patients with PLN variants.

RNA-BINDING MOTIF PROTEIN 20

Whereas the genes described above are generally involved in the structural integrity or contractile regulation of the myocyte, variants in RNA-binding motif protein 20 (RBM 20)—which is a regulator of pre-RNA splicing—have been identified as a cause of highly penetrant cardiomyopathy with a particularly aggressive arrhythmogenic course.[39,40] In vivo studies have suggested the mechanism of disease may be related to alterations in splicing of titin,[41] which is known to cause DCM, as well as of genes involved in intracellular calcium handling, which may explain the higher propensity for ventricular arrhythmia when compared with patients with titin variants alone.[42] Parikh and colleagues reported a registry of 74 patients with RBM20 variants.[43] Compared with patients with titin variants, these patients were much more likely to have an evidence of sustained ventricular arrhythmia and a family history of sudden cardiac arrest. Of the 22 patients with cMRI data, 50% had an evidence of LGE. There were no significant differences in rates of sustained ventricular arrhythmia or family history of sudden cardiac arrest when compared with a cohort of patients with lamin A/C cardiomyopathy. The investigators report that one-third of the patients with sustained ventricular arrhythmia had LVEF greater than 45%.

Hey and colleagues studied a cohort of 80 Danish patients with pathogenic RBM20 variants and reported that men developed LV dysfunction and ventricular arrhythmia at a younger age than women.[44] Nearly a third of patients developed malignant ventricular arrhythmia, and LV dysfunction was not significantly associated with risk of development.

These studies suggest that variants in RBM20 cause an aggressive LV ACM and that LV systolic function alone may be an insensitive predictor of malignant arrhythmia when traditional cutoffs are used. Future work is expected to define the longitudinal risk of life-threatening ventricular arrhythmias and atrial arrhythmias in the population with pathogenic RBM20 variants.

TRANSMEMBRANE PROTEIN 43

A highly penetrant and aggressive form of ARVC was identified in a family in Newfoundland, Canada in the 1980s, with a high incidence of SCD.[45] Linkage analysis revealed that the variant was on a region of chromosome 3 dubbed the "ARVD5" locus. On histology, TMEM43 localizes to the nuclear envelope in some tissues[46] and has been shown to interact with lamins,[47] though the protein function and mechanism of disease remain unknown. Other affected families with a common genetic ancestor by haplotype analysis were subsequently identified and found to have a decreased risk of death with prophylactic ICD placement when compared with historic age-matched controls.[48] Merner and colleagues identified a missense variant in the gene within the locus encoding transmembrane protein 43 (TMEM43), and they noted that LV enlargement was more common in affected individuals compared with other forms of ARVC.[49]

Dominguez and colleagues identified the same missense variant in 62 individuals from three Spanish families who were unrelated to the previously identified families by haplotype analysis.[50] Compared with unaffected family members (ie, who did not carry the TMEM43 variant), LVEF was significantly lower. Carriers were far more likely to have SCD with 24/62 (39%) of carriers affected. Male sex was a significant risk factor for SCD. This supported the notion that TMEM43 is associated with ALVC with a high incidence of SCD.

CHANNELOPATHIES

Channelopathies are a group of cardiac disorders that result from dysfunction of cardiac ion channels, which leads to increased risk of malignant ventricular arrhythmia. Whereas variants in ion channels were traditionally thought to lead to strictly arrhythmogenic phenotypes (ie, to occur in the absence of structural dysfunction), multiple variants in these genes have now been associated with broader phenotypes, including ventricular dilation and dysfunction. As an example, variants in the cardiac sodium channel protein type 5 subunit alpha (SCN5A) have been associated with multiple primary arrhythmia syndromes, including congenital long QT syndrome and Brugada syndrome.[51,52] However, variants in SCN5A have also been described in familial disease with a syndrome of atrial fibrillation and ventricular arrhythmia in the setting of ventricular dilation and dysfunction.[53–56] In addition to transmitting sodium current, SCN5A may also interact with cell-adhesion proteins, which is one possible mechanism for the observation of structural disease in patients harboring these variants.[57]

Similarly, variants in the potassium voltage-gated channel subfamily Q member 1—which is associated with congenital long QT syndrome type I—have been reported in individuals with left-sided structural heart disease and ventricular arrhythmia.[58,59] In addition, variants in the ryanodine receptor 2 (RYR2) calcium channel, which has been traditionally associated with familial catecholaminergic polymorphic tachycardia, have also been described in families with ventricular arrhythmia in the setting of right and/or LV dysfunction,[60,61] and molecular studies in vivo have suggested that RYR2 dysfunction leads to structural remodeling.[62,63]

These reports suggest that variants in cardiac ion channels have broader phenotypes which can include structural disease. More prospective data and genotypic-phenotypic correlation are needed to better characterize these patients and refine risk prediction.

SUMMARY AND FUTURE DIRECTIONS

We have presented an overview of the risk of malignant arrhythmia in gene-specific diagnoses of ALVC. A recurring theme is that severe LV systolic dysfunction is not a sensitive predictor of development of life-threatening arrhythmia in ALVC. For patients presenting with arrhythmia in the setting of relatively mild systolic dysfunction or patients with structural cardiac disease associated with non-severe LV dysfunction, genetic diagnosis can guide decisions around primary prevention ICD use. Furthermore, for family members in the presence of genetic diagnosis, understanding their risk based on their genotype as well as imaging and electrical phenotyping may prevent SCD.[63,64] In the current American Heart Association/American College of Cardiology/HRS guidelines on SCD prevention, the presence of non-missense variants in lamin A/C is the only gene-specific risk factor, which warrants ICD placement at higher LVEF.[64] The more recently published 2019 HRS Expert Consensus Statement on ACM also identifies variants in PLN and FLNC as risk factors warranting higher LVEF thresholds for ICD use,[7] and the 2022 European Society of Cardiology guidelines additionally identifies RBM20 variants.[65] As we have shown, variants in DSP and TMEM43 are also associated with a high risk of SCD beyond the LVEF; however, this has not been specifically recognized in guidelines yet.

Future studies that incorporate both genotype and cardiac MRI data such as LGE will be essential to further refine risk prediction in ALVC.[66] In a recent study of over 1000 patients with nonischemic cardiomyopathy (NICM) and cMRI, incorporation of LGE significantly improved risk prediction compared with the standard model of LVEF alone, but 90% of these patients did not have genetic testing.[67] Further data suggest that machine learning-enabled disease classification can identify patients at risk of specific outcomes including heart failure, SCD, and metabolic phenotypes.[68] Ongoing efforts to unify diverse multinational cohorts for definitive studies of genotype–phenotype interaction will lead the way to patient-specific sudden death risk stratification incorporating genetics and clinical data in ALVC.

DISCLOSURE

Y.B. Desai has no disclosures. V.N. Parikh is a consultant for Nuevocor and Viz.ai serves on the Scientific Advisory Board for BioMarin, Inc. and Lexeo Therapeutics and receives research funding from BioMarin, Inc.

REFERENCES

1. Thiene G, Nava A, Corrado D, et al. Right ventricular cardiomyopathy and sudden death in young people. N Engl J Med 1988;318(3):129–33.
2. Marcus FI, Fontaine GH, Guiraudon G, et al. Right ventricular dysplasia: a report of 24 adult cases. Circulation 1982;65(2):384–98.
3. McKenna WJ, Thiene G, Nava A, et al. Diagnosis of arrhythmogenic right ventricular dysplasia/cardiomyopathy. Task force of the working group myocardial and pericardial disease of the European Society of Cardiology and of the Scientific Council on cardiomyopathies of the International Society and Federation of Cardiology. Br Heart J 1994;71(3):215.
4. Sen-Chowdhry S, Syrris P, Ward D, et al. Clinical and genetic characterization of families with arrhythmogenic right ventricular dysplasia/cardiomyopathy provides novel insights into patterns of disease expression. Circulation 2007;115(13):1710–20.
5. Marcus FI, McKenna WJ, Sherrill D, et al. Diagnosis of arrhythmogenic right ventricular cardiomyopathy/dysplasia: proposed modification of the task force criteria. Circulation 2010;121(13):1533–41.
6. Sen-Chowdhry S, Syrris P, Prasad SK, et al. Left-dominant arrhythmogenic cardiomyopathy: an under-recognized clinical entity. J Am Coll Cardiol 2008;52(25):2175–87.
7. Towbin JA, McKenna WJ, Abrams DJ, et al. 2019 HRS expert consensus statement on evaluation, risk stratification, and management of arrhythmogenic cardiomyopathy. Heart Rhythm 2019;16(11): e301–72.
8. Rampazzo A, Nava A, Malacrida S, et al. Report Mutation in Human Desmoplakin Domain Binding to Plakoglobin Causes a Dominant Form of Arrhythmogenic Right Ventricular Cardiomyopathy. Am J Hum Genet 2002;71(5):1200–6.
9. Norgett EE, Hatsell SJ, Carvajal-Huerta L, et al. Recessive Mutation in Desmoplakin Disrupts Desmoplakin-Intermediate Filament Interactions and Causes Dilated Cardiomyopathy, Woolly Hair and Keratoderma. Vol 9. 2000.
10. Sen-Chowdhry S, Syrris P, McKenna WJ. Role of genetic analysis in the management of patients with arrhythmogenic right ventricular dysplasia/cardiomyopathy. J Am Coll Cardiol 2007;50(19):1813–21.
11. Norman M, Simpson M, Mogensen J, et al. Novel mutation in desmoplakin causes arrhythmogenic left ventricular cardiomyopathy. Circulation 2005; 112(5):636–42.
12. López-Ayala JM, Gómez-Milanés I, Muñoz JJ, et al. Desmoplakin truncations and arrhythmogenic left ventricular cardiomyopathy: Characterizing a phenotype. Europace 2014;16(12):1838–46.
13. Castelletti S, Vischer AS, Syrris P, et al. Desmoplakin missense and non-missense mutations in arrhythmogenic right ventricular cardiomyopathy: genotype-phenotype correlation. Int J Cardiol 2017;249:268–73.
14. van Tintelen JP, Entius MM, Bhuiyan ZA, et al. Plakophilin-2 mutations are the major determinant of familial arrhythmogenic right ventricular dysplasia/cardiomyopathy. Circulation 2006;113(13):1650–8.
15. Smith ED, Lakdawala NK, Papoutsidakis N, et al. Desmoplakin cardiomyopathy, a Fibrotic and Inflammatory form of cardiomyopathy Distinct from Typical dilated or arrhythmogenic right ventricular cardiomyopathy. Circulation 2020;141(23):1872–84.
16. Seidman JG, Seidman C. The Genetic Basis for Cardiomyopathy: Review from Mutation Identification to Mechanistic Paradigms. Vol 104. 2001.
17. Fatkin D, MacRae C, Sasaki T, et al. Missense mutations in the rod domain of the lamin A/C gene as causes of dilated cardiomyopathy and conduction-system disease. N Engl J Med 1999;341(23): 1715–24.
18. van Berlo JH, de Voogt WG, van der Kooi AJ, et al. Meta-analysis of clinical characteristics of 299 carriers of LMNA gene mutations: do lamin A/C mutations portend a high risk of sudden death? J Mol Med 2005;83(1):79–83.
19. Pasotti M, Klersy C, Pilotto A, et al. Long-term outcome and risk stratification in dilated Cardiolaminopathies. J Am Coll Cardiol 2008;52(15):1250–60.
20. van Rijsingen IAW, Arbustini E, Elliott PM, et al. Risk factors for malignant ventricular arrhythmias in Lamin A/C mutation carriers: a European cohort study. J Am Coll Cardiol 2012;59(5):493–500.
21. van Rijsingen IAW, Nannenberg EA, Arbustini E, et al. Gender-specific differences in major cardiac events and mortality in lamin A/C mutation carriers. Eur J Heart Fail 2013;15(4):376–84.
22. Kumar S, Baldinger SH, Gandjbakhch E, et al. Long-Term Arrhythmic and Nonarrhythmic Outcomes of Lamin A/C Mutation Carriers. 2016.

23. Hasselberg NE, Edvardsen T, Petri H, et al. Risk prediction of ventricular arrhythmias and myocardial function in Lamin A/C mutation positive subjects. Europace 2014;16(4):563–71.

24. Meune C, van Berlo JH, Anselme F, et al. Primary prevention of sudden death in patients with lamin A/C gene mutations. N Engl J Med 2006;354(2):209–10.

25. Wahbi K, ben Yaou R, Gandjbakhch E, et al. Development and validation of a new risk prediction score for life-threatening ventricular tachyarrhythmias in laminopathies. Circulation 2019;140(4):293–302.

26. Rootwelt-Norberg C, Christensen AH, Skjølsvik ET, et al. Timing of cardioverter-defibrillator implantation in patients with cardiac laminopathies—external validation of the LMNA-risk ventricular tachyarrhythmia calculator. Heart Rhythm 2023;20(3):423–9.

27. Peretto G, Barison A, Forleo C, et al. Late gadolinium enhancement role in arrhythmic risk stratification of patients with LMNA cardiomyopathy: results from a long-term follow-up multicentre study. Europace 2020;22(12):1864–72.

28. Otomo JUN, Kure S, Shiba T, et al. Electrophysiological and histopathological characteristics of progressive atrioventricular block accompanied by familial dilated cardiomyopathy caused by a novel mutation of lamin A/C gene. J Cardiovasc Electrophysiol 2005;16(2):137–45.

29. Stossel TP, Condeelis J, Cooley L, et al. Filamins as integrators of cell mechanics and signalling. Nat Rev Mol Cell Biol 2001;2(2):138–45.

30. Vorgerd M, van der Ven PFM, Bruchertseifer V, et al. A Mutation in the Dimerization Domain of Filamin C Causes a Novel Type of Autosomal Dominant Myofibrillar Myopathyband Alternatively Spliced PDZ Motif-Containing Protein (LDB3 MIM). Vol 77. 2005.

31. Ortiz-Genga MF, Cuenca S, Ferro MD, et al. Truncating FLNC Mutations Are Associated With High-Risk Dilated and Arrhythmogenic Cardiomyopathies. 2016.

32. Gigli M, Stolfo D, Graw SL, et al. Phenotypic expression, natural history, and risk stratification of cardiomyopathy caused by filamin C truncating variants. Circulation 2021;144(20):1600–11.

33. Akhtar MM, Lorenzini M, Pavlou M, et al. Association of left ventricular systolic dysfunction among carriers of truncating variants in filamin C with frequent ventricular arrhythmia and end-stage heart failure. JAMA Cardiol 2021;6(8):891–901.

34. MacLennan DH, Kranias EG. Phospholamban: a crucial regulator of cardiac contractility. Nat Rev Mol Cell Biol 2003;4(7):566–77.

35. Haghighi K, Kolokathis F, Gramolini AO, et al. A Mutation in the Human phospholamban gene, deleting Arginine 14, results in Lethal, Hereditary cardiomyopathy. Proc Natl Acad Sci U S A 2006;103(5):1388–93.

36. van der Zwaag PA, van Rijsingen IAW, Asimaki A, et al. Phospholamban R14del mutation in patients diagnosed with dilated cardiomyopathy or arrhythmogenic right ventricular cardiomyopathy: evidence supporting the concept of arrhythmogenic cardiomyopathy. Eur J Heart Fail 2012;14(11):1199–207.

37. van Rijsingen IAW, van der Zwaag PA, Groeneweg JA, et al. Outcome in phospholamban R14del carriers results of a large multicentre cohort study. Circ Cardiovasc Genet 2014;7(4):455–65.

38. Verstraelen TE, van Lint FHM, Bosman LP, et al. Prediction of ventricular arrhythmia in phospholamban p.Arg14del mutation carriers-reaching the frontiers of individual risk prediction. Eur Heart J 2021;42(29):2842–50.

39. Brauch KM, Karst ML, Herron KJ, et al. Mutations in ribonucleic acid binding protein gene cause familial dilated cardiomyopathy. J Am Coll Cardiol 2009;54(10):930–41.

40. Li D, Morales A, Gonzalez-Quintana J, et al. Identification of novel mutations in RBM20 in patients with dilated cardiomyopathy. Clin Transl Sci 2010;3(3):90–7.

41. Guo W, Schafer S, Greaser ML, et al. RBM20, a gene for hereditary cardiomyopathy, regulates titin splicing. Nat Med 2012;18(5):766–73.

42. van den Hoogenhof MMG, Beqqali A, Amin AS, et al. RBM20 mutations induce an arrhythmogenic dilated cardiomyopathy related to disturbed calcium handling. Circulation 2018;138(13):1330–42.

43. Parikh VN, Caleshu C, Reuter C, et al. Regional variation in RBM20 causes a highly penetrant arrhythmogenic cardiomyopathy. Circ Heart Fail 2019;12(3):e005371.

44. Hey TM, Rasmussen TB, Madsen T, et al. Pathogenic RBM20-variants are associated with a severe disease expression in male patients with dilated cardiomyopathy. Circ Heart Fail 2019;12(3):e005700.

45. Marshall W, Furey M, Larsen B, et al. Right ventricular cardiomyopathy and sudden death in young people. N Engl J Med 1988;319(3):174–6.

46. Christensen AH, Andersen CB, Tybjaerg-Hansen A, et al. Mutation analysis and evaluation of the cardiac localization of TMEM43 in arrhythmogenic right ventricular cardiomyopathy. Clin Genet 2011;80(3):256–64.

47. Bengtsson L, Otto H. LUMA interacts with emerin and influences its distribution at the inner nuclear membrane. J Cell Sci 2008;121(4):536–48.

48. Hodgkinson KA, Parfrey PS, Bassett AS, et al. The impact of implantable cardioverter-defibrillator therapy on survival in autosomal-dominant arrhythmogenic right ventricular cardiomyopathy (ARVD5). J Am Coll Cardiol 2005;45(3):400–8.

49. Merner ND, Hodgkinson KA, Haywood AFM, et al. Arrhythmogenic right ventricular cardiomyopathy

type 5 is a fully penetrant, lethal arrhythmic disorder caused by a missense mutation in the TMEM43 gene. Am J Hum Genet 2008;82(4):809–21.

50. Dominguez F, Zorio E, Jimenez-Jaimez J, et al. Clinical characteristics and determinants of the phenotype in TMEM43 arrhythmogenic right ventricular cardiomyopathy type 5. Heart Rhythm 2020;17(6): 945–54.

51. Wang Q, Shen J, Splawski I, et al. SCN5A mutations associated with an inherited cardiac arrhythmia, long QT syndrome. Cell 1995;80(5):805–11.

52. Chen Q, Kirsch GE, Zhang D, et al. Genetic basis and molecular mechanism for idiopathic ventricular fibrillation. Nature 1998;392(6673):293–6.

53. Olson TM, Michels V v, Ballew JD, et al. Sodium channel mutations and susceptibility to heart failure and atrial fibrillation. JAMA 2005;293(4):447–54.

54. McNair WP, Ku L, Taylor MRG, et al. SCN5A mutation associated with dilated cardiomyopathy, conduction disorder, and arrhythmia. Circulation 2004;110(15): 2163–7.

55. Shan L, Makita N, Xing Y, et al. SCN5A variants in Japanese patients with left ventricular noncompaction and arrhythmia. Mol Genet Metab 2008;93(4): 468–74.

56. Shi R, Zhang Y, Yang C, et al. The cardiac sodium channel mutation delQKP 1507–1509 is associated with the expanding phenotypic spectrum of LQT3, conduction disorder, dilated cardiomyopathy, and high incidence of youth sudden death. Europace 2008;10(11):1329–35.

57. te Riele ASJM, Agullo-Pascual E, James CA, et al. Multilevel analyses of SCN5A mutations in arrhythmogenic right ventricular dysplasia/cardiomyopathy suggest non-canonical mechanisms for disease pathogenesis. Cardiovasc Res 2017;113(1):102–11.

58. Xiong Q, Cao Q, Zhou Q, et al. Arrhythmogenic cardiomyopathy in a patient with a rare loss-of-function KCNQ 1 mutation. J Am Heart Assoc 2015;4(1): e001526.

59. Kharbanda M, Hunter A, Tennant S, et al. Long QT syndrome and left ventricular noncompaction in 4 family members across 2 generations with KCNQ1 mutation. Eur J Med Genet 2017;60(5):233–8.

60. Costa S, Medeiros-Domingo A, Gasperetti A, et al. Familial dilated cardiomyopathy associated with a novel heterozygous RYR2 early truncating variant. Cardiol J 2021;28(1):173–5.

61. Roux-Buisson N, Gandjbakhch E, Donal E, et al. Prevalence and significance of rare RYR2 variants in arrhythmogenic right ventricular cardiomyopathy/dysplasia: results of a systematic screening. Heart Rhythm 2014;11(11):1999–2009.

62. Yin L, Zahradnikova A Jr, Rizzetto R, et al. Impaired binding to junctophilin-2 and nanostructural alteration in CPVT mutation. Circ Res 2021;129(3): e35–52.

63. Hamilton S, Terentyev D. RyR2 Gain-of-function and not So sudden cardiac death. Circ Res 2021;129(3): 417–9.

64. Al-Khatib SM, Stevenson WG, Ackerman MJ, et al. 2017 AHA/ACC/HRS guideline for management of patients with ventricular arrhythmias and the prevention of sudden cardiac death: a report of the American College of Cardiology/American heart association task force on clinical practice guidelines and the heart Rhythm Society. J Am Coll Cardiol 2018;72(14):e91–220.

65. Zeppenfeld K, Tfelt-Hansen J, de Riva M, et al. 2022 ESC Guidelines for the management of patients with ventricular arrhythmias and the prevention of sudden cardiac death: developed by the task force for the management of patients with ventricular arrhythmias and the prevention of sudden cardiac death of the European Society of Cardiology (ESC) Endorsed by the Association for European Paediatric and Congenital Cardiology (AEPC). Eur Heart J 2022; ehac262.

66. Halliday BP, Cleland JGF, Goldberger JJ, et al. Personalizing risk stratification for sudden death in dilated cardiomyopathy: the past, present, and future. Circulation 2017;136(2):215–31.

67. di Marco A, Brown PF, Bradley J, et al. Improved risk stratification for ventricular arrhythmias and sudden death in patients with nonischemic dilated cardiomyopathy. J Am Coll Cardiol 2021;77(23):2890–905.

68. Tayal U, Verdonschot JAJ, Hazebroek MR, et al. Precision phenotyping of dilated cardiomyopathy using multidimensional data. J Am Coll Cardiol 2022; 79(22):2219–32.

Moving?

Make sure your subscription moves with you!

To notify us of your new address, find your **Clinics Account Number** (located on your mailing label above your name), and contact customer service at:

Email: journalscustomerservice-usa@elsevier.com

800-654-2452 (subscribers in the U.S. & Canada)
314-447-8871 (subscribers outside of the U.S. & Canada)

Fax number: 314-447-8029

Elsevier Health Sciences Division
Subscription Customer Service
3251 Riverport Lane
Maryland Heights, MO 63043

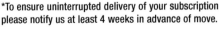

*To ensure uninterrupted delivery of your subscription, please notify us at least 4 weeks in advance of move.

ELSEVIER